MAKING SENSE of ECHOCARDIOGRAPHY

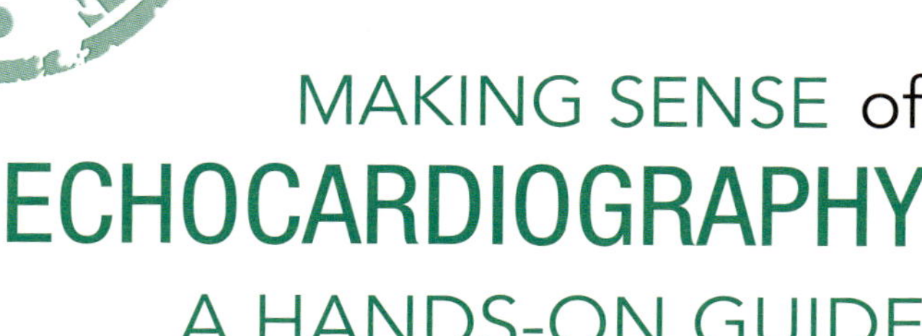

MAKING SENSE of ECHOCARDIOGRAPHY
A HANDS-ON GUIDE

Andrew R. Houghton
MA(Oxon) DM FRCP(Lond) FRCP(Glasg)
Consultant Cardiologist
Grantham and District Hospital
Grantham, UK
and
Visiting Fellow, University of Lincoln,
Lincoln, UK

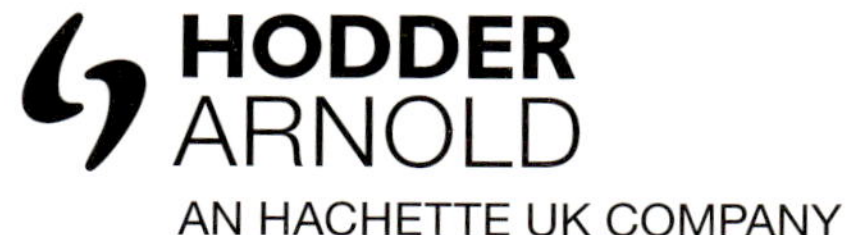

First published in Great Britain in 2009 by
Hodder Arnold, an imprint of Hodder Education,
an Hachette UK company, 338 Euston Road, London NW1 3BH

http://www.hoddereducation.com

British Library Cataloguing in Publication Data
A catalogue record for this book is available from the British Library

Library of Congress Cataloging-in-Publication Data
A catalog record for this book is available from the Library of Congress

ISBN-13 978 0 340 950 043

3 4 5 6 7 8 9 10

Commissioning Editor: Philip Shaw
Project Editor: Amy Mulick
Production Controller: Karen Tate
Cover Design: Helen Townson and Laura De Grasse

Typeset in 10/11 Chaparra MM250LT by Macmillan Publishing Solutions, Chennai, India
Printed and bound in India

This book is dedicated to the memory of Paul Michael Houghton (1952–2002).

Contents

FIGURE AND VIDEO LIBRARY

This book has a companion website available at: www.hodderplus.com/msecho

The website contains downloadable figures and video versions of many of the figures in this book, as well as supplementary clips providing further examples.

To access the video clips included on the website, please register on the website using the following access details:

Serial number: 892js92kd9dk

Foreword

Echocardiography underpins much of contemporary cardiology practice; far more echocardiograms are performed than coronary angiograms, myocardial perfusion studies or cardiac MR scans. Their unique simplicity and mobility lend themselves to emergency imaging in coronary care units, accident and emergency departments and cardiac catheterization laboratories, but contemporary echocardiography involves much more than rapid 2-dimensional imaging of the cardiac chambers and a quick look for valve pathology. Technology is evolving rapidly and the development of techniques such as harmonic imaging, tissue Doppler, speckle tracking and real time 3-dimensional imaging have expanded the role of echo to include sophisticated analysis of myocardial mechanics, the assessment of complex valvular pathology and guidance for the placement of intracardiac devices and other interventions.

With improved image quality has come an improved ability to quantify abnormalities. Gone are the days when the assessment of left ventricular function was limited to an eyeball estimate of ejection fraction. Measurement of left ventricular volumes and estimation of left atrial pressures are now performed routinely. Valvular stenosis and regurgitation may be quantified in the majority of patients and decisions made about reparability of valves or suitability for percutaneous interventions. Quantification demands rigorous standardization of technique and the adoption of accepted normal and pathological ranges. *Making Sense of Echocardiography* incorporates the reference ranges adopted by the British Society of Echocardiography and provides practical examples of how qualitative and quantitative data can be combined in an echo report.

The expanding role of echocardiography has provided new challenges for the echocardiographer. It has always been a subject requiring both sound theoretical knowledge and extensive practical experience, but this is even more the case as echo imaging becomes ever more sophisticated. More theoretical concepts need to be grasped and more techniques practiced. Echocardiographers need to understand which techniques to employ in a given clinical situation and how to interpret the resulting data to provide meaningful information for a clinician who cannot interpret the images themselves. This requires the ability to synthesize complex and sometimes conflicting information. Few echocardiographers are experts in all modalities and even the most experienced require occasional recourse to a reference text.

Most echocardiography books are either basic practical guides to scanning and reporting or lengthy and detailed reference texts. Excellent examples of both are mentioned in Appendix 1. *Making Sense of Echocardiography* differs in that it sets out to provide both a practical guide to routine scanning and sufficient detail to function as a first line reference text for the more experienced echocardiographer. Dr Houghton has succeeded in writing a book that fulfils these aims with clarity and simplicity and one that deserves a place in every echo reporting room.

Dr Simon Ray
President, British Society of Echocardiography
2009

Preface

Echocardiography is one of the most useful cardiac investigations – it is safe, painless, non-invasive, relatively inexpensive and provides key diagnostic information across a wide range of conditions. It does, however, require a high level of knowledge and experience – sonographers need a good understanding of ultrasound physics, anatomy, physiology and clinical cardiology, and need to undertake a substantial number of echo studies in order to attain (and maintain) their skills.

The aim of *Making Sense of Echocardiography* is to provide the echo trainee with a comprehensive yet readable introduction to echo, and to provide more experienced sonographers with an accessible handbook for reference when required. The approach to echo studies taken in this book is based on the guidelines published by national echo societies, in particular the British Society of Echocardiography (BSE), and I am particularly grateful to the BSE and the British Heart Foundation for their permission to use their recommended reference ranges throughout the book.

A good knowledge of clinical cardiology is important to appreciate the key features that need to be assessed in a particular echo study – for instance, knowing the indications for valve surgery makes it easier to know what information the referring clinician will want to see in an echo report on an abnormal valve. For this reason, the clinical aspects of disease management are interwoven with the information on how to perform echo studies throughout this book.

I am grateful to everyone who has taken the time to comment on draft copies of the text and to all those who have provided echo images for this book. Finally, I would like to thank all of the staff at Hodder Arnold who have contributed to the success of the *Making Sense . . .* series of books.

Andrew R. Houghton

2009

Acknowledgements

I would like to thank everyone who provided suggestions and constructive criticism while I prepared *Making Sense of Echocardiography*. I am particularly grateful to Stephanie Baker, Lawrence Green, Daniel Law and Cara Mercer for their invaluable help in the preparation of this book and for their comments on draft copies of the text.

I would also like to thank the following for assisting me in acquiring the images that illustrate this book:

Mookhter Ajij
Denise Archer
Hannah Clark
Nigel Dewey
Jeffrey Khoo
Diane Lunn
Lisa McAdam
Jane Robinson
Nimit Shah
Upul Wijayawardhana
Bernadette Williamson

I am indebted to the British Society of Echocardiography (BSE) and the British Heart Foundation (BHF) for their permission to quote their recommended echo reference ranges which, where applicable, form the basis of the reference ranges used in this book. Further details of the BSE/BHF reference ranges can be found at the end of the book (see 'Echo resources').

I am also grateful to Philips for allowing me to reproduce echo images from its clinical image collection, and to the BMJ Publishing Group and to Elsevier for permission to reproduce images from their journals.

I would also like to thank my wife, Kathryn Ann Houghton, for her support and patience during the preparation of this book.

Finally, I would also like to express my gratitude to everyone at Hodder Arnold for their guidance and support.

Abbreviations

2-D	two-dimensional
3-D	three-dimensional
A	peak A-wave velocity
ACE	angiotensin-converting enzyme
A_{dur}	duration of atrial reversal in pulmonary vein flow
A_{dur}	duration of A wave in left ventricular inflow
AF	atrial fibrillation
A_m	atrial contraction velocity on tissue Doppler imaging of mitral annulus (also known as A′)
Ao	aorta
AR	aortic regurgitation
ARVC	arrhythmogenic right ventricular cardiomyopathy
AS	aortic stenosis
ASD	atrial septal defect
ASE	American Society of Echocardiography
AV	aortic valve *or* atrioventricular
BSA	body surface area
BCS	British Cardiovascular Society
BHF	British Heart Foundation
BSE	British Society of Echocardiography
CI	cardiac index
CO	cardiac output
CRT	cardiac resynchronization therapy
CSA	cross-sectional area
CW	continuous wave (Doppler)

Cx	circumflex (coronary) artery
DCM	dilated cardiomyopathy
E	peak E-wave velocity
EAE	European Association of Echocardiography
ECG	electrocardiogram
EF	ejection fraction
E_m	early myocardial velocity on tissue Doppler imaging of mitral annulus (also known as E′)
EDV	end-diastolic volume
ESC	European Society of Cardiology
ESV	end-systolic volume
ET	ejection time
FS	fractional shortening
HCM	hypertrophic cardiomyopathy
HFPEF	heart failure with preserved ejection fraction
HFREF	heart failure with reduced ejection fraction
HID	half-intensity depth
HOCM	hypertrophic obstructive cardiomyopathy
HR	heart rate
ICD	implantable cardioverter defibrillator
ICT	isovolumic contraction time
INR	international normalized ratio
IRT or IVRT	isovolumic relaxation time
IV	intravenous
IVC	inferior vena cava
IVNC	isolated ventricular non-compaction
IVS	interventricular septum
IVSd	interventricular septal wall dimension – diastole
IVSs	interventricular septal wall dimension – systole
JVP	jugular venous pressure
LA	left atrium
LAA	left atrial appendage

LAD	left anterior descending (coronary artery)
LCA	left coronary artery
LCC	left coronary cusp
LLPV	left lower pulmonary vein
LMS	left main stem
LUPV	left upper pulmonary vein
LV	left ventricle
LVEDV	left ventricular end-diastolic volume
LVEF	left ventricular ejection fraction
LVESV	left ventricular end-systolic volume
LVH	left ventricular hypertrophy
LVIDd	left ventricular internal dimension – diastole
LVIDs	left ventricular internal dimension – systole
LVOT	left ventricular outflow tract
LVPW	left ventricular posterior wall
LVPWd	left ventricular posterior wall dimension – diastole
LVPWs	left ventricular posterior wall dimension – systole
MI	mechanical index *or* myocardial infarction
MR	mitral regurgitation
MS	mitral stenosis
MV	mitral valve
NCC	non-coronary cusp
NSTEMI	non-ST elevation myocardial infarction
OM	obtuse marginal (coronary artery)
P½T	pressure half-time
P_{max}	peak pressure
P_{mean}	mean pressure
PA	pulmonary artery
PADP	pulmonary artery diastolic pressure
PASP	pulmonary artery systolic pressure
PBMV	percutaneous balloon mitral valvuloplasty
PDA	persistent ductus arteriosus *or* posterior descending artery

PFO	patent foramen ovale
PG	pressure gradient
PISA	proximal isovelocity surface area
PR	pulmonary regurgitation
PRF	pulse repetition frequency
PS	pulmonary stenosis
PV	pulmonary valve *or* pulmonary vein
PV_a	peak atrial reversal ('A' wave) velocity in pulmonary vein
PV_D	peak diastolic ('D' wave) velocity in pulmonary vein
PV_S	peak systolic ('S' wave) velocity in pulmonary vein
PW	pulsed-wave (Doppler)
RA	right atrium
RAP	right atrial pressure
RCA	right coronary artery
RF	regurgitant fraction
RLPV	right lower pulmonary vein
RUPV	right upper pulmonary vein
RVDP	right ventricular diastolic pressure
RVSP	right ventricular systolic pressure
RV	regurgitant volume *or* right ventricle
RVOT	right ventricular outflow tract
SD	stroke distance
SV	stroke volume
STEMI	ST elevation myocardial infarction
SVC	superior vena cava
SVI	stroke volume index
TAVI	transcatheter aortic valve implantation
TDI	tissue Doppler imaging
TGC	time-gain compensation
TIA	transient ischaemic attack
TOE	transoesophageal echo
ToF	tetralogy of Fallot

TR	tricuspid regurgitation
TS	tricuspid stenosis
TTE	transthoracic echo
V_{max}	peak velocity
V_{mean}	mean velocity
VSD	ventricular septal defect
VTI	velocity time integral
WHO	World Health Organization

PART 1

Essential Principles

1 History of echocardiography

The first application of diagnostic ultrasound in medicine was in the late 1930s, when Karl Dussik, an Austrian psychiatrist and neurologist, became interested in the potential use of ultrasound for brain imaging. Ultrasound was already in use at that time, by mariners for underwater imaging and also by engineers for flaw detection in metals. The piezoelectric effect was already well known, having been discovered more than half a century earlier, and the concept of using a piezoelectric crystal both to transmit and receive ultrasound was described in 1917.

Dussik's brain imaging technique was different to today's ultrasound, in that it was based on the transmission of ultrasound waves *through* an object, rather than detecting waves *reflected from* an object. His technique, which, he called hyperphonography, involved placing a transmitter on one side of the head and a receiver on the other, and using this apparatus he was able to produce images of the ventricles of the brain. Echotransmission was also the first ultrasound technique used for cardiac imaging, by the German physiologist Wolf-Dieter Keidel, in order to make measurements of the heart and thorax.

Echoreflection was first used by Inge Edler and Carl Hellmuth Hertz in Sweden. One weekend in 1953 they borrowed an industrial device, used to detect flaws in metals by the Kockum shipyard in Malmö, to conduct their work on human subjects. By a fortunate coincidence the frequency of the echo transducer happened to be one that was suitable for cardiac imaging. The image of the heart they produced was known as an A-mode scan and was thought to show the posterior wall of the left ventricle (LV). They were soon granted an ultrasound machine of their own and began to produce M-mode scans, with which they were able to examine the mitral valve and also detect atrial thrombus, myxoma and pericardial effusion.

Nonetheless, it was not until the early 1960s that the potential value of cardiac ultrasound became more widely recognized. The first dedicated cardiac ultrasound machine, developed by Jack Reed and Claude Joyner, appeared at this time and the term 'echocardiography' was coined for the first time.

Real-time 2-D echo followed in the 1960s, spurred on by advances in electronics, and by the early 1970s mechanical transducers were available that could produce 2-D images by steering the transducer back and forth, sweeping the ultrasound beam across the heart. Phased-array transducers soon followed, in which the mechanical beam-steering mechanism was replaced by solid-state electronics.

The 1970s also saw rapid developments in the use of Doppler techniques and by the early 1980s colour Doppler imaging was becoming a common feature of echo studies. During the 1980s, the technique of transoesophageal echo started to enter clinical practice, initially with monoplane probes but later with biplane probes, multiplane probes and, more recently, the use of 3-D transoesophageal imaging.

The 1990s saw a gradual change in archiving methods, with a move away from recording studies on videotape towards more versatile digitally based archiving. There were also refinements in the quality of echo, with the introduction of harmonic imaging and the growing use of echo contrast agents to enhance endocardial border definition. Tissue Doppler imaging entered mainstream practice towards the end of the 1990s, adding a new modality that has proven particularly valuable in the assessment of LV diastolic function.

Continuing technological advances are making echo more widely accessible, with small and highly portable echo machines now available that nevertheless offer a wide range of imaging modalities. The growing use of echo has reinforced the need for professional regulation, and the past few years have seen the publication of many key national and international guidelines that set clear quality standards for the performance of echo in the twenty-first century.

FURTHER READING

An excellent and detailed overview of the history of medical ultrasound can be accessed at: www.ob-ultrasound.net/history.html

Coman IM. Christian Andreas Doppler – the man and his legacy. *Eur J Echocardiogr* 2005; **6**: 7–10.

Edler I, Hertz CH. The use of ultrasonic reflectoscope for the continuous recording of the movement of heart walls. *Kungl Fysiografiska Sällskapets i Lund Förhandlingar* 1954; **24**: 40–58.

Fraser AG. Inge Edler and the origins of clinical echocardiography. *Eur J Echocardiogr* 2001; **2**: 3–5.

Roelandt JRTC. Seeing the invisible: A short history of cardiac ultrasound. *Eur J Echocardiogr* 2000; **1**: 8–11.

2 Cardiac anatomy and physiology

The heart lies within the thorax, to the left of the midline, protected by the rib cage and lying in close proximity to the lungs and, underneath, the diaphragm (Fig. 2.1). The ribs and lungs can provide a challenge for the sonographer trying to obtain clear images of the heart, as ultrasound does not penetrate bone or aerated lung well.

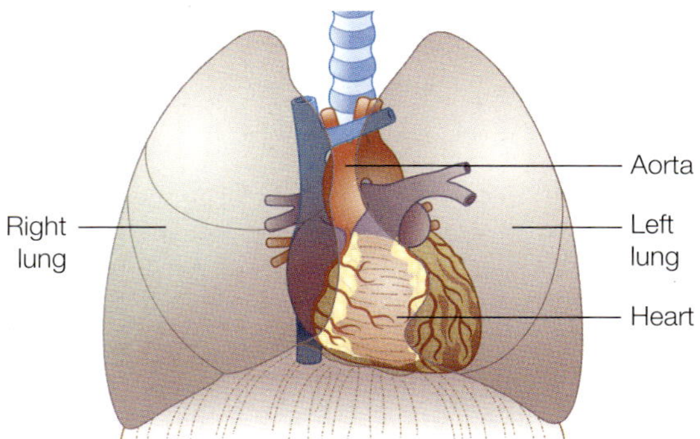

Fig. 2.1 The heart and its relation to the rest of the thorax

The heart consists of four main chambers (left and right atria, and left and right ventricles) and four valves (aortic, mitral, pulmonary and tricuspid). Venous blood returns to the right atrium (RA) via the superior and inferior vena cavae, and leaves the right ventricle (RV) for the lungs via the pulmonary artery. Oxygenated blood from the lungs returns to the left atrium (LA) via the four pulmonary veins, and leaves the left ventricle (LV) via the aorta (Fig. 2.2).

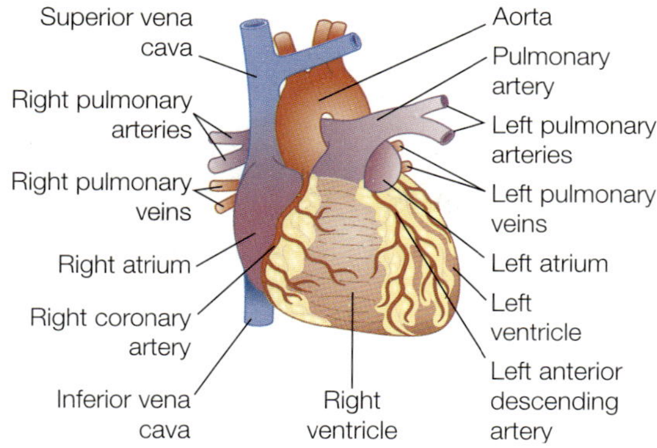

Fig. 2.2 The heart and major vessels

Cardiac chambers and valves

The aortic valve

The aortic valve lies between the left ventricular outflow tract (LVOT) and aortic root (Fig. 2.3) and has three cusps, which open widely during systole. In diastole, the valve closes and, in the parasternal short axis view (aortic valve level), has a Y-shaped appearance (sometimes referred to as resembling a 'Mercedes-Benz badge'; Fig. 6.5).

Upstream of the aortic valve are the sinuses of Valsalva, an expanded region of the aortic root, from which the coronary arteries originate. Each of the sinuses

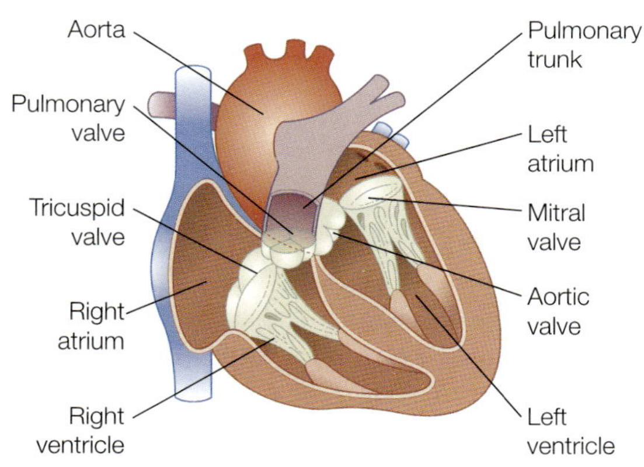

Fig. 2.3 The heart valves and chambers

and aortic valve cusps is named according to its relationship to these coronary arteries: hence the right coronary cusp lies adjacent to the sinus giving rise to the right coronary artery (RCA), and the left coronary cusp to the sinus giving rise to the left coronary artery (LCA). The third sinus does not have a coronary artery, and the adjacent cusp is named the non-coronary cusp.

Where the valve cusps attach to the aortic root is often termed the aortic valve annulus, although the annulus is not a discrete structure (unlike the mitral valve annulus). The point where adjacent cusps meet is called the commissure. Each cusp has a small nodule at its centre, called the nodule of Arantius, which is more prominent in older patients. The ventricular surface of a cusp sometimes carries small mobile filaments, called Lambl's excrescences, arising from the edge of the cusp. Lambl's excrescences are of no clinical significance, but should not be mistaken for vegetations (Chapter 17) or papillary fibroelastoma (Chapter 21).

Below the aortic valve lies the LVOT, which includes the membranous part of the interventricular septum (IVS) and the anterior mitral valve leaflet. The fibrous tissue of the aortic root is continuous with the anterior mitral valve leaflet.

The left ventricle

The normal LV is an approximately symmetrical structure, which is cylindrical at its base (the mitral annulus) and tapers towards its apex. It is the main pumping chamber of the heart and its wall is thicker (and myocardial mass greater), although less trabeculated, than that of the RV. The LV myocardium is conventionally subdivided into 16 or 17 segments, the function of each of which should be assessed individually (Chapter 12).

The mitral valve

The mitral valve lies between the left atrium and ventricle and has two leaflets that open during diastole and close in systole, to prevent regurgitation of blood from the LV back into the LA. The mitral valve needs to be thought of as more than just two leaflets, however, because the mitral annulus, papillary muscles and chordae tendineae are all essential to the valve's structure and function (Fig. 2.4).

The mitral leaflets are termed anterior and posterior and attach around their base to the fibrous mitral annulus, an elliptical ring separating the

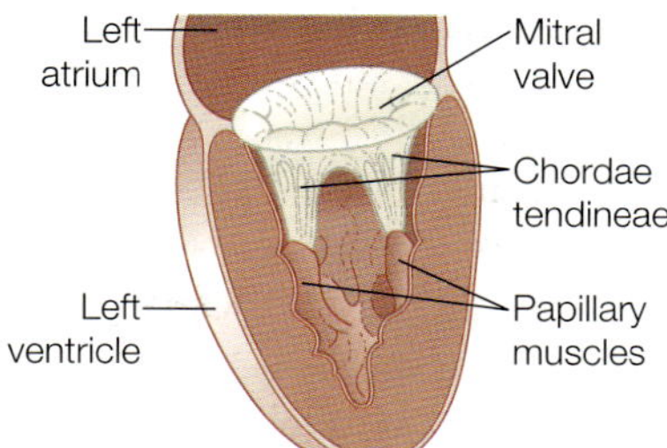

Fig. 2.4 Mitral valve anatomy

LA and LV. The anterior mitral leaflet is longer (from base to tip) than the posterior leaflet, but the length of its attachment to the annulus is shorter and so the surface area of both leaflets is about equal. Each leaflet is divided into three segments, or scallops, which are named A1, A2 and A3 (anterior leaflet) and P1, P2 and P3 (posterior leaflet), with the numbering running from the anterolateral commissure (A1/P1) to the posteromedial commissure (A3/P3) (Fig. 14.2).

There are two papillary muscles, named anterolateral and posteromedial (after the location of their attachment to the LV), and which are attached to the mitral leaflets via the chordae tendineae. Although there are two leaflets and two papillary muscles, each papillary muscle supplies chordae to *both* leaflets – it is not a 1:1 relationship. Chordae from the medial aspects of both leaflets attach to the posteromedial papillary muscle and from the lateral aspects to the anterolateral papillary muscle.

The chordae keep the mitral leaflets under tension during systole, preventing prolapse of the leaflets back into the LA. They are categorized into three groups:

- first order or marginal chordae, which attach to the free edges of the mitral leaflets
- second order or strut chordae, which attach to the ventricular surface of the leaflets (away from the free edges)
- third order or basal chordae, which run directly from the ventricular wall (rather than the papillary muscles) to the ventricular surface of the posterior leaflet, usually near the annulus.

The mitral leaflets are normally thin and open widely during diastole, with the anterior leaflet almost touching the IVS. As the leaflets close (coapt) they overlap at their tips by several millimetres (apposition). A reduced degree of apposition results in poor coaptation and can cause mitral regurgitation.

The left atrium

The LA is situated at the back of the heart, in front of the oesophagus (and it is therefore the chamber immediately adjacent to the probe in the mid-oesophageal transoesophageal echo view). The LA is a relatively smooth-walled structure, but does have an appendage which can act as a focus for thrombus formation. It is entered by four pulmonary veins carrying oxygenated blood from the lungs – two from the right lung and two from the left.

The LA is not just a passive conduit between the pulmonary veins and the LV, but contracts during atrial systole (immediately after the onset of the P wave) to provide additional diastolic filling of the LV (the 'atrial kick'). This is particularly important when diastolic filling is impaired, in the presence of elevated LV filling pressures.

The LA is separated from the RA by the interatrial septum, but there can be a communication between the two in the form of a patent foramen ovale or atrial septal defect (ASD) (Chapter 22).

The pulmonary valve

The pulmonary valve lies between the right ventricular outflow tract (RVOT) and pulmonary artery, opening during systole to allow blood to pass from the ventricle into the pulmonary circulation, and closing in diastole to prevent regurgitation (a small amount of 'physiological' pulmonary regurgitation is normal). The valve itself is structurally similar to the aortic valve, having three cusps (called anterior, left and right).

The right ventricle

The RV is more complex to assess by echo than the left, forming a crescent-shaped structure around the LV. It is more heavily trabeculated, but thinner-walled than the LV, and contains a moderator band that stretches between the free wall and the septum. The RVOT is not trabeculated and leads to the pulmonary valve. The RV acts as the pumping chamber for deoxygenated blood returning from the body en route to the lungs.

The tricuspid valve

The tricuspid valve lies between the RA and RV, opening during diastole to allow blood to pass from the atrium to the ventricle, and closing in systole to prevent regurgitation (although a small amount of 'physiological' tricuspid regurgitation is commonly seen in normal individuals).

As its name suggests, the tricuspid valve has three cusps – in order of decreasing size, these are called the anterior, posterior and septal cusps. There are also three papillary muscles, which, in a similar way to the mitral valve, are attached to the cusps via chordae tendineae. The orifice area of the tricuspid valve is greater than that of the mitral valve, normally $>7.0\,\text{cm}^2$.

The right atrium

The RA receives blood returning to the heart via the superior and inferior vena cavae. It also receives blood draining from the myocardium via the coronary sinus, which enters the RA posteriorly, just superior to the tricuspid valve. The coronary sinus is often visible on echo, particularly when it is dilated (Fig. 21.4).

The Eustachian valve, an embryological remnant, may be seen in the RA near the junction with the inferior vena cava.

The coronary arteries

The coronary circulation normally arises as two separate vessels from the sinuses of Valsalva – the LCA from the left coronary sinus, and the RCA from the right coronary sinus (Fig. 2.5).

The initial portion of the LCA is the left main stem, which soon divides into the left anterior descending (LAD) and circumflex (Cx) arteries. The LAD artery runs down the anterior interventricular groove giving rise to diagonal branches, which course towards the lateral wall of the LV, and septal perforators that supply the IVS. The Cx artery runs in the left atrioventricular groove, giving rise to obtuse marginal branches which extend across the lateral surface of the LV.

The RCA runs in the right atrioventricular groove, and in most people gives rise to the posterior descending artery which runs down the posterior interventricular groove. This defines 'dominance' – most people therefore

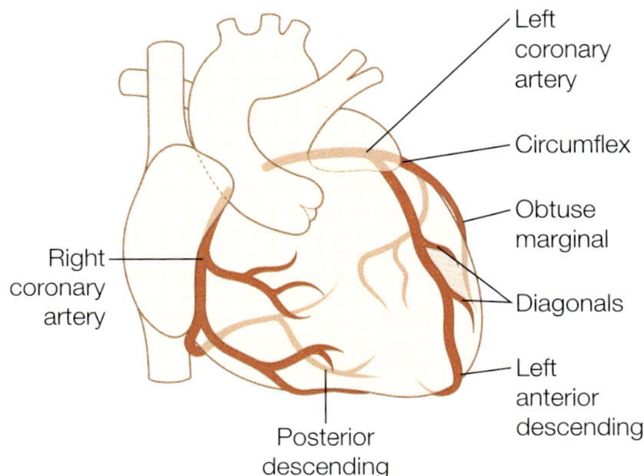

Fig. 2.5 The coronary circulation

have a 'dominant' RCA, but in some people the Cx gives rise to the posterior descending artery and they are said to have a 'dominant' Cx.

The pericardium

The pericardium is a sac-like structure that surrounds most of the heart. There is an outer fibrous layer – the *fibrous pericardium* – which blends with the diaphragm inferiorly, and an inner layer – the *serous pericardium* – which itself has two layers (the parietal pericardium, continuous with the fibrous outer layer, and the visceral pericardium, which is the epicardium of the heart).

The pericardium contains 'gaps' where vessels enter and leave the heart, and the pericardium forms a small sleeve around these vessels. As a result, there is a small pocket of pericardium around the aorta/pulmonary artery (transverse sinus) and between the four pulmonary veins (oblique sinus).

The pericardial cavity is a potential space between the parietal and visceral layers, and normally contains less than 50 mL of fluid. Inflammation of the pericardium (pericarditis) can lead to the accumulation of a larger volume of fluid – a pericardial effusion. If this affects the normal functioning of the heart, cardiac tamponade can result. In the longer term, inflammation of the pericardium can lead to thickening of pericardium and pericardial constriction.

The cardiac cycle

The events that occur during each heartbeat are termed the cardiac cycle, commonly represented in diagrammatic form (Fig. 2.6). The cardiac cycle has four phases:

1. isovolumic contraction
2. ventricular ejection
3. isovolumic relaxation
4. ventricular filling.

These phases apply to both left and right heart, but we will focus on the left heart here for clarity. Phases 1–2 correspond with ventricular systole and phases 3–4 with ventricular diastole.

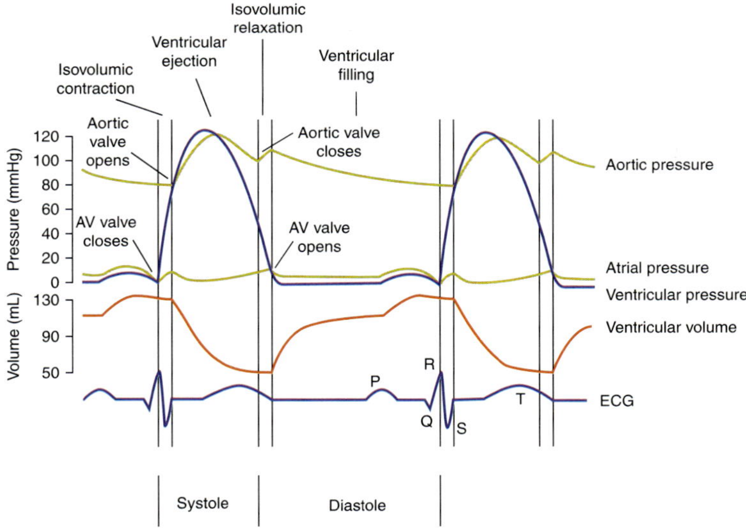

Fig. 2.6 The cardiac cycle. (AV = atrioventricular; ECG = electrocardiogram)

Isovolumic contraction begins with closure of the mitral valve, caused by the rising LV pressure at the start of ventricular systole. After the mitral valve has closed, pressure within the LV continues to rise but the LV volume remains constant (hence 'isovolumic') until the point when the aortic valve opens.

Ventricular ejection commences when the aortic valve opens and blood is ejected from the LV into the aorta. The LV volume falls during the ejection phase, as blood is expelled from the LV, but pressure continues to rise until it peaks and then starts to fall.

Isovolumic relaxation commences with closure of the aortic valve. Pressure within the LV falls during this phase (but volume remains constant), until the LV pressure falls below LA pressure. At this point, the pressure difference between LA and LV causes the mitral valve to open and isovolumic relaxation ends.

Ventricular filling begins as the mitral valve opens and blood flows into the LV from the LA. This phase ends when the mitral valve closes at the start of ventricular systole. Towards the end of the ventricular filling phase, atrial systole (contraction) occurs, coinciding with the P wave on the ECG, and this augments ventricular filling.

As shown in Fig. 2.6, the pressures within the cardiac chambers vary throughout the cardiac cycle. Table 2.1 lists the typical pressures found within each chamber. A pressure difference between two chambers causes the valve between them to open or close. For example, when LA pressure exceeds LV pressure the mitral valve opens, and when LV pressure exceeds LA pressure the mitral valve closes.

Table 2.1 Normal intracardiac pressures

	Pressure (mmHg)
Right atrium	Mean 0–5
Right ventricle	Systolic 15–25/diastolic 0–5
Pulmonary artery	Systolic 15–25/diastolic 5–12
Left atrium	Mean 5–12
Left ventricle	Systolic 100–140/diastolic 5–12
Aorta	Systolic 100–140/diastolic 60–90

Closure of the mitral and tricuspid valves can be heard with a stethoscope as the first heart sound (S_1). Closure of the aortic and pulmonary valves causes the second heart sound (S_2). During expiration S_2 occurs as a single sound, but during inspiration the return of venous blood to the right heart makes the pulmonary valve close slightly later than the aortic valve, causing normal physiological splitting of S_2 with the pulmonary component (P_2) occurring just after the aortic component (A_2). The presence of an ASD removes this respiratory variation in S_2, so that the slight gap between A_2 and P_2 is there all the time ('fixed splitting').

FURTHER READING

Anderson RH, Ho SY, Brecker SJ. Anatomic basis of cross-sectional echocardiography. *Heart* 2001; **85**: 716–20.

Anderson RH, Webb S, Brown NA *et al*. Development of the heart: (2) Septation of the atriums and ventricles. *Heart* 2003; **89**: 949–58.

Anderson RH, Webb S, Brown NA *et al*. Development of the heart: (3) Formation of the ventricular outflow tracts, arterial valves, and intrapericardial arterial trunks. *Heart* 2003; **89**: 1110–18.

Moorman A, Webb S, Brown NA *et al*. Development of the heart: (1) Formation of the cardiac chambers and arterial trunks. *Heart* 2003; **89**: 806–14.

3 Physics and instrumentation

Echocardiography uses ultrasound to examine the structure and function of the heart. A firm understanding of the physics of ultrasound gives the sonographer:

- an understanding of the capabilities and limitations of their echo machine
- the confidence to adjust the machine's controls to optimize the images.

Elementary physics

Sound travels as a longitudinal mechanical wave, and can be thought of as a series of vibrating particles in a line. Unlike electromagnetic waves (e.g. light waves, radio waves), sound waves need the presence of particles to be transmitted – sound cannot travel though a vacuum but instead requires a medium such as air, water or a solid. When a sound wave travels through a medium, there are areas of compression (high pressure and density, where the particles are closer together) and rarefaction (low pressure and density, where they are further apart). Sound can be represented as a sine wave, showing the variation in pressure through the medium (Fig. 3.1).

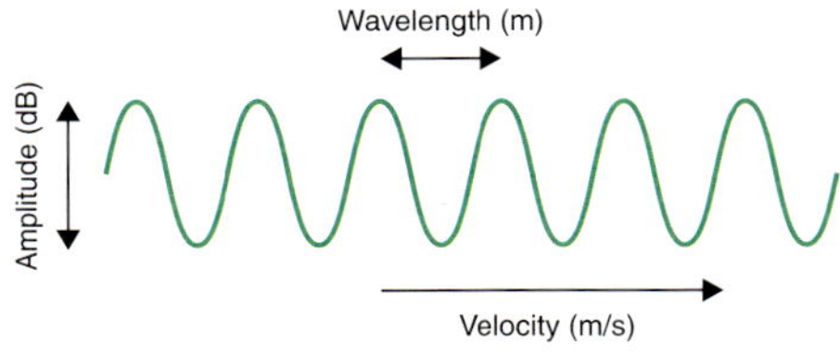

Fig. 3.1 An ultrasound wave

The **amplitude** of a sound wave indicates its strength, measured as the difference between the peak pressure in the medium and the average pressure. The unit of measurement is decibels (dB), using a logarithmic scale such that a difference of 6 dB represents a doubling in amplitude. Amplitude can be adjusted by the sonographer by changing the echo machine's power output (transmit power).

The **wavelength** of a sound wave is the distance between two successive waves – we normally measure this between the peak (or trough) of one wave and the identical point on the next wave. Wavelength is measured in appropriate units of length, such as metres (m) or millimetres (mm).

The **frequency** of a sound wave is the number of wave cycles (or oscillations) per second, and this is measured in Hertz (Hz). A sound wave with 100 oscillations per second has a frequency of 100 Hz. For high frequencies, the units of kiloHertz (kHz $= 10^3$ Hz) or MegaHertz (MHz $= 10^6$ Hz) can be used.

Audible sound lies in the frequency range 20 Hz to 20 000 Hz (20 kHz). Sound with a frequency below 20 Hz is called infrasound, and sound with a frequency greater than 20 kHz is called **ultrasound**. Ultrasound used for echocardiography usually lies in the frequency range 1.5–7 MHz.

The **propagation velocity** of a sound wave refers to the speed at which the wave propagates through the medium. This varies from one medium to another, depending both on the density and the stiffness of the medium. Propagation velocities for different body tissues are listed in Table 3.1. The average propagation velocity for the heart (and for soft tissues in general) is 1540 m/s.

Table 3.1 Propagation velocities in various body tissues

Medium	Speed (m/s)
Air	330
Fat	1450
Soft tissue (average)	1540
Blood	1570
Muscle	1580
Bone	3500

Wavelength, frequency and velocity are linked by the following equation:

$$\text{Propagation velocity} = \text{frequency} \times \text{wavelength}$$

For the heart, the propagation velocity of sound waves is fixed at approximately 1540 m/s – this cannot be altered by the sonographer. The sonographer can, however, choose the frequency of the sound waves being transmitted towards the heart. Choosing different frequencies will therefore influence the wavelength of the sound waves as they are transmitted through the heart (and the surrounding tissues). If, for instance, the sonographer was to choose a frequency of just 5 kHz, then the wavelength of the sound waves would be:

$$\text{Wavelength} = \frac{\text{Propagation velocity}}{\text{Frequency}}$$

$$\text{Wavelength} = \frac{1540\text{m/s}}{5000\text{Hz}}$$

$$\text{Wavelength} = 0.308\,\text{m}$$

Such a long wavelength, of just over 30 cm, would give very little spatial resolution and would be of little use for cardiac imaging. The higher the frequency chosen, the shorter the wavelength. As shorter wavelengths provide better resolution (see later), higher frequencies of between 1.5 MHz and 7 MHz are used for echo imaging.

So why not use even higher frequencies and get even better image resolution? One reason is that there is a trade-off between resolution and penetration – the higher the ultrasound frequency, the better the resolution but the poorer the penetration of the ultrasound into the body. The ultrasound frequencies used for echo offer a good balance between resolution and penetration. Paediatric echo uses higher frequencies (typically 5–10 MHz) than adult echo as the patient's smaller body size means that less penetration is required. Similarly, in intravascular ultrasound (p. 98), where high resolution but little penetration is required, frequencies of 20–50 MHz are used.

Ultrasound propagation

As an ultrasound pulse is transmitted from a transducer and into the body, it will encounter a number of different tissues, each of which has a different **acoustic impedance** ('resistance' to ultrasound transmission). These differences in acoustic impedance are particularly important at the boundaries between tissues. When an ultrasound pulse crosses a boundary between two tissues with very different acoustic impedances, a large proportion of the energy within the pulse will be **reflected** back towards the transducer.

This effect is most marked at the boundary between the air and the skin, where almost all of the ultrasound energy will be reflected back to the transducer and less than 1 per cent will enter the body. This would be a major drawback to performing medical ultrasound, so to get around this problem sonographers use gel to bridge the gap between the transducer and the skin. By excluding the air between the transducer and the skin, the gel reduces the impedance mismatch and allows much more of the ultrasound energy to enter the body. Similarly, echo can be challenging in patients with hyperinflated lungs (e.g. emphysema), where views of the heart can be obscured by air-filled lung tissue causing a large impedance mismatch.

As the ultrasound pulse is transmitted through the body, it will meet further boundaries where different degrees of reflection occur. There are two types of reflection (Fig. 3.2):

- specular reflection
- backscatter.

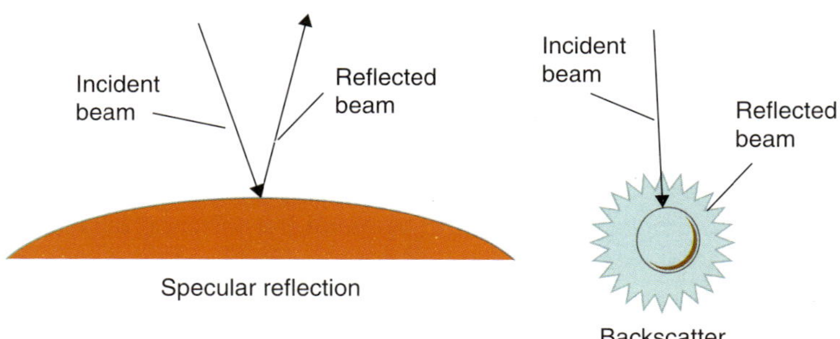

Fig. 3.2 Specular reflection and backscatter

Specular ('mirror-like') reflection occurs at tissue boundaries where the reflector is relatively large (at least two wavelengths in diameter) and smooth – structures such as the heart valves and the walls of the heart chambers and major vessels are examples of specular reflectors. The proportion of ultrasound energy reflected by a specular reflector is highly dependent on the angle of incidence of the incoming ultrasound beam – in order to maximize the amount of energy reflected, the incoming beam should be as perpendicular (i.e. as close to 90°) to the reflector as possible.

Backscatter occurs with small and/or rough-surfaced structures, where the reflected ultrasound will scatter in many different directions. The returning signal will be weaker than from a specular reflector, but will not be dependent on the angle of the incident (incoming) ultrasound beam. An example of a scatter reflector is the tissue within the myocardium. Red blood cells also cause scatter, and as this scatter is equal in all directions they are referred to as a special group known as **Rayleigh scatterers**.

As an ultrasound pulse travels through tissue, it will gradually lose energy, a process known as **attenuation**. Attenuation results from reflection and backscatter, and also from the absorption of energy by the tissues themselves (where the sound energy is converted into heat). This loss of energy can be quantified in decibels, and in soft tissues a change of –3 dB equates to a fall in signal intensity of 50 per cent. The **half-intensity depth** (HID) is the depth (in cm) in soft tissue in which the intensity of the ultrasound is reduced by 50 per cent, and depends upon the frequency (f) of the ultrasound emitted by the transducer, measured in MHz:

$$\text{HID (soft tissue)} = \frac{6}{f}$$

Thus the ultrasound emitted by a 4 MHz transducer would lose 50 per cent of its intensity after travelling through just 6/4 = 1.5 cm of soft tissue. Attenuation is therefore greater at higher frequencies.

Refraction is the change in direction of an ultrasound pulse as it passes across a boundary between two tissues (or materials) of different acoustic impedance. Although refraction can be useful (for instance, refraction is used to focus the ultrasound beam with an acoustic lens) it can also be a source of artefact (p. 27).

Ultrasound transducers

In transthoracic echo, ultrasound is generated by a transducer (commonly called a probe) which is held on the patient's chest. For other imaging techniques (e.g. transoesophageal echo (TOE), intravascular ultrasound), the transducer may be passed into the oesophagus or even into the heart itself. The transducer is both a transmitter and a receiver – it transmits ultrasound into the chest, and also detects the return of the reflected ultrasound back to the probe.

Ultrasound transducers work using the **piezoelectric effect**. Piezoelectric crystals change shape when an electrical voltage is applied, and so an alternating voltage can make them oscillate rapidly, thereby generating ultrasound. In addition, if the crystals are themselves caused to oscillate by a *returning* ultrasound wave, they *generate* an electrical voltage which can be detected as a signal. Thus the crystals both generate and detect ultrasound.

Contemporary **phased-array transducers** consist of an array of piezoelectric elements (typically 128 for a 2-D echo probe, several thousand for a 3-D probe). The ultrasound beam can be 'steered' and focused electronically by altering the timing of activation (or 'phasing') of the individual elements. Older mechanical transducers used a motor within the transducer to move the piezoelectric elements but had limited Doppler capabilities, and were prone to mechanical failure.

The key components of a transducer are shown in Figure 3.3. The **piezoelectric elements** are mounted on **a backing layer**, which has high impedance and is designed to absorb ultrasound and 'damp down' reverberation ('ringing') of the piezoelectric elements. In front of the elements is **a matching layer**, which improves the impedance matching between the elements and the body.

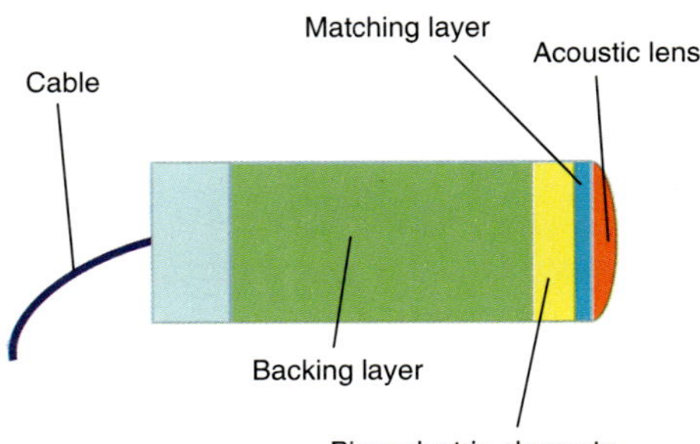

Fig. 3.3 Structure of an ultrasound transducer

The ultrasound beam remains cylindrical for a short distance after it leaves the transducer (the **near field** or Fresnel zone), but then diverges (the **far field** or Fraunhofer zone). Imaging quality is best within the near field, and maximizing the depth of the near field (i.e. the distance travelled by the ultrasound beam before it diverges) is important for image optimization. The length of the near field is greater at higher transducer frequencies and wider transducer diameters.

Focusing the ultrasound beam does *not* affect the length of the near field, but it does produce a narrower beam (and higher resolution) within the near field, albeit at the expense of making the beam wider in the far field (Fig. 3.4). A plastic **acoustic lens** at the front of the transducer helps to focus the ultrasound beam. A phased-array transducer also offers electronic focusing, which allows the sonographer to control the depth at which ultrasound beam is most tightly focused.

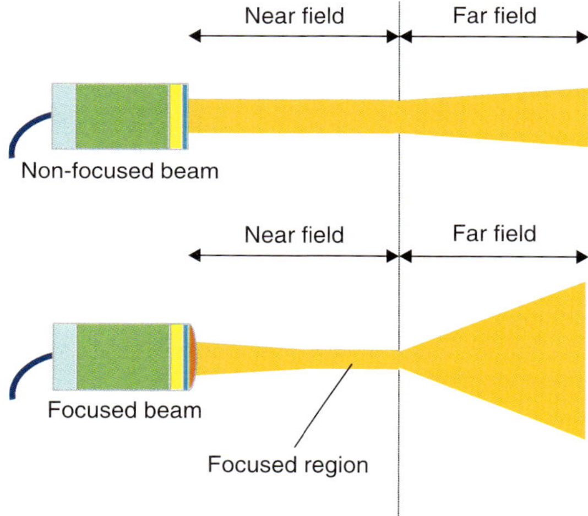

Fig. 3.4 Effect of focusing on near and far field

A transducer will transmit short bursts of ultrasound (lasting just a few microseconds), and then wait for a few hundred microseconds for the reflected ultrasound to return before transmitting the next bursts of ultrasound. A small amount of the ultrasound energy will be reflected back to the transducer each time the ultrasound pulse reaches an interface, and as the transducer detects these returning pulses it measures the time taken between the pulse being emitted and returning to the transducer ('round trip time'). From this, and from a knowledge of the propagation velocity of ultrasound in soft tissue, the echo machine can calculate the distance between the transducer and the reflector. The transducer can also determine the intensity of the returning signal, and use this information in building up the image display. Other features of the returning signal, such as its frequency and any frequency shift compared to the transmitted signal, are discussed in relation to Doppler principles in Chapter 4.

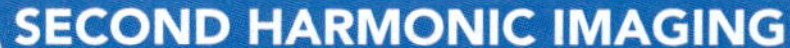

SECOND HARMONIC IMAGING

The reflected echo signal that returns to the transducer contains not just ultrasound at the original (fundamental) frequency of the transmitted signal, but also harmonics (multiples of the original frequency). These harmonics originate mainly from the central portion of the beam and also from deeper structures. Second harmonic imaging filters the returning signal to remove the fundamental frequency and build up an image using the second harmonic components of the signal. In so doing, the image resolution improves (because of the higher frequency), particularly for far field structures. Disadvantages of second harmonic imaging are that it requires a higher power output, and it does slightly alter the appearance of myocardial texture and also the apparent thickness of structures such as valve leaflets compared with fundamental imaging.

Imaging modalities

The earliest echo modality was amplitude mode (A-mode) imaging, which simply plotted the amplitude of the reflected ultrasound (as a 'spike' with a certain amplitude) versus the distance of the reflected signal from the transducer. Brightness mode (B-mode) imaging was similar in principle, but rather than plotting the returning signals as a row of spikes of varying sizes, it represented the amplitude of the returning signal by the brightness of a dot. A-mode and B-mode imaging have been superseded by M-mode and 2-D imaging.

M-mode imaging

M-mode (or motion-mode) imaging records motion along a single 'line of sight', selected by careful positioning of the on-screen cursor across a region of interest (Fig. 3.5). Once the cursor is in place, activation of M-mode imaging produces a scrolling display of movement (along the vertical y axis), as it occurs along the cursor line, plotted against time (along the horizontal x axis). A typical M-mode trace for a normal mitral valve is shown in Figure 3.6.

The very narrow field of view of M-mode imaging – essentially a single scan line, represented by the on-screen cursor – means that a very high pulse repetition frequency can be used, giving a sampling rate of around 1800 times per second. This is very useful in visualizing rapid motion, such as the

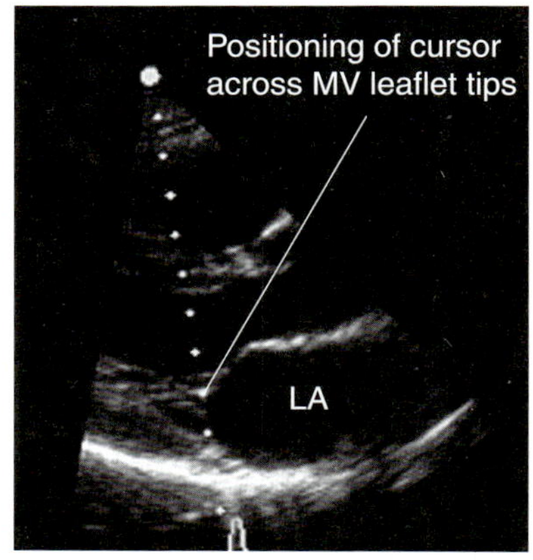

View	Parasternal long axis
Modality	2-D (with M-mode cursor)

Fig. 3.5 Positioning of the cursor for an M-mode study of the mitral valve (LA = left atrium; MV = mitral valve)

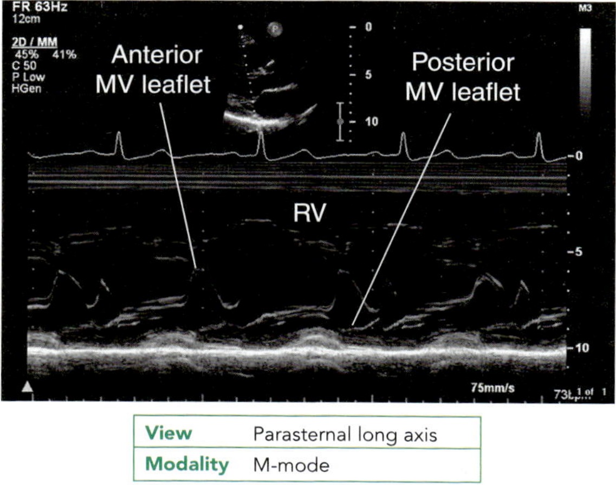

View	Parasternal long axis
Modality	M-mode

Fig. 3.6 M-mode study of the mitral valve (MV = mitral valve; RV = right ventricle)

movement of valve leaflets, and permits accurate timing of events as well as measurement of cardiac dimensions.

2-D imaging

Whereas in M-mode imaging the heart is imaged along just a single scan line, in 2-D imaging a picture of the heart is built up from a series of scan lines side by side. In 2-D imaging the ultrasound probe sweeps a beam across the heart around 20–30 times per second, creating a series of scan lines (usually around 120) each time it makes a sweep, in order to build up a 2-D image (Fig. 3.7).

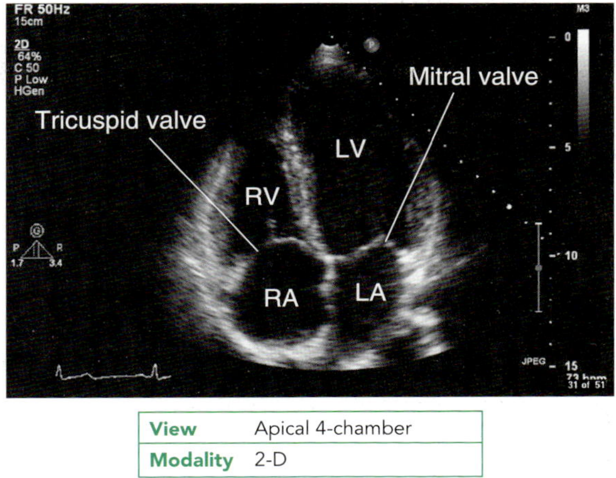

View	Apical 4-chamber
Modality	2-D

Fig. 3.7 Normal 2-D echo (LA = left atrium; LV = left ventricle; RA = right atrium; RV = right ventricle)

The probe has to transmit and receive an ultrasound pulse for each scan line of the image and there is therefore a limit on how many image 'frames' can be generated each second, determined by the number of scan lines that make up the image (the sector width) and the depth of the image. Reducing the sector width and/or depth will reduce the time taken to generate an image frame, increasing the number of image frames that can be generated each second ('frame rate'). It is therefore important to optimize image quality by narrowing down the size of the image sector to cover just the key area of interest.

Echo machine instrumentation

At first sight, the number of controls on an echo machine can appear daunting. In reality, the controls are relatively simple to understand and to use, and it is important to know how to optimize their settings to obtain the best possible image quality. In this section the controls that affect M-mode and 2-D imaging will be discussed. Controls for the spectral and colour Doppler modalities are discussed in Chapter 4.

Transmit power controls the amount of ultrasound energy delivered to the patient, and to minimize the risk of adverse mechanical or thermal effects it is important to use the lowest setting possible (p. 29).

Gain refers to the amplification of the received signal to increase the brightness of the displayed images. Gain can be adjusted for the whole image (overall gain) or for part of the image (see time-gain compensation (TGC) below). While a high gain setting can be useful for detecting weaker signals that might otherwise not be visible, it reduces lateral resolution and also increases noise.

The **depth** setting determines how far the ultrasound beam 'looks' into the patient and is an important determinant of frame rate. The greater the depth setting, the longer the transducer will have to wait for the ultrasound pulse to make its round trip before repeating the pulse, and so the lower the frame rate. The depth setting should be chosen so that the whole area of interest can be seen, but not so deeply that it includes irrelevant structures beyond the region of interest.

Sector width determines the field of view across which the ultrasound beam sweeps. As with depth, sector width is an important determinant of frame rate and should be optimized for each view to include the region of interest but no more.

Focus can be fine-tuned with phased-array transducers and should be adjusted for each view so that the beam is focused on the region of interest.

TGC is also known as depth compensation, and corrects for the attenuation of the ultrasound signal that occurs with increasing distance from the transducer. TGC boosts the gain of the signals returning from the far field to ensure an even 'echo brightness' across the whole depth of the image. The TGC controls can be fine-tuned by the sonographer using slider-bars.

Grey scale compression (dynamic range) adjusts the number of shades of grey that are displayed in the image. This allows the sonographer to choose the degree of contrast in the image.

Resolution

Resolution refers to the ability to discriminate between two objects that are close together in space (spatial resolution) or two events that occur close together in time (temporal resolution). Spatial resolution has two components:

- axial resolution
- lateral resolution.

Axial resolution relates to objects that lie along the axis of the ultrasound beam, and is mainly determined by transducer frequency (higher frequency = better axial resolution) and pulse length (shorter pulse length = better axial resolution). Axial resolution is typically around 3 mm.

Lateral resolution, also known as azimuthal resolution, relates to objects that lie side by side, perpendicular to the ultrasound beam, and varies according to how far the objects lie from the transducer. The narrower the beam, the better the lateral resolution. The width of the beam can be optimized by focusing it on the region of interest (see Fig. 3.4, p. 22). Lateral resolution is also affected by gain settings – the higher the gain, the worse the lateral resolution. Lateral resolution is typically around 1 mm.

Temporal resolution, or frame rate, is important in trying to distinguish events that occur close together in time. Frame rate depends upon the time taken to collect all the data required to create one image, which in turn depends upon the sector width and depth. M-mode imaging offers very high sampling rates, typically 1800 times per second, because of the very narrow field of view (see above). 2-D echo has a much slower frame rate, typically 20–30 frames per second, because of the much greater amount of ultrasound data that must be collected to create a single frame.

Imaging artefacts

Imaging artefacts occur when 'structures' and/or distortions are seen on the echo image that are not actually present in the heart (or, at least, not at the apparent location), or when structures that *are* present seem to be absent on the image.

Acoustic shadowing occurs when a highly echo-reflective structure (e.g. a mechanical valve prosthesis) blocks ultrasound from penetrating any further, causing echo drop-out in the far field. This can pose a particular problem when assessing the structure and function of prosthetic valves.

Reverberation occurs when ultrasound rebounds several times between two strong specular reflectors before returning to the transducer. The time spent 'rebounding' delays the return of the signal to the transducer, and so the processing software misinterprets the returning signal as having originated further away that it really has. This leads to 'ghost' images occurring in the far field, which can be recognized because they move in tandem with the structure that caused the reverberation.

Beam width artefact arises because the ultrasound beam has a finite width (especially in the far field) and the machine is unable to discriminate whether a returning echo signal has arisen from the centre of the beam and/or the edge. Strong reflectors at the edge of the beam are therefore displayed by the echo machine as though they arise from the centre of the beam, 'smearing' the displayed echo. Beam width artefact can be reduced by focusing the ultrasound beam to minimize its diameter.

Side lobe artefact is similar in its mechanism to beam width artefact, but arises from unwanted but unavoidable 'side lobe' beams (which are additional beams surrounding the main ultrasound beam). Signals returning from the side lobe beams are interpreted by the echo machine as having arisen from the central beam, and can be displayed some distance away from the true location of the structure in question.

Display and recording methods

The returning echo signal at the transducer undergoes a series of initial processing steps which include amplification, TGC and filtering. The video signal is then sent to a scan converter, which converts the signal into a 'rectangular' format suitable for display. The resulting data undergo further processing ('post-processing') and can then be stored in a digital format and/or can undergo digital-to-analogue conversion to create a video signal for display on a monitor (and/or archiving onto videotape). This process occurs so rapidly that the acquired data can be displayed on a monitor almost in 'real time'.

Storage of echo studies can be on videotape, which is relatively inexpensive, although it rapidly becomes cumbersome to store (and to review) studies when large numbers are archived in this way. Digital archiving is now more commonly used, with storage on hard drives or optical disks. This makes accessing studies easier and allows greater flexibility in image processing after the study has been completed. However, the quantity of digital data generated by an echo study can be considerable, so high-volume storage media (and 'lossless' data compression techniques) are required if large numbers of studies are to be archived.

Safety of ultrasound

Ultrasound involves the delivery of external energy to body tissues and so it is important to consider the potential adverse biological effects that this could entail. The intensity of exposure to ultrasound is expressed as power per unit of area (watts/cm^2) expressed as the maximum intensity within the ultrasound beam (the spatial peak) averaged over the duration of exposure (temporal average), the **spatial peak temporal average** (SPTA). There are two main biological effects of exposure to ultrasound energy: thermal (heating) and mechanical (e.g. cavitation).

Thermal effects are caused by conversion of the mechanical energy of the ultrasound into heat energy as it passes though the tissues. The amount of heating is hard to predict but relates to several factors including transducer frequency, transmit power, focus and depth. Thermal effects are most relevant to TOE where the probe may remain stationary in the oesophagus for long periods, particularly during intraoperative studies. Heat may be generated not just by the ultrasound but also directly by the probe itself. It is prudent to keep imaging time to a minimum and to ensure that the TOE probe is repositioned regularly, and to monitor the temperature of the probe.

Mechanical effects include cavitation, in which gas bubbles are created as ultrasound passes through the tissues. It is not thought to be a problem during standard transthoracic studies, but is important when bubble contrast agents are used as it can cause resonance and even disruption of the bubbles (p. 95). Mechanical effects of ultrasound can also be measured by **mechanical index** (MI), which is the peak negative (rarefactional) pressure divided by the square root of the transducer frequency. An MI of <1 is considered safe.

Although echo has an excellent safety record, it is nevertheless prudent to minimize risk by:

- only performing echo for appropriate clinical indications
- keeping the power output as low as possible
- keeping the exposure time to a minimum.

M-mode and 2-D echo have the lowest ultrasound intensity, and pulsed-wave Doppler has the highest intensity (with colour Doppler having an intermediate value).

Ensuring safety also requires an awareness of more general hazards such as:

- risk of electrical shock from damaged or poorly maintained equipment
- risk of injury from trips and falls, particularly when transferring onto the examination couch
- risk of infection from inadequate infection control measures.

Echo departments should have appropriate risk assessment tools and protocols in place to minimize risks to patients and staff.

FURTHER READING

Adeyemi B. *British Society of Echocardiography Distance Learning Module 14: Physics of transducers for imaging and Doppler.* Accessible from the BSE website (www.bsecho.org).

Monaghan MJ. Second harmonic imaging: a new tune for an old fiddle? *Heart* 2000; **83**: 131–2.

Reynolds T. *Ultrasound Physics: A Registry Exam Preparation Guide*. School of Cardiac Ultrasound, Arizona Heart Institute Foundation, Phoenix, 1996.

4 Doppler physics

Echo can be used to examine not just the heart's anatomical structure but also the flow of blood through the heart. This in turn provides valuable information about valvular function, intracardiac shunts and so forth. The study of the heart's fluid dynamics is made possible by the Doppler principle, discussed in this chapter. As well as allowing the assessment of blood flow, the Doppler principle has also, more recently, been applied to the study of myocardial function (tissue Doppler imaging).

Doppler principles

The Doppler effect describes how an observer perceives a change in the wavelength or frequency of a sound (or light) wave if the source is moving relative to them. A classic example is that of a moving ambulance sounding its siren – as the ambulance approaches an observer, its siren sounds higher pitched than when it is moving away. Figure 4.1 shows how sound waves from a source, moving towards Observer A, shorten in wavelength (and therefore increase in frequency) in the direction of movement. Observer A

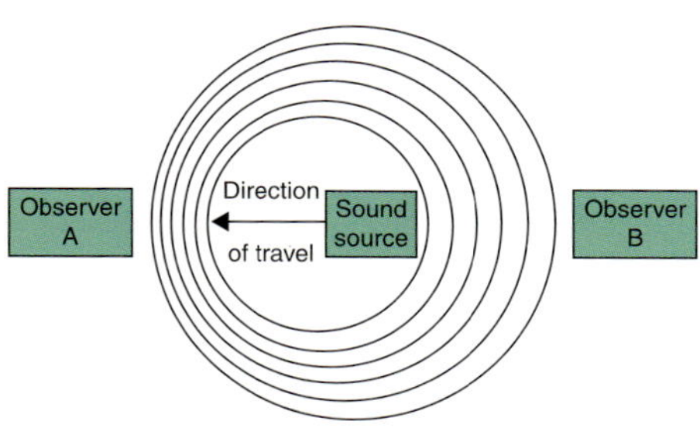

Fig. 4.1 The Doppler effect

would therefore hear a higher pitch, and observer B a lower pitch, than if the source was stationary.

The same phenomenon occurs with ultrasound waves when they are reflected from moving red blood cells. The frequency of the returning ultrasound is increased if the red blood cells are moving towards the ultrasound transducer, or decreased if they are moving away. This change in frequency between the transmitted and returning ultrasound signal is the Doppler shift, from which the velocity (V) of the red blood cells can be calculated:

$$V = \frac{c \times f_d}{2 \times f_t \times \cos\theta}$$

where c is the speed of sound in blood, f_d is the Doppler shift in frequency between transmitted and returning signals, f_t is the frequency of the transmitted signal, and θ is the angle between the ultrasound beam and the direction of blood flow.

It follows from this equation that a large angle between the direction of blood flow and the ultrasound beam will lead to an underestimation of flow velocity, and this is particularly marked for angles >20°. For this reason, when undertaking echo Doppler studies it is important to align the ultrasound beam with the direction of blood flow as closely as possible.

Spectral Doppler

When the ultrasound beam returns to the transducer, the difference in frequency between the transmitted and returning beams is compared to calculate the Doppler shift. This is a complex process as the returning signal contains a spectrum of frequencies, and a mathematical technique called a fast Fourier transform is used to undertake the necessary spectral analysis.

A spectral Doppler display can then be produced (Fig. 4.2). These displays conventionally plot frequency shifts (shown as velocities) on the vertical axis against time on the horizontal axis. A zero line is shown, and flow towards the transducer is plotted above the line (and flow away from the transducer, as in Fig. 4.2, is plotted below the line). For each time point the grey pixels show the blood flow velocity detected, and the density of the signal (i.e. the shade of grey plotted at each point in the spectrum) represents the amplitude of the signal at that particular velocity (i.e. the proportion of red blood cells moving at that particular velocity). The overall brightness of the greyscale display can also be adjusted by the sonographer, using the Doppler gain setting. Such spectral displays form the basis of continuous wave (CW) and pulsed-wave (PW) Doppler techniques (see below).

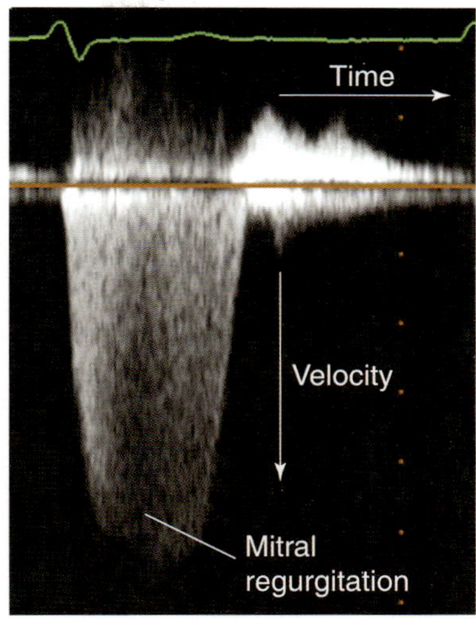

Fig. 4.2 Spectral Doppler display (showing mitral regurgitation)

Spectral (CW and PW) Doppler controls on an echo machine include:

Transmit power, which controls the amount of ultrasound energy delivered to the patient.

Gain, which amplifies the received signal to increase the brightness of the displayed spectral trace. High gain settings amplify weaker signals that might otherwise not be visible, but increase noise.

Baseline shift, which shifts the 'zero point' of the display up or down.

Velocity range, which alters the vertical velocity scale to a higher or lower range.

The frequency range seen with Doppler shift (−10 to +10 kHz) falls within the audible range of the human ear, so it is possible to listen to blood flow via the loudspeaker on the echo machine, adjusting the volume as appropriate, and to use the audible 'quality' of the sound to guide fine adjustments in the alignment of the ultrasound beam with the blood flow, in order to obtain the best possible signal.

Continuous wave Doppler

CW Doppler uses *continuous* transmission and receiving of ultrasound (unlike the intermittent pulses used in 2-D imaging). Two crystals in the transducer are used, one to transmit an ultrasound signal and the other to receive the returning signal. A dedicated CW Doppler probe ('pencil probe') can also be used; this contains two crystals specifically for performing CW Doppler.

A typical CW Doppler display, obtained by interrogating flow across the mitral valve in the apical 4-chamber view, is shown in Figure 4.3. This shows a positive spectral trace above the zero line which corresponds to forward flow across the valve during diastole, and a negative trace below the line corresponding to regurgitant flow during systole. The 2-D image/colour Doppler image in the upper part of the figure shows the positioning of the cursor to align the ultrasound beam with the mitral valve flow.

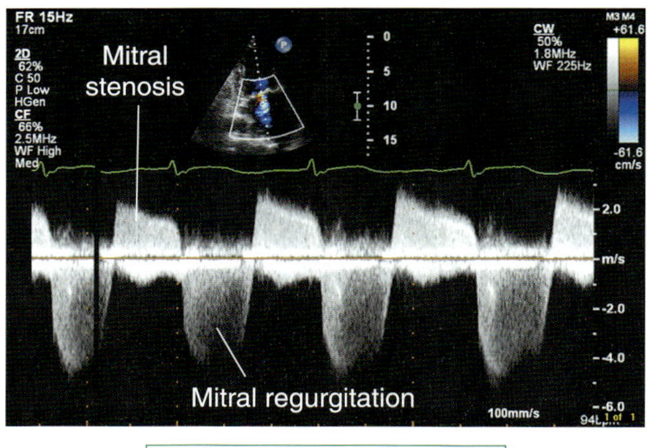

View	Apical 4-chamber
Modality	CW Doppler

Fig. 4.3 Continuous wave Doppler imaging, showing mitral stenosis and regurgitation

It is important to appreciate that, in CW Doppler, the echo machine obtains signals along the *entire length* of the ultrasound beam (or cursor line) – the resulting spectral trace therefore reflects the direction and velocity of movement of red blood cells at every point along the beam, and so CW Doppler is unable to assess flow at any one specific point in the heart. The spectral display reflects the full range of red blood cell velocities detected along the beam at any particular time point, usually ranging from zero up to the peak velocity demarcated by the edge of the spectral trace.

Although the inability to discriminate flow velocity at any specific point puts CW Doppler at a disadvantage in comparison to the specific sampling ability of PW Doppler, CW Doppler has the advantage of being able to measure higher velocities without aliasing (see below).

Pulsed-wave Doppler

PW Doppler measures blood flow velocity at a specific location, which the sonographer chooses by placing a **sample volume** (indicated by two parallel lines perpendicular to the main cursor line) at the point of interest (Fig. 4.4). The length of the sample volume can be adjusted by the sonographer – typically a length of 3 mm is used.

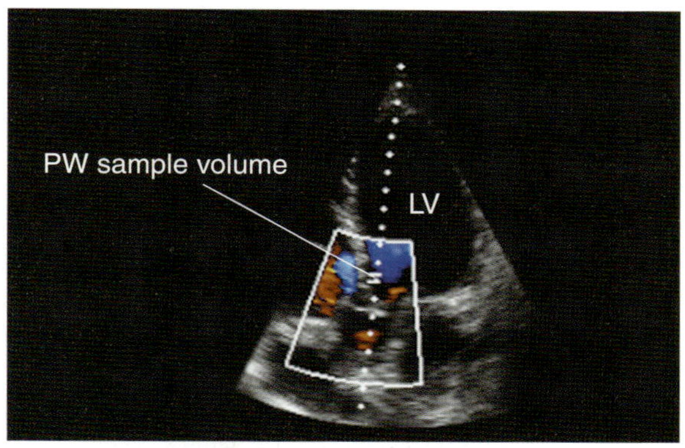

View	Apical 5-chamber
Modality	PW Doppler

Fig. 4.4 Pulsed-wave (PW) Doppler imaging, showing sample volume (LV = left ventricle)

In order to measure Doppler shift (and hence flow velocity) within the boundaries of the sample volume, the transducer cannot use continuous transmission/reception of ultrasound. Instead, the transducer transmits an ultrasound pulse and then only samples the reflected signal as it returns from the point of interest – the machine can calculate how long the signal will take to make the return journey between the transducer and the sample volume, and 'listens out' for the returning signal at that time point. In doing so, the machine 'ignores' the returning ultrasound from all other points along the beam.

The fact that the echo machine has to transmit a pulse and then wait for it to return places a limit on how rapidly it can send out consecutive pulses – the

pulse repetition frequency (PRF). The further away the sample volume is from the transducer, the longer the 'round trip time' of the ultrasound pulse and so the lower the PRF. This gives rise to the phenomenon known as aliasing, which is one of the main limitations to the usefulness of PW Doppler.

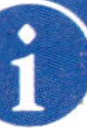

ALIASING

The concept of aliasing is traditionally explained in terms of a movie film of a rotating spoked wheel. If the wheel is rotating 30 times per second, and the film is running at 30 frames per second, then every time the wheel is captured (or 'sampled') on a movie frame it will have made one full rotation and will have returned to the same orientation. When the film is played back, the wheel will look as though it is stationary. In order to capture the rotation of the wheel the movie frame rate (or 'sampling rate') needs to be higher – with regard to sampling ultrasound, in order to unambiguously measure wavelength a waveform must be sampled at least twice in each cycle (**Nyquist's theorem**). This places an upper limit on the Doppler shift that can be measured using PW Doppler (**Nyquist limit**), which equals half the PRF. Once the blood velocity exceeds this limit, the spectral trace will appear with the top of the waveform 'missing' (in fact, transposed to the opposite side of the baseline). Shifting the baseline can help reduce the problem of aliasing to some extent, but the phenomenon nevertheless places a significant limitation on the maximum velocity that can be assessed with PW Doppler. Aliasing can also be reduced by:

- adjusting the Doppler velocity scale (as far as possible)
- sampling at the lowest possible distance from the transducer
- decreasing the transmitted frequency
- increasing the angle of incidence.

Ultimately it may prove necessary to switch to CW Doppler instead, where possible. One further alternative is to use high-PRF PW Doppler, in which a higher PRF is used, which means that sampling now occurs at two or more distinct sites along the ultrasound beam but a higher velocity can be measured before aliasing occurs. Careful placement of the sample volumes so that one lies in the region of interest and all the others lie in low-velocity regions means that high-PRF PW Doppler can sometimes be a useful way round the aliasing problem.

An example of a PW Doppler spectral display is shown in Figure 4.5, with the sample volume placed in the left ventricular outflow tract (LVOT). Note that a PW Doppler spectral display typically has a more distinct 'border' to the spectral envelope, with less 'filling in' within the lower-velocity regions of the envelope, compared with CW Doppler. This is because the limited sample volume of PW Doppler means that the red blood cells sampled have a narrower range of velocities than those sampled along the whole length of the ultrasound beam with CW Doppler.

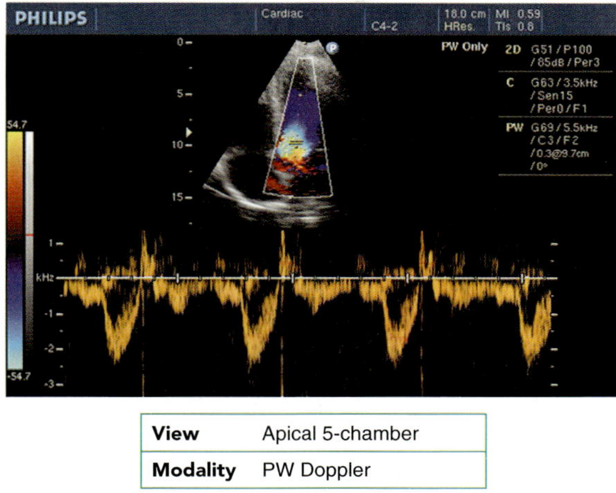

View	Apical 5-chamber
Modality	PW Doppler

Fig. 4.5 Pulsed-wave Doppler imaging in the left ventricular outflow tract (Figure reproduced with permission of Philips)

Fluid dynamics

Normal intracardiac blood flow is described as laminar, in which a column of blood flows in parallel (or concentric) streams, each having a uniform flow velocity. Turbulent flow occurs when this breaks down, for instance when passing through an area of stenosis, causing blood to flow in multiple directions and at different velocities (Fig. 4.6).

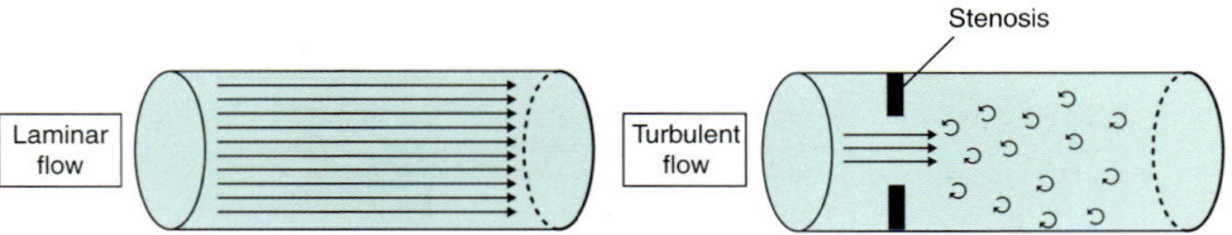

Fig. 4.6 Laminar and turbulent flow

The point at which laminar flow along a vessel becomes turbulent is described by the Reynolds equation, in which turbulent flow is more likely when blood with high density and low viscosity flows at high velocity through a wide-calibre vessel.

Blood flow is pulsatile, increasing (and then decreasing) in velocity with time during each cardiac cycle. A number of velocity measurements can be made from a spectral Doppler display. The outermost edge of the spectral trace represents the **peak velocity** at any particular time point. The brightest portion of the spectral display represents the velocity of the majority of the red blood cells (**modal velocity**). The average velocity of the red blood cells is expressed as the **mean velocity**.

Stroke distance and volume

Measurement of flow volume in a tube can, *for a constant flow rate*, be calculated simply by multiplying the cross-sectional area of the tube by the flow velocity. However, blood flow is pulsatile, not constant, so to calculate flow volume (mL per heartbeat) it is necessary to measure the cross-sectional area of the region of interest and to measure the **velocity time integral** (VTI) of flow in that region. VTI is measured by integrating the area under the spectral envelope – this can easily be achieved by tracing the outline of the spectral Doppler envelope and allowing the echo machine software to calculate the VTI. VTI is measured in cm and represents the **stroke distance** – the distance travelled by a column of blood in the region of interest during one flow period (Fig. 4.7). To measure cross-sectional area (CSA), measure the diameter of the region where the spectral Doppler trace was obtained:

$$\text{CSA} = 0.785 \times (\text{diameter})^2$$

Flow volume, in mL per flow period, can now be calculated from:

$$\text{Flow volume} = \text{CSA} \times \text{VTI}$$

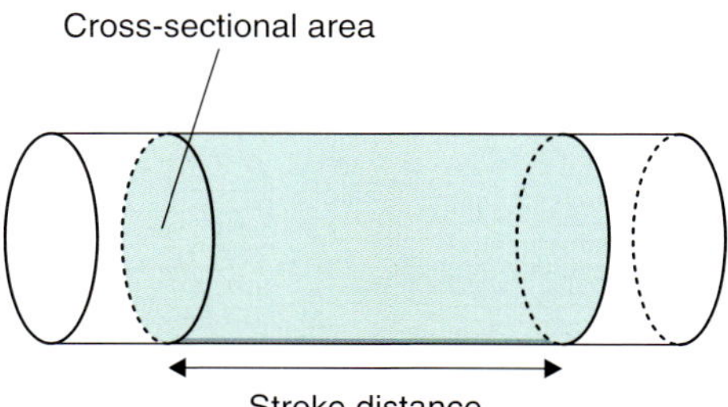

Fig. 4.7 Calculation of blood flow volume

This method is commonly used to calculate **stroke volume** using CSA and VTI measurements taken in the LVOT.

Continuity equation

The law of conservation of mass states that volume flow through the cardiovascular system is constant (assuming that blood is incompressible and that the chamber or vessel carrying the blood is not elastic). Thus the flow rate in one area is equal to the flow rate in another, assuming a closed circuit (i.e. no loss of blood between the two regions of measurement). Thus:

$$\text{Flow volume in region A} = \text{Flow volume in region B}$$

$$CSA_A \times VTI_A = CSA_B \times VTI_B$$

This means that if CSA and VTI can be measured in region A, and VTI measured in region B, then the CSA of region B can be calculated:

$$CSA_B = CSA_A \times \frac{VTI_A}{VTI_B}$$

This is the **continuity equation**. If a particular cross-sectional area (e.g. the orifice of a stenosed aortic valve) is difficult to measure directly, then the continuity equation can be used to calculate it by measuring the VTI in that area together with the VTI and CSA of a different area (where CSA is easier to measure).

A typical example is the measurement of CSA and VTI (using PW Doppler) in the LVOT, and VTI (using CW Doppler) through the aortic valve (AV), and using these data to calculate aortic valve orifice area:

$$CSA_{AV} = CSA_{LVOT} \times \frac{VTI_{LVOT}}{VTI_{AV}}$$

Pressure gradient

Doppler measurements of blood flow velocity can be used to calculate pressure gradients between two regions, for instance the pressure gradient between left ventricle (LV) and aorta in aortic stenosis. The relationship between pressure gradient and velocity is expressed by the Bernoulli equation:

$$\Delta P = 4 \times (V_2^2 - V_1^2)$$

where ΔP is the pressure gradient between the two regions, V_1 is the velocity proximal to the stenosis and V_2 is the velocity distal to the stenosis.

If V_2 is significantly greater than V_1, then V_1 can be ignored and an even simpler version (the simplified Bernoulli equation) can be used:

$$\Delta P = 4 \times V^2$$

where V is the peak velocity of the jet flowing between the two regions. A typical example is the calculation of aortic valve gradient in aortic stenosis – if the peak velocity of flow through the aortic valve is 4 m/s, measured using CW Doppler, then the peak pressure gradient across the valve is:

$$\Delta P = 4 \times V^2$$
$$\Delta P = 4 \times 4^2$$
$$\Delta P = 64 \text{ mmHg}$$

Colour Doppler

Colour flow mapping, or colour Doppler, is based upon the principle of PW Doppler. However, rather than measuring blood flow at just a single sample volume, in colour Doppler the blood flow is assessed at multiple points within a pre-selected area. The sonographer chooses the area in which to display colour Doppler data by overlaying a 'box' on the 2-D image. The size and position of this box can be adjusted so that it covers the region of interest (Fig. 4.8).

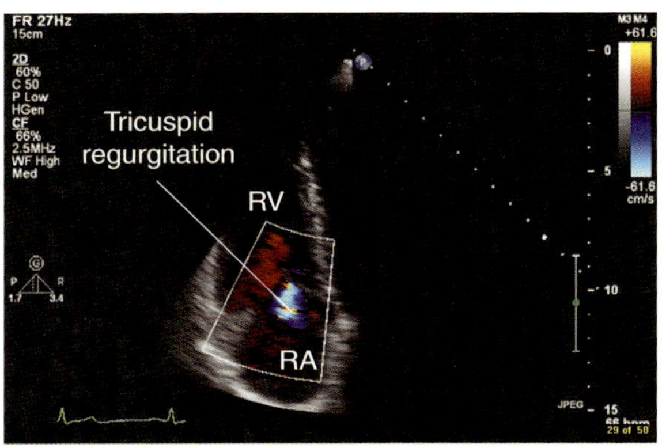

View	Apical 4-chamber
Modality	Colour Doppler

Fig. 4.8 Colour Doppler imaging, showing tricuspid regurgitation (RA = right atrium; RV = right ventricle)

A colour Doppler display colour-codes blood flow according to its direction and the *mean* velocity within each sample volume. Flow away from the transducer is traditionally shown as blue, and towards the transducer is shown as red (BART – Blue Away, Red Towards). Turbulent flow, in which there are rapid changes in the flow velocity (high 'variance') in a particular region, is colour-coded green.

At the edge of the display is a velocity scale, correlating the shade of colour with the measured flow velocity. As it is based upon PW Doppler, colour Doppler suffers the same limitation of aliasing and so once flow exceeds the upper measurable limit it will be coded in the 'opposite' colour. The numbers at the top and bottom of the velocity scale indicate the maximum velocities towards/away from the transducer that can be measured before aliasing occurs (Nyquist limit). To optimize the image by maximizing frame rates, the size of the colour Doppler 'box' should be kept as small as possible.

Colour Doppler M-mode

Colour Doppler M-mode uses the same principles as colour Doppler, but instead of overlaying the colour data on a 2-D display it instead overlays it on an M-mode display (Fig. 4.9). It can be useful for precisely timing the occurrence of colour jets, and is commonly used for measuring the width of a jet of aortic regurgitation in relation to the diameter of the LVOT (p. 160).

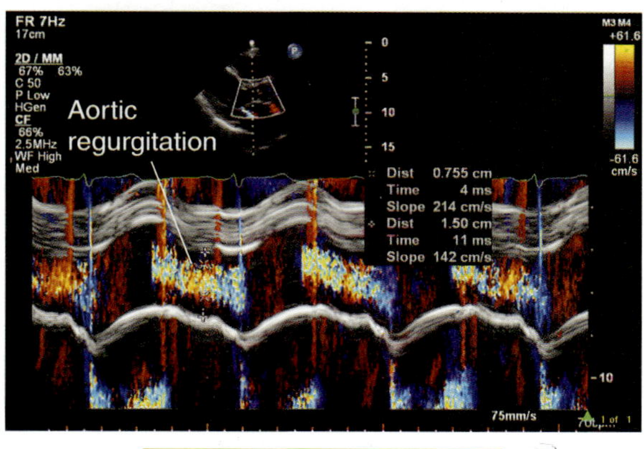

View	Parasternal long axis
Modality	Colour M-Mode

Fig. 4.9 Colour Doppler M-mode imaging, showing aortic regurgitation

Tissue Doppler imaging

For many years Doppler techniques were principally used for assessing the movement of blood in the heart and great vessels. Although other structures, including the myocardium, move as well, filtering techniques were used to remove the Doppler signals returning from myocardium in order to optimize the signals relating to blood flow.

However, since the 1990s there has been growing interest in Doppler assessment of the myocardium (tissue Doppler imaging, TDI). The Doppler signals returning from myocardium are distinct from signals from blood (myocardial motion generates a stronger but lower-velocity signal) and so can be selected with appropriate filtering. The resulting signals can be displayed as colour Doppler images to show myocardial motion (Fig. 4.10) or as spectral PW Doppler traces to assess motion in specific myocardial regions (see Fig. 11.15, p. 135).

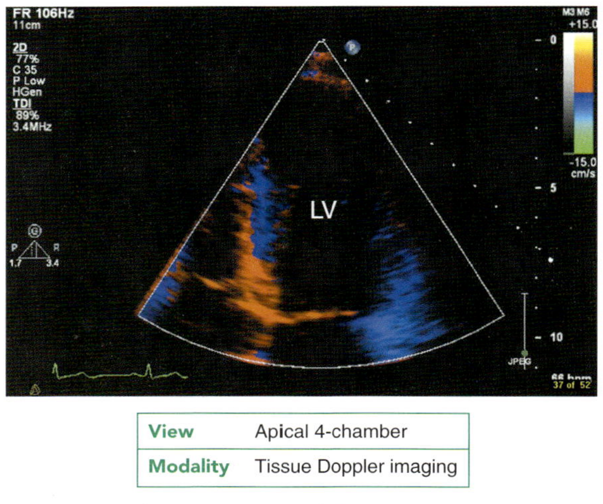

View	Apical 4-chamber
Modality	Tissue Doppler imaging

Fig. 4.10 Tissue Doppler imaging (LV = left ventricle)

TDI can play a significant role in the assessment of LV function (systolic and diastolic), in myocardial ischaemia, in distinguishing between constrictive pericarditis and restrictive cardiomyopathy, and in the assessment of ventricular dyssynchrony for cardiac resynchronization therapy.

FURTHER READING

Adeyemi B. British Society of Echocardiography Distance Learning Module 14: Physics of transducers for imaging and Doppler. Available at: www.bsecho.org.

Reynolds T. *Ultrasound Physics: A Registry Exam Preparation Guide*. Phoenix: School of Cardiac Ultrasound, Arizona Heart Institute Foundation, 1996.

Van de Veire NR, De Sutter J Bax JJ, et al. Technological advances in tissue Doppler imaging echocardiography. Heart 2008; **94**: 1065–74.

5 Service provision

In addition to the technicalities of performing and reporting an echo study, there are wider issues to consider in relation to providing an echo service. This chapter looks at service provision in terms of the departmental and staffing issues involved, and also examines the question of quality control.

Departmental issues

The British Society of Echocardiography (BSE) sets out standards for departmental accreditation in the UK, which include (but are not limited to) the following:

- An echo department should have both a technical head and a clinical head.
- The department should have agreed indications and minimum standards for echo studies and a system for the review of uncertain studies.
- Studies should be triaged according to urgency and systems should be in place to alert clinicians to important abnormalities.
- Studies should be reported on the day they are performed and should be archived for future reference.
- A database of echo reports should be maintained.
- Echo rooms should be of adequate size (at least $20\,m^2$ if used for inpatient studies).
- Equipment maintenance must be carried out regularly, with echo machines being replaced (or having a major upgrade) at least every 5 years.
- A period of 30–40 min should be allowed for routine studies and up to 1 h for complex studies.

- A patient information leaflet should be available.
- Chaperones should be available.

Staffing issues

Training and accreditation

Echo trainees should have at least one (and ideally two) protected half-day tutorial sessions each week and have access to appropriate training materials (books, CD-ROMs, internet access) and echo meetings. Sonographers who undertake and report echo studies unsupervised should have appropriate accreditation.

Undertaking a recognised accreditation programme provides the sonographer with a structured means of attaining a minimum standard in echo. Although gaining accreditation does not in itself guarantee competence, it nonetheless provides a foundation on which to build one's knowledge and skills. The process of learning about echo does not end with accreditation, but must continue to develop with continuing professional education and ongoing experience in performing echo studies, and by seeking reaccreditation at regular intervals.

Several national societies provide accreditation programmes. The BSE offers accreditation in:

- adult transthoracic echo (TTE)
- transoesophageal echo (TOE)
- community echo.

The European Association of Echocardiography (EAE) offers accreditation in:

- adult TTE
- adult TOE
- congenital heart disease echo.

Further details can be obtained from the relevant society's website (BSE: www.bsecho.org; EAE: www.escardio.org/COMMUNITIES/EAE).

Workforce requirements

In 1995 the Cardiac Workforce Committee of the British Cardiac Society (now the British Cardiovascular Society) published a report on cardiac workforce requirements in the UK. With regard to echo, the report found that the annual requirement for echo studies was as follows:

- TTE 42 800–47 700 per million population
- stress echo 6000 per million population
- TOE 2000 per million population.

In terms of staffing levels, the report's authors calculated that the requirements were as follows:

- sonographers (full-time equivalent) 28–40 per million population
- consultants specialising in echo 10.3–13 per million population.

Echo departments need to pay careful attention to health and safety, particularly with regard to musculoskeletal and eye problems, liaising with local occupational health and risk management departments as appropriate. Sonographers should not perform more than 2000 echo studies per year.

Quality control

It should be the aim of every sonographer, and every echo department, to provide a high-quality echo service. This chapter has already covered the key staffing and departmental issues that have to be addressed in order to lay the foundations of a high-quality service, However, ensuring that all the foundations are in place is only half the story – it's also essential to monitor whether the echo service is performing as well as it should with an ongoing audit programme.

Audit is one of the cornerstones of clinical governance, the process by which healthcare organizations are accountable for continually improving the quality and safety of their services. Clinical governance is described as having seven key foundations or 'pillars', all of which have some relevance to running an echo service:

- audit
- risk management
- clinical effectiveness and research
- education and training
- patient and public involvement
- staffing and staff management
- clinical information.

Audit is a systematic way of assessing the quality of healthcare and is often described in terms of an 'audit cycle'. The cycle begins with the selection of a topic or 'question' to be looked at: with regard to echo, an example might be whether a department's echo reports meet agreed reporting criteria. Next, an appropriate 'gold standard' must be chosen, against which the department's performance will be compared (e.g. national standards on the minimum dataset for an echo report). A method of collecting the data is then chosen, and then the necessary data are collected and analysed. The results are then presented and discussed, comparing the department's performance against the agreed standard. Any deficiencies should be identified (while at the same time recognizing areas of good performance), and a mechanism agreed by which improvements can be made. Any changes should then be implemented and, after an appropriate timescale, the audit cycle should be repeated to see whether the changes have led to the expected improvements.

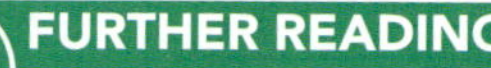

FURTHER READING

The BSE has several useful documents on its website relating to service provision (www.bsecho.org). These include:

- *What is an Echocardiogram?*
- *Clinical Indications for Echocardiography*
- *Recommendations for Standard Adult Transthoracic Echocardiography*
- *A Minimum Dataset for a Standard Adult Transthoracic Echocardiogram*
- *Cardiac Workforce Requirements in the UK*
- *Community Echo Services and Guidance on Commissioning Echo Services*
- *Chaperones and Echocardiography*

PART 2

Cardiac Imaging Techniques

6 The transthoracic echo study

Indications for transthoracic echo

The versatility of transthoracic echo (TTE) means that it can play a useful role in a diverse range of clinical situations. The British Society of Echocardiography (BSE) has published guidance on the appropriate indications for TTE on its website (see Further Reading). The American College of Cardiology has also produced guidance (jointly with a number of other societies). The two sets of guidelines are broadly similar and describe echo as being an appropriate investigation in the assessment of patients with:

- symptoms, signs or previous tests that indicate possible structural heart disease
- heart murmurs when associated with symptoms or when structural heart disease is suspected, and the follow-up of those with known significant valvular stenosis or regurgitation
- prosthetic valves (except asymptomatic patients with mechanical valves or those in whom no further intervention would be undertaken)
- suspected or proven infective endocarditis
- known or suspected ischaemic heart disease (e.g. diagnostic stress echo, assessment following myocardial infarction)
- known or suspected cardiomyopathy
- suspected pericarditis or pericardial effusion, and follow-up of patients with known moderate or large pericardial effusions (or small effusions if there has been a clinical change)
- suspected or possible cardiac masses (and follow-up of patients following surgical excision of a cardiac mass)
- pulmonary disease (with cardiac involvement)
- pulmonary hypertension

- thromboembolism
- neurological disorders (with cardiac involvement)
- arrhythmias (with suspected/possible structural heart disease)
- syncope (with suspected/possible structural heart disease)
- hypertension (if left ventricular hypertrophy (LVH)/dysfunction or aortic coarctation are suspected)
- aortic disease (e.g. monitoring of aortic root dimensions in Marfan syndrome)
- known or suspected congenital heart disease.

It is essential that echo requests contain adequate clinical data both to judge the appropriateness of the request and also to allow the sonographer to place the echo findings into an appropriate clinical context (see the box 'Sensitivity, specificity and Bayesian analysis'). Echo requests should therefore carry appropriate clinical details and must contain information about known cardiac diagnoses or previous cardiac interventions/surgery (e.g. prosthetic valves). Clinicians requesting echo studies should be encouraged to include specific questions with their request (e.g. 'Does this patient have pulmonary hypertension?'), as this provides a clear focus for the echo study and ensures that the sonographer can address the specific concerns of the clinician.

SENSITIVITY, SPECIFICITY AND BAYESIAN ANALYSIS

A perfect diagnostic test would always detect an abnormality when present ('true positive') or rule out an abnormality when absent ('true negative'). However, as with virtually every clinical test, echo has its limitations and can sometimes produce an erroneous result. Detecting an abnormality when in fact none is present is called a 'false positive', and missing an abnormality that *is* present is a 'false negative'. The terms sensitivity and specificity are often used to describe the accuracy of a test:

- **Sensitivity** is the degree to which a test will identify all those who have a particular disease – if 100 people with disease 'X' undergo a test with 90 per cent sensitivity, the test will detect the disease in 90 of them (but will produce a false negative in 10)
- **Specificity** is the degree to which a test will identify all those without a particular disease – if 100 people *without* disease 'X' undergo a test with 90 per cent specificity, the test will be normal in 90 of them (but will produce a false positive in 10).

The number of people who receive false positive/negative results is determined not only by the sensitivity and specificity of the test, but also by the population prevalence of the disease in question. Screening a large number of normal individuals for a rare disease using a test with imperfect specificity will produce a relatively large number of false positive results.

The technique of **Bayesian analysis** takes this into account by considering how likely it is that the patient has the disease in question (the pretest probability) in order to predict how likely it is that a positive or negative test result is genuinely positive or negative. In general terms, a positive test result for disease 'X' is more likely to be a true positive if the patient already had a high probability of having disease 'X' before the test was done – it is therefore important to know a patient's full clinical details before performing a test such as an echo in order to judge the likely significance of any abnormalities that you find.

Triage of inpatient echo requests

Echo should be performed **immediately** if acute cardiac tamponade is suspected following an interventional procedure or if a patient presents with massive pulmonary embolism and echo is likely to help in deciding whether to administer thrombolysis.

Urgent echo (within 24 hours, or even sooner depending on the clinical situation) is required for patients who are unstable with infective endocarditis, who have a new murmur following recent myocardial infarction, who are persistently hypotensive (and not responding to treatment) for unknown reasons, have suspected pericardial effusion/bleeding/tamponade or have suspected aortic dissection.

Other inpatient echo requests can be performed more routinely, but should nevertheless be undertaken on an inpatient basis as soon as practicable. If circumstances do not permit this, the request should be discussed with the referring clinician to see if the study can be deferred and performed on an outpatient basis once the patient is discharged from hospital.

Patient preparation

Patients attending for an echo study may feel anxious, not only about having the test itself but also about any abnormalities that it may reveal. To help reduce anxiety the test should be described to patients in clear and reassuring terms – patients should have an explanation of why they are having an echo, whether any special preparation is needed before they attend, what happens during the scan and how long it will take. Patients should be reassured that having an echo is safe and painless. Patients can eat and drink normally before attending for a standard TTE, and they can take their medication as usual.

It is good practice to offer patients an information leaflet before they attend (and to make available large print/Braille and translated versions as appropriate). The patient information leaflet and/or appointment letter can also invite the patient to bring a friend or relative if they wish to have someone accompany them during the echo. If a friend or relative does not accompany the patient when they attend, the patient should be offered a chaperone in line with hospital policy.

Once the patient is in the echo room and you have checked that they understand the test that is about to be performed, you should ask them to undress to the waist for the echo study. Female patients should always be offered a gown to wear during the echo (even if the sonographer is female). Ask the patient to sit on the echo couch and recline at 45°, rolling on to their left side. The patient should then raise their left arm and place their left hand behind their head. Be sure to check if the patient has any physical limitations that may make it difficult or uncomfortable for them to adopt this position. If so, you may need to adapt the patient's position until they are comfortable. Sonographers who prefer to scan left-handed will also need to adapt the patient's positioning accordingly.

When the patient is in a comfortable position, apply the ECG electrodes and ensure that a clear ECG tracing is visible on the screen of the echo machine. You may need to adjust the electrodes and/or the ECG gain setting to obtain a good trace. Ensure that the correct patient identification and clinical details are entered into the echo machine, and then perform and report the study as described in the sections that follow. At the end of the study, explain to the patient that you will be writing a report which will be sent to the referring clinician. Patients may ask you what the study has shown, but you should not discuss the study findings at this stage and it is usually better to redirect persistent requests for information to the referring clinician.

Standard windows and views

There are five TTE windows (Fig. 6.1), each providing one or more views of the heart. Windows and views listed in brackets are optional and can be used when other views are suboptimal or when additional information is needed:

- Left parasternal window
  - Parasternal long axis view
  - (Parasternal right ventricular (RV) inflow view)
  - (Parasternal RV outflow view)
  - Parasternal short axis view
- (Right parasternal window)
- Apical window
  - Apical 4-chamber view
  - Apical 5-chamber view
  - Apical 2-chamber view
  - Apical 3-chamber (long axis) view
- Subcostal window
  - Subcostal long axis view
  - Subcostal short axis view
- Suprasternal window
  - Aorta view.

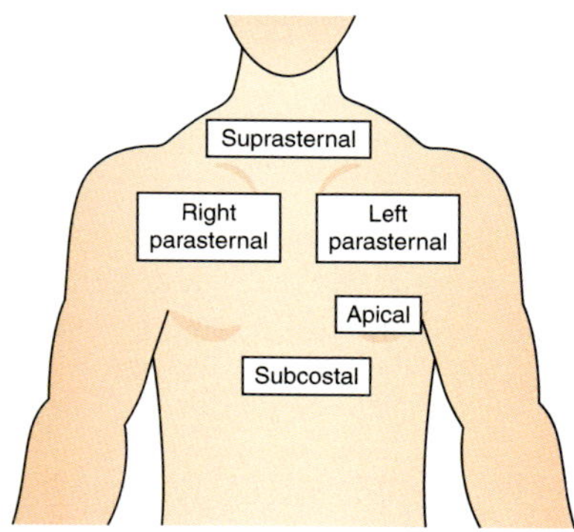

Fig. 6.1 Transthoracic echo windows

Left parasternal window

The left parasternal window is located to the left of the sternum, usually in the third or fourth intercostal space, but in some patients you may need to adjust the position to optimize the image by moving the probe up/down a rib space or further towards/away from the sternum. From the left parasternal window a number of views can be obtained.

Parasternal long axis view

The parasternal long axis (LAX) view is shown in Fig. 6.2. To obtain the view with the probe in the left parasternal window, rotate the probe so that the probe's 'reference point' (sometimes a 'dot') is pointing towards the patient's right shoulder.

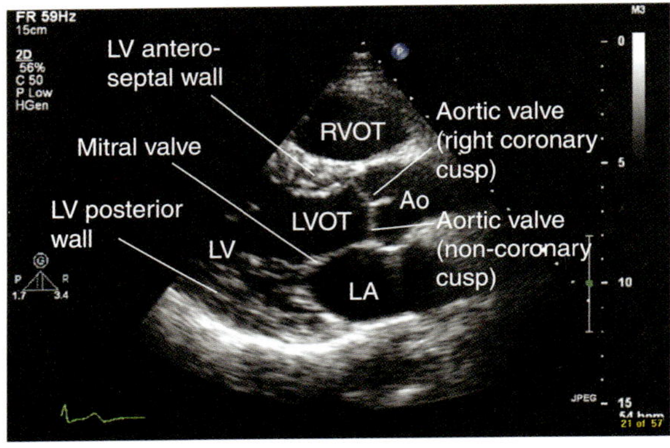

View	Parasternal long axis
Modality	2-D

Fig. 6.2 Normal parasternal long axis view (Ao = aorta; LA = left atrium; LV = left ventricle; LVOT = left ventricular outflow tract; RVOT = right ventricular outflow tract)

For an optimal view, aim to position the probe so that the view cuts through the centre of mitral and aortic valves, without foreshortening the left ventricle (LV) or ascending aorta. In this view:

- Use 2-D ± M-mode to:
  - assess structure and mobility of the aortic valve. The right and non-coronary cusps are visible and normally have a central closure line – an eccentric closure line suggests bicuspid aortic valve
  - measure the aortic root dimensions and inspect the ascending aorta; do not forget to look at the descending aorta as it runs behind the left atrium (LA) – this is a useful landmark for assessing a pericardial/pleural effusion
  - assess structure and mobility of the mitral valve – in this view, the A2 and P2 segments are visible
  - measure LA dimensions

- measure LV dimensions and assess function (anteroseptum and posterior (also known as inferolateral) wall)
- measure RV dimensions and assess function
- assess the pericardium and check for any pericardial (or pleural) effusion.

- Use colour Doppler to:
  - assess the aortic valve for stenosis or regurgitation
  - examine mitral valve inflow and check for regurgitation
  - check for flow acceleration in the left ventricular outflow tract (LVOT) in association with septal hypertrophy
  - check the integrity of the interventricular septum (IVS).

Parasternal right ventricular inflow view

This 'optional' view is obtained from the left parasternal window by tilting the probe so that it points more medially and towards the patient's right hip, bringing the right atrium (RA), tricuspid valve and RV into view (Fig. 6.3).

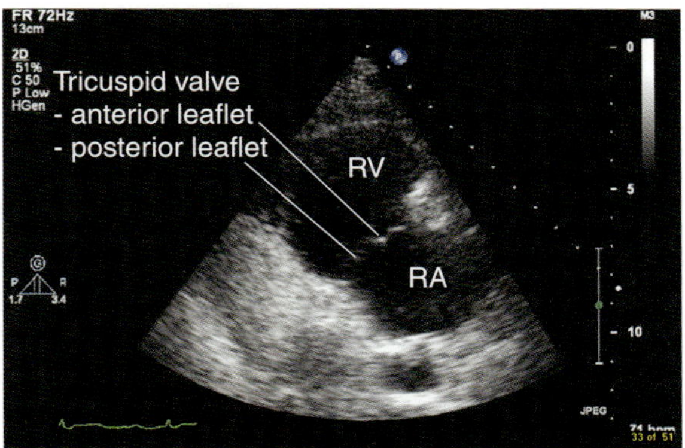

View	Parasternal right ventricular inflow
Modality	2-D

Fig. 6.3 Normal right ventricular inflow view (RA = right atrium; RV = right ventricle)

- Use 2-D ± M-mode to:
  - assess structure and mobility of the tricuspid valve (the two leaflets seen are the anterior and posterior leaflets)

  - assess the structure of the RA. In this view it may be possible to see the coronary sinus and the inferior and superior vena cavae as they join the RA. There may be a prominent Eustachian valve at the junction with the inferior vena cava (IVC)
  - assess the size and function of the RV.
- Use colour Doppler to examine tricuspid valve inflow and check for regurgitation.
- Use continuous wave (CW) and pulsed wave (PW) Doppler to assess tricuspid valve function. If tricuspid regurgitation is present, measure the maximum velocity to assess RV systolic pressure.

Parasternal right ventricular outflow view

This 'optional' view is obtained from the left parasternal window by tilting the probe so that it points more laterally and towards the patient's left shoulder, bringing the right ventricular outflow tract (RVOT), pulmonary valve and pulmonary artery into view (Fig. 6.4). It may be possible to see the pulmonary artery bifurcation.

- Use 2-D ± M-mode to:
  - assess structure and mobility of the pulmonary valve
  - assess the structure of the RVOT and main pulmonary artery; check for the presence of thrombus (pulmonary embolus).

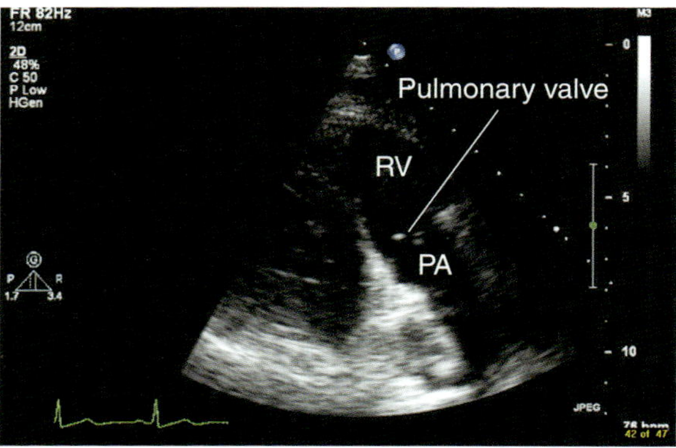

View	Parasternal right ventricular outflow
Modality	2-D

Fig. 6.4 Normal right ventricular outflow view (PA = pulmonary artery; RV = right ventricle)

- Use colour Doppler to examine the pulmonary valve for stenosis or regurgitation.

It may be possible to detect the abnormal jet of a patent ductus arteriosus by examining the pulmonary artery with colour Doppler in this view.

- Use CW and PW Doppler to:
  - assess flow in the RVOT
  - assess the pulmonary valve for stenosis or regurgitation.

Parasternal short axis view

To obtain the parasternal short axis (SAX) view, keep the probe in the left parasternal window and rotate it so that the 'dot' is pointing towards the patient's left shoulder. There are actually three SAX views, obtained by tilting the probe along the axis of the heart from the level of the aortic valve down to the apex. The standard SAX views are:

- aortic valve level
- mitral valve level
- papillary muscle level.

At the **aortic valve level** (Fig. 6.5):

- Use 2-D ± M-mode to:
  - assess structure and mobility of the aortic valve; all three cusps should be visible
  - inspect the LA and RA and interatrial septum
  - assess structure and mobility of the tricuspid valve (the two leaflets seen are the septal and anterior leaflets)
  - assess RV size and function
  - assess size of the RVOT
  - assess structure and mobility of the pulmonary valve
  - assess morphology of the main pulmonary artery up to its bifurcation.

You may be able to inspect the origins of the left main stem and right coronary arteries arising just above the aortic valve cusps.

- Use colour Doppler to:
  - check the integrity of the interatrial septum
  - examine the aortic valve for regurgitation
  - examine tricuspid valve inflow and check for regurgitation
  - examine the pulmonary valve for stenosis or regurgitation

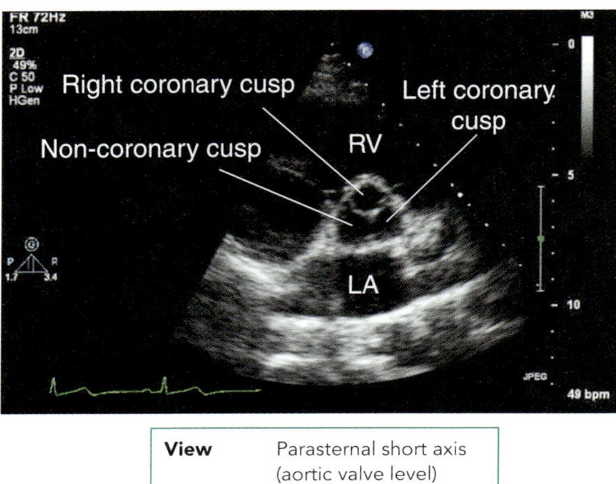

View	Parasternal short axis (aortic valve level)
Modality	2-D

Fig. 6.5 Normal parasternal short axis view (aortic valve level) (LA = left atrium; RV = right ventricle)

- it may be possible to detect the abnormal jet of a ventricular septal defect (VSD) or a persistent ductus arteriosus with colour Doppler in this view.

- Use CW and PW Doppler to:
  - assess tricuspid valve function. If tricuspid regurgitation is present, assess RV systolic pressure
  - assess flow in the RVOT
  - assess the pulmonary valve for stenosis or regurgitation.

At the **mitral valve level** (Fig. 6.6), use 2-D ± M-mode to:

- assess structure and mobility of the mitral valve. The anterior and posterior leaflets are visible as is the classical mitral valve orifice, which can be planimetered to measure orifice area
- assess LV function and look for any regional wall motion abnormalities at the basal level
- assess RV size and function.
- Use colour Doppler to:
  - examine mitral valve inflow
  - check for mitral regurgitation and identify precisely where it occurs in relation to the leaflet scallops
  - check the integrity of the IVS.

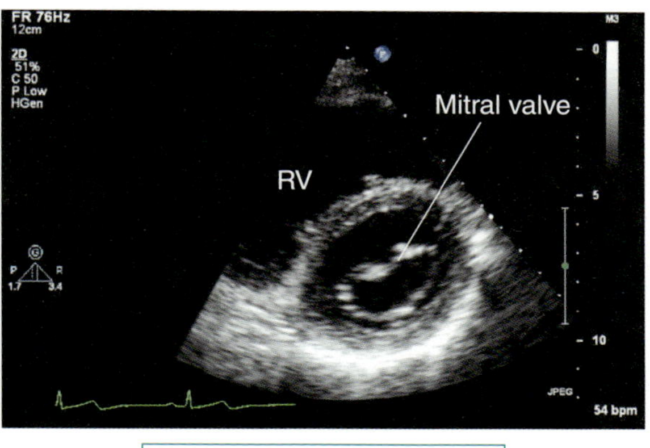

View	Parasternal short axis (mitral valve level)
Modality	2-D

Fig. 6.6 Normal parasternal short axis view (mitral valve level) (RV = right ventricle)

- At the **papillary muscle level** (Fig. 6.7), use 2-D ± M-mode to:
  - assess structure of the posteromedial and anterolateral papillary muscles

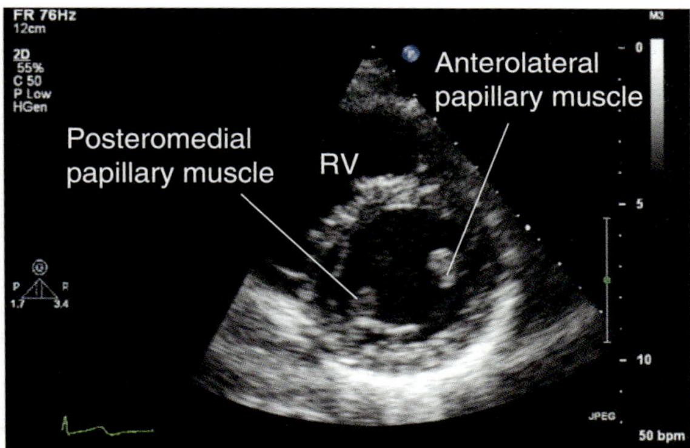

View	Parasternal short axis (papillary muscle level)
Modality	2-D

Fig. 6.7 Normal parasternal short axis view (papillary muscle level) (RV = right ventricle)

  - measure LV wall thickness
  - assess LV function and look for any regional wall motion abnormalities at the mid-ventricle level
  - assess RV size and function.
- Use colour Doppler to check the integrity of the IVS.

Right parasternal window

The right parasternal window is 'optional' but can be useful for assessing flow in the ascending aorta. With the patient lying on their right-hand side, place the probe to the right of the sternum in the third intercostal space (some adjustment may be required, as with the left parasternal window) and angle the probe downwards and pointing towards the heart. It is a challenging view, but it may be possible to visualize the ascending aorta and assess colour Doppler within it. This view is most useful for undertaking CW Doppler assessment of the aortic valve, particularly with a standalone pencil probe.

Apical window

The apical window is located at the LV apex. This is normally in the mid-clavicular line and the fifth intercostal space, but may be displaced downwards and to the left if the heart is enlarged. From the apical window a number of views can be obtained.

Apical 4-chamber view

To obtain this view, place the probe in the apical position with the 'dot' pointing towards the patient's left. For an optimal view, aim to position the probe exactly at the apex to avoid distortion or foreshortening of the cardiac structures. The interatrial and interventricular septa should be in line with the probe and lie vertically on the screen (Fig. 6.8). In this view:

- Use 2-D to:
  - assess structure and mobility of the mitral valve – in this view, the P1, A2 and A3 segments are visible
  - assess structure and mobility of the tricuspid valve
  - assess (LV) dimensions and function (inferoseptum and lateral – also known as anterolateral – wall)
  - assess RV dimensions and function
  - assess LA dimensions
  - assess RA dimensions
  - assess the pericardium and check for any pericardial (or pleural) effusion.

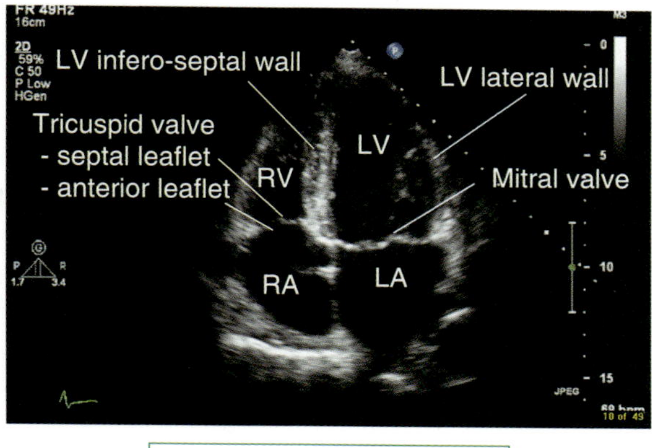

View	Apical 4-chamber
Modality	2-D

Fig. 6.8 Normal apical 4-chamber view (LA = left atrium; LV = left ventricle; RA = right atrium; RV = right ventricle)

- Use colour Doppler to:
  - examine mitral valve inflow and check for regurgitation
  - examine tricuspid valve inflow and check for regurgitation
  - check the integrity of the interatrial and ventricular septa.
- Use CW and PW Doppler to:
  - assess the pattern of LV inflow
  - assess mitral valve function
  - assess tricuspid valve function; if tricuspid regurgitation is present, assess RV systolic pressure
  - if any of the pulmonary veins are visible, assess pulmonary vein inflow.

Apical 5-chamber view

From the apical 4-chamber view, maintain the same window but angulate the probe anteriorly so that the aortic valve and aortic root (the 'fifth chamber') come into view (Fig. 6.9). This view is used principally to assess the LVOT and aortic valve, and it is important to align these with the ultrasound beam so that reliable Doppler traces can be obtained.

Use 2-D to:

- assess LV dimensions and function
- assess the appearance of the LVOT (any signs of asymmetrical hypertrophy?)
- assess structure and mobility of the aortic valve.

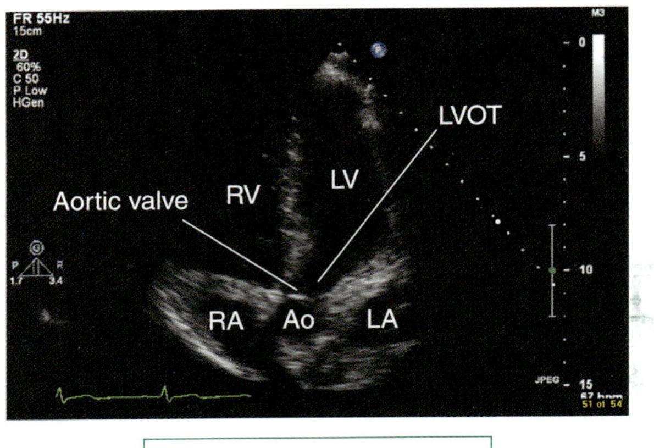

View	Apical 5-chamber
Modality	2-D

Fig. 6.9 Normal apical 5-chamber view (Ao = aorta; LA = left atrium; LV = left ventricle; LVOT = left ventricular outflow tract; RA = right atrium; RV = right ventricle)

Use colour Doppler to:

- check for flow acceleration in the LVOT in association with septal hypertrophy
- examine the aortic valve for stenosis or regurgitation
- check for a perimembranous VSD.

Use CW and PW Doppler to:

- assess aortic valve function
- assess flow in the LVOT.

Apical 2-chamber view

Return to the apical 4-chamber view and maintain the same window but rotate the probe about 60° anticlockwise so that the 'dot' points approximately towards the patient's left shoulder. Stop rotating the probe before the LVOT comes into view, and ensure that the mitral valve is centred in the image (Fig. 6.10).

- Use 2-D to:
  - assess LV dimensions and function (anterior and inferior walls)
  - assess structure and mobility of the mitral valve – in this view, the P1, A2 and P3 segments are visible

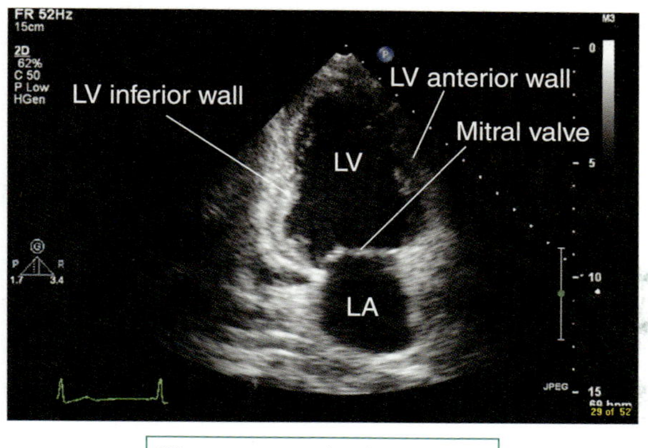

View	Apical 2-chamber
Modality	2-D

Fig. 6.10 Normal apical 2-chamber view (LA = left atrium; LV = left ventricle)

- the LA appendage may be visible as a small 'pocket' to the right of the mitral valve
- the coronary sinus may be visible as a circular structure to the left of the mitral valve.

- Use colour Doppler to examine mitral valve inflow and check for regurgitation.
- Use CW and PW Doppler to assess mitral valve function.

Apical 3-chamber (long axis) view

From the apical 2-chamber view, maintain the same window but rotate the probe a further 60° anticlockwise so that the 'dot' now points approximately towards the patient's right shoulder. Stop rotating the probe once the LVOT comes into view, and ensure that the mitral and aortic valves are centred and not foreshortened (Fig. 6.11). This view is the apical equivalent of the parasternal LAX view.

- Use 2-D to:
  - assess LV dimensions and function (anteroseptum and posterior – also known as inferolateral – walls)
  - assess the appearance of the LVOT (any signs of asymmetrical hypertrophy?)

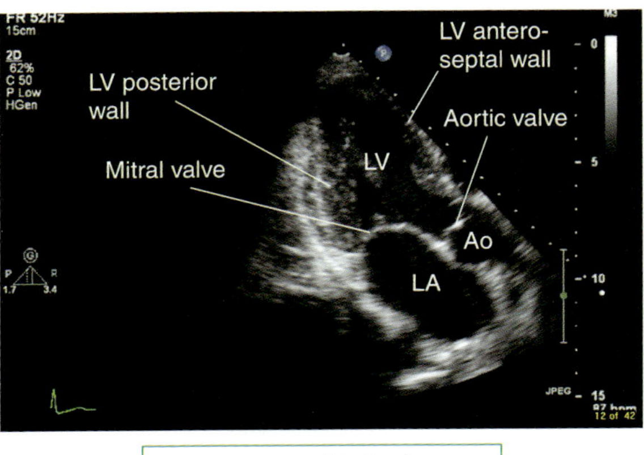

View	Apical 3-chamber
Modality	2-D

Fig. 6.11 Normal apical 3-chamber view (Ao = aorta; LA = left atrium; LV = left ventricle)

- assess structure and mobility of the aortic valve
- assess structure and mobility of the mitral valve – in this view, the A2 and P2 segments are visible.
- Use colour Doppler to:
  - examine mitral valve inflow and check for regurgitation
  - check for flow acceleration in the LVOT in association with septal hypertrophy
  - examine the aortic valve for stenosis or regurgitation.
- Use CW and PW Doppler to:
  - assess mitral valve function
  - assess flow in the LVOT
  - assess aortic valve function.

Subcostal window

The subcostal window is obtained with the patient lying supine with their arms by their sides. It is important that the abdominal wall is relaxed, and asking the patient to lie with their knees bent can help this. The probe should be placed just below the xiphisternum and angled up towards the heart, with the 'dot' to the patient's left. From the subcostal window a number of views can be obtained.

Subcostal long axis view

To optimize this view, ensure that the interatrial septum is perpendicular to the ultrasound beam (i.e. lies horizontally across the screen) with no foreshortening of the chambers (Fig. 6.12).

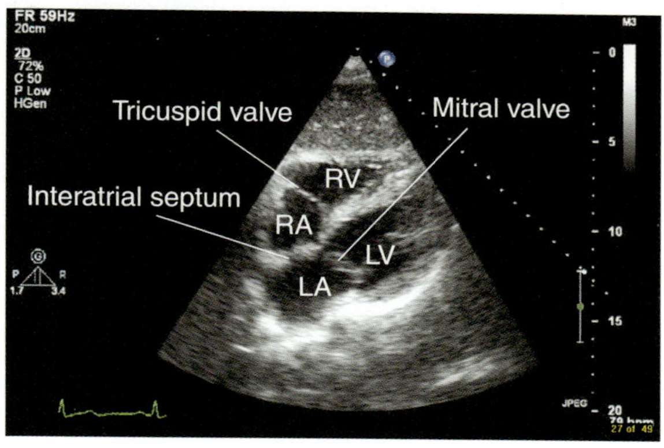

View	Subcostal long axis
Modality	2-D

Fig. 6.12 Normal subcostal long axis view (LA = left atrium; LV = left ventricle; RA = right atrium; RV = right ventricle)

- Use 2-D to:
  - assess RV dimensions and function
  - assess RA dimensions
  - assess LV dimensions and function
  - assess LA dimensions
  - assess structure and mobility of the tricuspid valve
  - assess the pericardium and check for any pericardial effusion.
- Use colour Doppler to:
  - examine the tricuspid valve for regurgitation
  - examine the mitral valve for regurgitation
  - check the integrity of interatrial and interventricular septa.
- Use CW and PW Doppler to assess flow across any septal defect.

Subcostal short axis view

Keeping the probe in the subcostal window rotate the probe 90° to obtain a SAX view (Fig. 6.13).

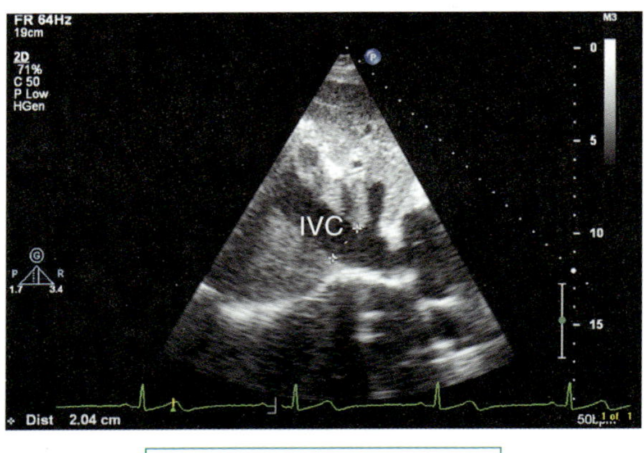

View	Subcostal short axis (inferior vena cava)
Modality	2-D

Fig. 6.13 Normal subcostal short axis (inferior vena cava (IVC)) view

- Use 2-D ± M-mode to:
  - assess IVC dimensions (check for respiratory variation by taking measurements in inspiration and expiration)
  - assess hepatic veins (congested?)
  - assess LV dimensions and function
  - assess RV dimensions and function
  - assess the interatrial septum
  - assess the descending aorta (modified view).
- Use colour Doppler to:
  - assess flow in the IVC and hepatic veins
  - check the integrity of the interatrial septum.
- Use PW Doppler to:
  - assess flow in the hepatic veins
  - assess flow in the descending aorta.

Suprasternal window

The suprasternal window is located in the suprasternal notch. Ask the patient to lie supine and to raise their chin. Place the probe in the notch and angle it downwards into the chest. Be mindful that some patients find this uncomfortable. This view shows the aortic arch in LAX (Fig. 6.14). A similar view can, if needed, be obtained from the right supraclavicular position.

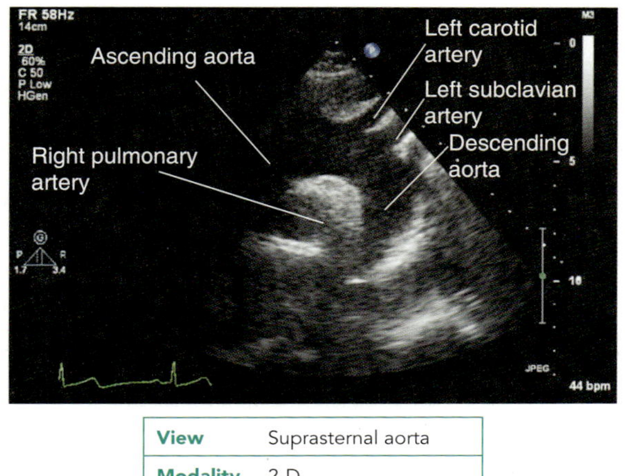

View	Suprasternal aorta
Modality	2-D

Fig. 6.14 Normal suprasternal aorta view

Aorta view

- Use 2-D to assess the appearances and dimensions of the aortic arch.
- Use colour Doppler to assess flow in the aorta, looking in particular for evidence of coarctation or persistent ductus arteriosus.
- Use CW and PW Doppler to:
  - assess flow in the ascending aorta in the presence of aortic stenosis
  - assess flow in the descending aorta in the presence of a coarctation.

The transthoracic echo report

Once you've completed the echo study, ensure that the report is written up on the same day. In writing your report, follow the reporting guidelines of the BSE and/or American Society of Echocardiography (ASE) (see Further Reading). Your echo report should be clearly and systematically structured and contain:

- patient identifying and demographic information
- detailed findings
- study summary.

Patient identifying and demographic information

It is essential that the report contains adequate information to allow correct identification of the patient. The report should therefore begin with the patient's name and a unique identifier (in the UK, this would be the patient's National Health Service (NHS) number). The patient's age (or date of birth) and gender should be stated. The report must also identify the referring clinician and the sonographer and state the indication for the echo request and the date on which the study was performed.

It may also be appropriate to include the patient's location (e.g. outpatient or name of ward), where the study was performed (e.g. echo department, coronary care unit), when the echo was requested and whether it was performed as an emergency/urgent/routine study. It is helpful to include details of the patient's height, weight and blood pressure (e.g. for indexing measurements to body surface area). You may also wish to include any details that will assist in retrieving the archived echo images for review (e.g. computer disk or videotape number).

Detailed findings

The main body of your echo report should contain systematic descriptions of each of the main cardiac structures (chambers, valves, great vessels and pericardium). For each structure you need to describe its appearance and also its function, grading any abnormalities as mild, moderate or severe where possible (and supporting these statements with measurements where appropriate).

It is usually easiest to set out your study findings by anatomical structure (e.g. mitral valve, LV, etc.) rather than by echo window or modality (which can make the report confusing and repetitive). You can simply describe the findings relating to each anatomical structure in turn, or you may prefer to adapt the list of findings so that the most significant abnormalities appear at the start. Any relevant measurements (M-mode, 2-D and Doppler) and calculations can be included in the descriptive text of each anatomical structure, or if you prefer as a separate section.

The BSE Minimum Dataset for a Standard Adult Transthoracic Echocardiogram describes the essential information you need to include in a standard echo report (see Further Reading). It is important to use standardized terminology in your report to minimize variability between studies performed at different times and by different sonographers. The BSE and ASE reporting guidelines contain tables of recommended descriptive terms and diagnostic statements and it can be very helpful to use these guidelines as a reference when writing up your study findings.

Study summary

The study summary should sum up the key findings of the echo study and place the findings in a clinical context, with particular reference to the clinical question(s) posed by the referring clinician. The summary should not contain any information about the study that hasn't already been included in the detailed technical report, but it can include reference to previous studies performed on the same patient where a comparison is useful. Any technical limitations of the study (such as suboptimal imaging windows) should be mentioned, and if any structures could not be adequately assessed this must be highlighted so that the referring clinician can consider alternative imaging as necessary. Clinical advice should not normally be offered in the study summary.

FURTHER READING

Douglas PS, Khandheria B, Stainback RF, *et al.* ACCF/ASE/ACEP/ASNC/SCAI/SCCT/SCMR Appropriateness criteria for transthoracic and transesophageal echocardiography. *J Am Coll Cardiol* 2007; **50**: 187–204.

The British Society of Echocardiography has several useful documents relating to TTE on its website (www.bsecho.org). These include:

A Minimum Dataset for a Standard Adult Transthoracic Echocardiogram

Chaperones and Echocardiography

Clinical Indications for Echocardiography

Recommendations for Standard Adult Transthoracic Echocardiography

The ASE has published *Recommendations for a Standardized Report for Adult Transthoracic Echocardiography*, which is available on its website (www.asecho.org).

7 The transoesophageal echo study

It is beyond the scope of this textbook to provide a comprehensive overview of transoesophageal echo (TOE), but for anyone performing transthoracic echo (TTE) it is important to know how it fits into the cardiac imaging armamentarium.

Indications for transoesophageal echo

The key difference between TTE and TOE is that for a TOE study the echo probe views the heart from within the patient's oesophagus rather than via the chest wall (Fig. 7.1). The advantage of this is that it allows for superior image quality – the proximity of the probe to the heart means that the ultrasound does not need to penetrate so deeply, and so higher ultrasound frequencies can be used (giving higher image resolution). The fact that the TOE probe lies behind the back of the heart also means that certain structures – such as the left atrial (LA) appendage and pulmonary veins – can be seen more clearly than with a transthoracic study.

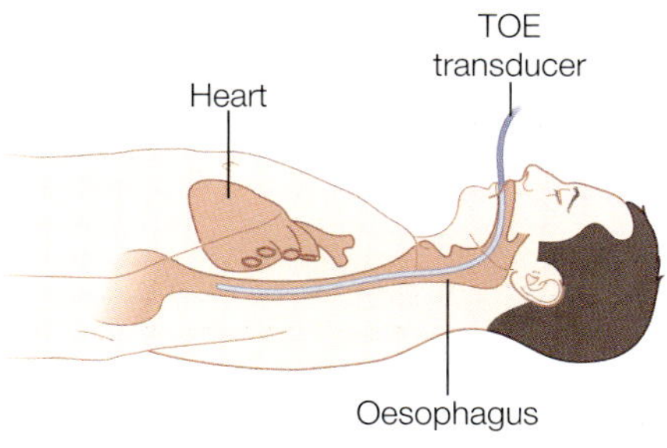

Fig. 7.1 Transoesophageal echo (TOE)

The superior image quality of TOE means that it is generally indicated in situations where TTE is unable to deliver the image quality required to make a diagnosis. The commonest indications for a TOE study include assessment of:

- cardiac source of emboli
- atrial fibrillation/flutter, to judge thromboembolic risk (and thus guide decisions on anticoagulation and cardioversion)
- suspected or proven infective endocarditis
- aortic diseases (e.g. aortic dissection/trauma)
- regurgitant heart valves, to judge suitability for surgical repair
- prosthetic valves (especially those in the mitral position)
- cardiac masses
- congenital heart disease and intracardiac shunts, e.g. atrial septal defect (ASD), patent foramen ovale (PFO).

TOE plays a major role in the cardiothoracic intraoperative setting, particularly in relation to valve repair and replacement, and also in the cardiac catheter laboratory for guiding device closure of ASD or PFO. TOE can also be useful in the intensive care unit, where the image quality of TTE is often limited in ventilated patients, and as well as being a diagnostic tool it can also help in haemodynamic monitoring.

CONTRAINDICATIONS TO A TOE STUDY

Any history of difficulty in swallowing should be investigated before a TOE study can be considered. A TOE study is contraindicated by:

- patient refusal
- cervical spine instability
- any abnormality posing a risk of oesophageal or gastric perforation, e.g. oesophageal obstruction (e.g. stricture, tumour), oesophageal trauma, oesophageal fistula or diverticulum.

Relative contraindications include the presence of clotting disorders, large hiatus hernia (apposition of the probe to the oesophageal wall can be difficult), oesophageal varices or upper gastrointestinal haemorrhage.

Patient preparation

As with any investigation, patients should receive a clear explanation of what a TOE study entails and be offered an information leaflet. Inform the patient that a TOE study involves passing a probe into the oesophagus, in a similar manner to having an endoscopy for stomach ulcers, in order to obtain clear ultrasound pictures of the heart.

Inform the patient about the need for local anaesthetic throat spray and the departmental policy on sedation (some units provide sedation routinely, others make it optional) and the consequent need for an escort as appropriate. Discuss the risks of the procedure. TOE is regarded as a low-risk procedure, but complications can occur and these include:

- oesophageal or oropharyngeal trauma
- laryngospasm
- arrhythmias
- risks associated with sedation (e.g. respiratory depression).

Ensure the patient is aware of the need to be nil by mouth on the day of the procedure, having nothing to eat for 6 h (and nothing to drink for 4 h) prior to the test. In view of the need to be nil by mouth, patients with diabetes mellitus should receive appropriate advice about any adjustments that may be needed to their medication to avoid hypoglycaemia.

The transoesophageal echo probe

The earliest TOE probes were **monoplane** probes, in which the echo transducer was fixed in a single plane at the end of the probe. To obtain views of different planes through the heart the probe had to be advanced/withdrawn and/or rotated within the oesophagus, and the tip of the probe could be flexed to different angles. Nevertheless, monoplane probes could be challenging to use. The next generation were **biplane** probes, in which a second transducer, perpendicular to the first, was added to the tip of the probe. This allowed imaging in two planes at 90° to each other and made it easier to get certain views.

Multiplane TOE probes contain a transducer at the tip of the probe that can be rotated through an angle of 180° (using a control situated in the handle of the probe). Rotating the transducer changes the angle of the imaging plane and so a 'cut' through the heart can be obtained in just about any plane. Combining this with the ability to advance/withdraw the probe up and down the oesophagus (and stomach), to rotate the probe to the left or right, and to flex the tip of the probe to the left/right and anteriorly/posteriorly, means that a comprehensive study can be undertaken utilizing a wide range of imaging planes.

Performing the transoesophageal echo study

A standard diagnostic TOE study is usually performed by a team of staff including a clinician sonographer, a technician sonographer and a nurse experienced in airway management. The study is performed in a room containing a couch for the patient, an echo machine and TOE probe (with facilities for cleaning/sterilizing the probe between studies), a supply of oxygen, suction apparatus, a pulse oximeter, blood pressure monitoring, appropriate drugs for the procedure, and a fully equipped resuscitation trolley.

Prior to undertaking the TOE study, ensure that the patient understands what is planned and has given informed consent, and check that they have been nil by mouth for the required period. Review the patient's history and prior investigation findings and check for contraindications or anything that may increase the risk of complications (e.g. respiratory disorders). Obtain intravenous access and check the blood glucose of patients with diabetes, and the international normalized ratio (INR) of patients taking warfarin.

Attach the ECG electrodes of the echo machine and use these to monitor the patient's heart rate and rhythm during the study. Use an automated cuff to check blood pressure at regular intervals, and monitor arterial oxygen saturations continuously using pulse oximetry, providing the patient with inspired oxygen via nasal cannulae as appropriate.

Check if the patient has any loose teeth, and check for (and remove) dentures. Administer local anaesthetic throat spray and allow up to 5 min for it to take full effect. Before giving sedation (where necessary), ask the patient to lie on the couch on their left-hand side, facing towards the sonographer. Follow local protocols with regard to sedation – many units offer midazolam, the effects of which can be reversed with flumazenil (which must be available for immediate use in case of respiratory depression). Before giving sedation, check that appropriate transport/escort arrangements are in place for the patient's discharge after the procedure.

When you are ready to begin the study, place a bite guard in the patient's mouth and flex their neck slightly, with the chin towards the chest. Flex the tip of the TOE probe and apply gel for lubrication. Next, pass the tip of the

CONSCIOUS SEDATION

Where sedation is given, the aim is to achieve *conscious* sedation – the patient should still be able to respond to verbal instructions (such as 'open your eyes') from the sonographer. Oversedation to the point of unconsciousness carries a significant risk of respiratory depression for the patient (and litigation for the sonographer!).

probe into the patient's mouth and, gently advancing it, ask the patient to swallow. Once the probe has passed round the back of the throat, start to straighten the tip of the probe and gently advance it to mid-oesophagus level, usually 30–40 cm (distances are marked along the side of the probe). **Never advance the probe against resistance**. When the patient has got used to the probe (some retching is common initially), commence the study while keeping a careful watch on their pulse, blood pressure and oxygen saturations.

The 'standard' transoesophageal echo study

There is no fixed 'routine' to performing a TOE study and many operators will begin a study by assessing the most relevant pathology first. This is because the study may need to be cut short if the patient is unable to tolerate it or if there are arrhythmias and/or haemodynamic instability. Once the main aim of the study has been addressed, you should move on to look at the rest of the heart in a systematic manner, being sure not to overlook any coexistent pathology.

Mid-oesophageal views

With the probe in mid-oesophagus a wide range of views can be obtained. Starting with the transducer at an angle of 40° (all angles quoted are approximate), the aortic valve is seen in short axis together with surrounding structures (Fig. 7.2). Rotating a little further to 60° brings the pulmonary and tricuspid valves into view, and then further rotation to 130° provides a long-axis view of the left heart with clear views of both the aortic and mitral valves (Fig. 7.3).

Centring the image on the mitral valve, rotation of the transducer back to 90° provides a 2-chamber view of the left heart (usually including a good view of the LA appendage), and rotating further back to 60° reveals a bicommissural view of the mitral valve. Returning to a transducer angle of

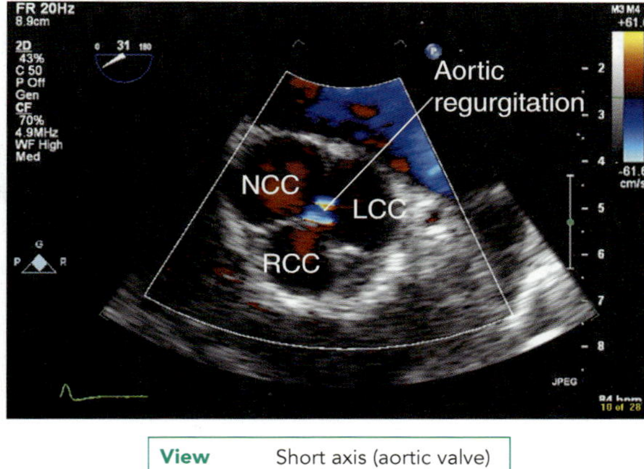

View	Short axis (aortic valve)
Modality	TOE colour Doppler

Fig. 7.2 Transoesophageal echo short axis view of aortic valve showing central jet of mild aortic regurgitation (LCC = left coronary cusp; NCC = non-coronary cusp; RCC = right coronary cusp)

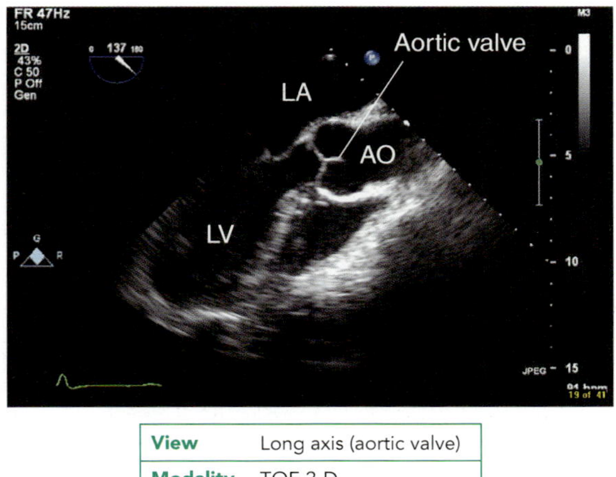

View	Long axis (aortic valve)
Modality	TOE 2-D

Fig. 7.3 Transoesophageal echo long axis view of normal aortic valve (Ao = aorta; LA = left atrium; LV = left ventricle)

90° and rotating the probe towards the patient's right produces the bicaval view, showing the interatrial septum, LA and right atrium (RA), and superior and inferior vena cavae (Fig. 7.4).

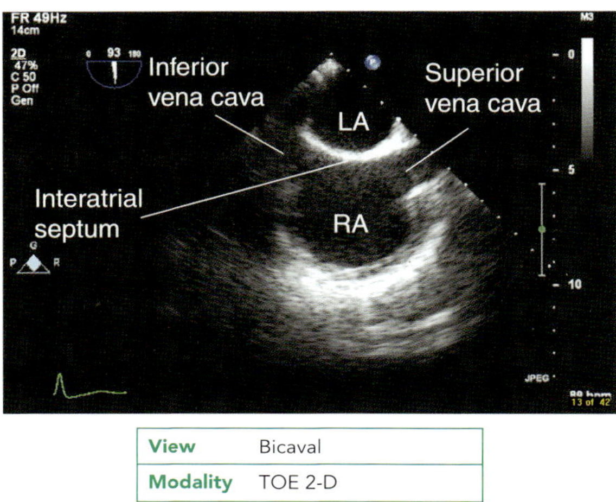

View	Bicaval
Modality	TOE 2-D

Fig. 7.4 Bicaval view (LA = left atrium; RA = right atrium)

Advancing the probe slightly further down the oesophagus, and maintaining a transducer angle of 0°, produces a 4-chamber view (Fig. 7.5)

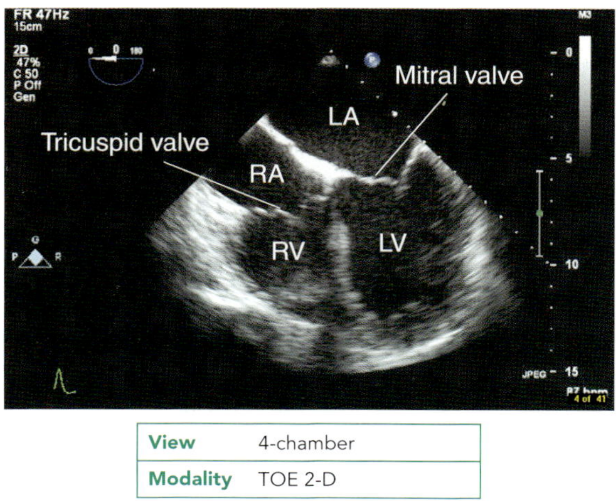

View	4-chamber
Modality	TOE 2-D

Fig. 7.5 The 4-chamber view (LA = left atrium; LV = left ventricle; RA = right

The ascending aorta can be inspected at the mid-oesophageal level both in short axis (with the pulmonary artery looping around it) and long axis, and by rotating the entire probe by 180° (so that the transducer points posteriorly), the descending aorta can also be imaged in short and long axis.

Transgastric views

Advancing the probe into the stomach allows for a series of transgastric views. With the transducer set at 0° you can obtain a short axis view of the left ventricle (LV) at the level of the mitral valve and the papillary muscles (Fig. 7.6). Rotating the transducer to 90° provides a 2-chamber view with a particularly clear view of the papillary muscles and chordae tendineae. Further rotation of the transducer to 120° brings the left ventricular outflow tract and aortic valve into view. Remaining at an angle of 120° but rotating the probe towards the patient's right brings the right ventricle, tricuspid valve and RA into view.

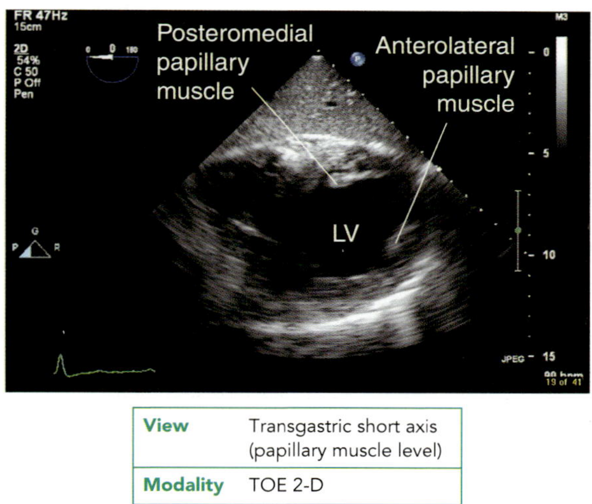

View	Transgastric short axis (papillary muscle level)
Modality	TOE 2-D

Fig. 7.6 Transgastric short axis view (papillary muscle level) (LV = left ventricle)

Advancing the probe further into the stomach, with the transducer angle at 0°, provides a **deep transgastric** view, with the transducer lying close to the apex of the LV. This view provides a good alignment with the aortic valve for Doppler studies.

Upper oesophageal views

With the probe facing posteriorly in the upper oesophagus, the aortic arch can be studied in long axis (transducer angle 0°) and short axis (transducer angle 90°).

After the transoesophageal echo study

Once you have withdrawn the TOE probe, check it for any signs of bleeding (or for any damage) before sending it for sterilization. Be sure too to check the patient's mouth for any trauma. Once the patient has recovered from the procedure (and any sedation) discuss the results and management plan with them. Ensure they receive appropriate verbal and written instructions before going home, including:

- to remain nil by mouth for an hour after the procedure (until the local anaesthetic throat spray wears off)
- not to drive, operate machinery or sign any legal documents until the next day
- to seek advice if they feel unwell or if a sore throat persists for more than 48 h.

FURTHER READING

Douglas PS, Khandheria B, Stainback RF, *et al.* ACCF/ASE/ACEP/ASNC/SCAI/SCCT/SCMR Appropriateness criteria for transthoracic and transesophageal echocardiography. *J Am Coll Cardiol* 2007; **50**: 187–204.

Flachskampf FA, Decoodt P, Fraser AG, *et al.* Recommendations for performing transoesophageal echocardiography. *Eur J Echocardiogr* 2001; **2**: 8–21.

Sengupta PP, Khandheria BK. Transoesophageal echocardiography. *Heart* 2005; **91**: 541–7.

Shanewise JS, Cheung AT, Aronson S, *et al.* ASE/SCA guidelines for performing a comprehensive intraoperative multiplane transesophageal echocardiography examination: Recommendations of the American Society of Echocardiography Council for Intraoperative Echocardiography and the Society of Cardiovascular Anesthesiologists Task Force for Certification in Perioperative Transesophageal Echocardiography. *J Am Soc Echocardiogr* 1999; **12**: 884–900.

8 The stress echo study

Stress echo is based upon the principle that an abnormality in myocardial perfusion leads to a change in myocardial function. Stress echo therefore plays a valuable role in the assessment of myocardial perfusion (and, therefore, of underlying coronary artery disease). It also can make an important contribution to the assessment of certain patients with aortic and mitral stenosis. This chapter will consider each of these indications.

Principles of stress echo

The principal role of stress echo is in the detection of regional wall motion abnormalities – areas of left ventricular (LV) myocardium that show abnormal function at rest and/or during stress. Each region of the myocardium is supplied with blood (and therefore oxygen) by one of the coronary arteries (see Chapter 12), and an imbalance between supply and demand will cause myocardial ischaemia.

Even a relatively severe stenosis in one of the major epicardial coronary arteries does not cause myocardial ischaemia at rest, as the myocardial vasculature compensates to maintain resting blood flow by dilating the arterioles downstream of the stenosis. However, this is inadequate to prevent ischaemia with stress, as the increase in myocardial oxygen demand exceeds the ability of the arterioles to dilate further. Thus a patient with a significant coronary stenosis will usually have normal myocardial perfusion (and therefore contractility) at rest, but will develop myocardial ischaemia (and abnormal wall motion) with stress.

The myocardium can be 'stressed' by increasing myocardial oxygen demand, either with physical exercise or pharmacologically using an intravenous (IV) infusion of dobutamine. Alternatively, an IV infusion of a vasodilator (e.g. dipyridamole, adenosine) can be used as the stressor. Vasodilators work by redistributing coronary blood flow, causing dilatation of normal coronary arteries but not of abnormal ones. This increases blood flow down the normal arteries but leads to a reduction in blood flow to areas supplied by stenosed coronaries, via a 'steal' mechanism, leading to ischaemia.

For the purposes of a stress echo study, the LV is subdivided into 16 or 17 myocardial segments, and the function of each segment is assessed at rest and with stress. A number of distinct patterns of response can be identified.

- A **normal response** is indicated by normal contractility (normokinetic) at rest, with normal or increased contractility (hyperkinetic) with stress.
- An **ischaemic response** is indicated by normokinetic myocardium at rest, but worsening function on stress, shown by reduced (hypokinetic), absent (akinetic) or paradoxical (dyskinetic) contractility. This is usually due to a stenosis in the supplying coronary artery.
- A **necrotic response** is indicated by abnormal contractility (akinetic, hypokinetic) at rest which remains unchanged with stress. This is usually due to an area of myocardial infarction (scar tissue) resulting from an occlusion in the supplying coronary artery.
- A **viability response** is indicated by abnormal contractility (akinetic, hypokinetic) at rest which improves with stress:
  - If the improvement is sustained throughout stress, the myocardium is said to be **stunned**. Stunned myocardium can result from a brief period of coronary occlusion and gradually improves with time.
  - If the improvement only occurs at low level stress, and the myocardium worsens again at higher levels of stress ('biphasic response'), it is said to be **hibernating**. Hibernating myocardium will not recover spontaneously but may improve following coronary revascularization.

All stress studies (exercise, dobutamine, dipyridamole and adenosine) permit the identification of normal, ischaemic and necrotic myocardium. To assess viability, a dobutamine stress study (using low-dose as well as higher doses of dobutamine) is necessary, in order to assess wall motion at different levels of stress.

Indications for stress echo

Because it can provide valuable information about the presence and extent of coronary artery disease, the indications for a stress echo study include:

- diagnosis of suspected coronary artery disease
- risk assessment of patients with known coronary artery disease

- identification of viable myocardium prior to revascularization
- localization of myocardial ischaemia ('culprit coronary lesion' identification prior to revascularization)
- assessment of myocardial perfusion following revascularization.

Stress echo is reported as having a sensitivity of 88 per cent and a specificity of 83 per cent in the detection of coronary artery disease (coronary stenosis >50 per cent). This is similarly sensitive to, but more specific than, nuclear myocardial perfusion imaging (p. 102). Stress echo does not, however, involve exposure to ionizing radiation.

In addition to its role in the assessment of myocardial ischaemia, stress echo can be useful in assessing:

- low-gradient aortic stenosis with LV dysfunction
- mitral stenosis where there is disparity between severity and symptoms.

CONTRAINDICATIONS TO A STRESS ECHO STUDY

For all forms of stress:

- acute coronary syndrome in first 24–72 h (high-dose dobutamine should not be used for 7 days after myocardial infarction)
- known left main stem coronary artery stenosis
- LV failure with symptoms at rest
- recent life-threatening arrhythmias
- severe dynamic or fixed left ventricular outflow tract obstruction
- severe systemic hypertension (systolic blood pressure >220 mmHg and/or diastolic blood pressure >120 mmHg)
- recent pulmonary embolism or infarction
- thrombophlebitis or active deep vein thrombosis
- hypokalaemia
- active endocarditis, myocarditis, or pericarditis.

For atropine:

- closed-angle glaucoma
- severe prostatic disease.

For vasodilator (dipyridamole, adenosine) stress:

- suspected or known severe bronchospasm
- sick sinus syndrome, second or third degree atrioventricular block (unless a functioning pacemaker is present)
- hypotension (systolic blood pressure <90 mmHg)
- xanthine (e.g. caffeine, aminophylline) use in the last 12 h or dipyridamole use in the last 24 h.

Vasodilator stress is relatively contraindicated by bradycardia of <40 beats/min, equivocal left main stem coronary artery stenosis, recent cerebral ischaemia or infarction.

Patient preparation

Patients should receive a clear explanation of what a stress echo study entails and be offered an information leaflet. Ensure that patients taking beta-blockers are informed, where necessary, to omit the beta-blocker for 48 h prior to the stress echo. Patients should be advised to bring a companion to drive them home.

A minimum of two personnel should be present throughout the stress echo study, one of whom should be trained in advanced life support and the other in basic life support. The sonographer should be experienced in stress echo, and a physician should be immediately available if not present during the study. Appropriate cardiopulmonary resuscitation equipment must be available.

Prior to undertaking the stress echo study, ensure that the patient understands what is planned and has given informed consent. Review the patient's history and prior investigation findings and check for contraindications or anything that may increase the risk of complications.

A 12-lead ECG must be recorded (and reviewed) at baseline and every minute during the stress study. Attach the ECG electrodes in their standard positions, although these may need to be modified slightly to allow access to the appropriate echo imaging windows. There must also be continuous ECG monitoring (usually via the ECG electrodes of the echo machine) to monitor for arrhythmias. Use an automated cuff to check blood pressure at baseline and again at each stress stage.

Acquiring the stress echo images

The key to a successful stress echo study is to obtain clear definition of the LV endocardial border. It is important to spend adequate time acquiring the rest images before starting the stress part of the study to ensure that image quality is **optimal** and that the imaging views will be **reproducible** when a set of images is acquired at each stage of the stress study – it is essential to compare 'like with like' at each stage.

Endocardial border definition can be enhanced using:

- harmonic imaging (p. 23)
- ultrasound contrast agents (p. 95).

The use of an ultrasound contrast agent is appropriate if two or more myocardial segments cannot be seen clearly on the rest images.

Imaging of the LV must show each of the myocardial segments in at least one and, where possible, two views. The standard stress echo windows and views are:

- left parasternal window
  - parasternal long axis view
  - parasternal short axis view
- apical window
  - apical 4-chamber view
  - apical 2-chamber view.

The apical 3-chamber (long axis) view can be used as an alternative to the parasternal long axis view where necessary. With conventional 2-D echo each view has to be obtained in turn. However 3-D echo, where available, offers an opportunity to image *all* of the LV myocardial segments at once, which can make image acquisition faster and also allows more flexible 'slicing' of the LV to permit better alignment between views obtained at different levels of stress.

Take your time in acquiring the baseline images – these are the benchmark for comparison with the stress images, so it is important that they are as good as they can be. Make a mental note of the position and angulation of the probe that you used for each view – when you repeat the images during the stress part of the study, you'll be under pressure to find the same views in a much shorter time. The baseline echo should also include an assessment of:

- chamber dimensions (including the aortic root)
- overall left and right ventricular function
- valvular structure and function.

Images should be acquired digitally, rather than on video tape, so that images acquired from the same view (but at different stages of the study) can later be displayed side by side for direct comparison, making identification of any regional wall motion abnormalities easier. This comparison is typically done in a 'quad screen' view, with images acquired at baseline, low level stress, peak stress and recovery displayed side by side (Fig. 8.1).

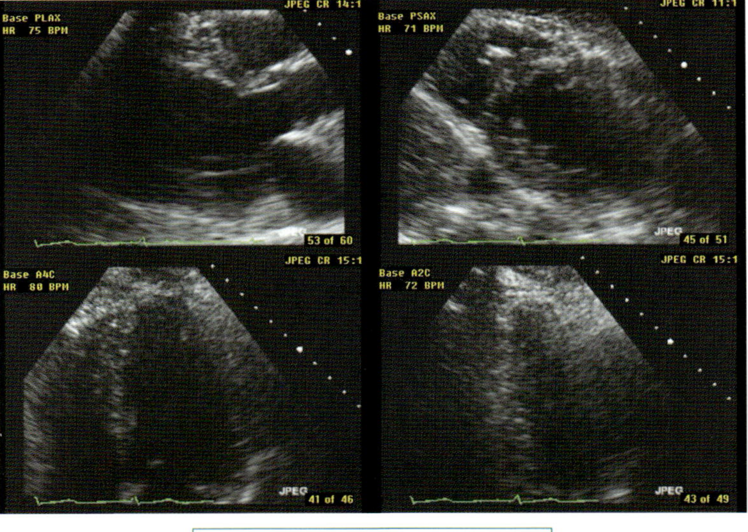

View	Stress echo quad screen
Modality	2-D

Fig. 8.1 Stress echo 'quad screen' view

As you acquire the images, the wall motion of each myocardial segment should be assessed and scored appropriately. Some departments use a 16-segment model, others a 17-segment model (see Chapter 12 for more details); be sure to use the standard model adopted by your department. The wall motion of each segment should be described using one of the following terms:

- X = unable to interpret (suboptimal image quality)
- 1 = normokinetic
- 2 = hypokinetic
- 3 = akinetic
- 4 = dyskinetic
- 5 = aneurysmal.

Wall motion is assessed according to the degree of excursion of the endocardium and in particular by the degree of wall thickening – normal segments should have an excursion of >5 mm and thicken by >50 per cent during systole. Each segment should be assessed at baseline, low-level stress (where appropriate), peak stress and in recovery. The clearest way to summarize the scores is in the form of a chart, as shown for a 16-segment model in Figure 8.2.

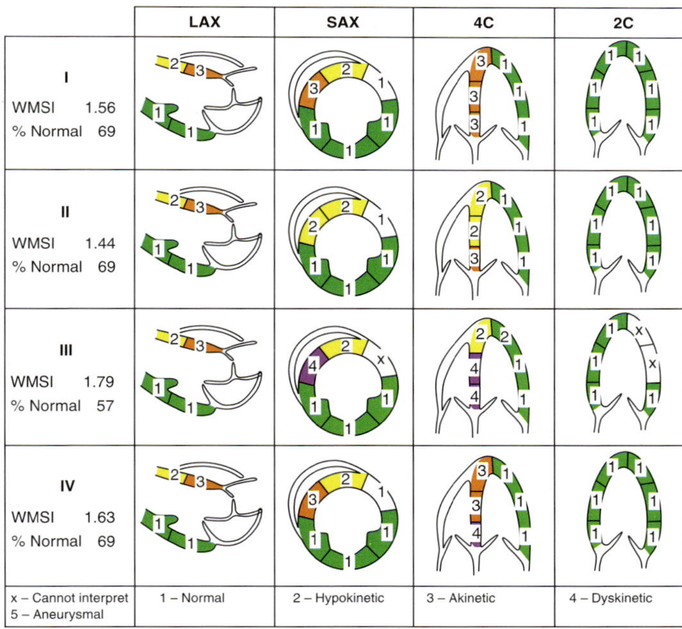

Fig. 8.2 Stress echo wall motion scores (WMSI = wall motion score index)

The stress echo study should be terminated if:

- target heart rate (85 per cent of age-predicted maximum) is attained
- maximal exercise workload or pharmacological dose are attained
- the patient experiences severe chest pain or intolerable symptoms
- there are new (or worsening) regional wall motion abnormalities in ≥2 adjacent myocardial segments, or with ventricular dilatation
- there is a global reduction of LV systolic function
- there is clear ECG evidence of ischaemia (new ST segment depression >2 mm)

- systolic blood pressure falls by >20 mmHg below baseline or from a previous level
- blood pressure increases >220/120 mmHg
- there are supraventricular or complex ventricular arrhythmias.

When each myocardial region has been scored, the **wall motion score index** (WMSI) can be calculated at baseline and for each level of stress. This is calculated by adding together the total wall motion score (i.e. the individual scores for all the segments that can be scored), and then dividing this by the number of scored segments. If all the segments are normokinetic, the WMSI will be 1.0. If any regional wall motion abnormalities are present, the WMSI will be greater than 1.0. An additional quantitative measure is the percentage of scored segments that are normokinetic.

If the study has confirmed myocardial ischaemia, you should note the heart rate at which ischaemia was first evident (this is only possible with dobutamine or bicycle stress echo, where repeated imaging occurs at different levels of stress). **Ischaemic threshold** is the heart rate at which ischaemia first occurred and is calculated as a percentage, using the equation:

$$\text{Ischaemic threshold} = \frac{\text{heart rate when ischaemia first occurred}}{220 - \text{patient's age (in years)}} \times 100$$

Ischaemic threshold is particularly useful in assessing cardiovascular risk in patients due to undergo non-cardiac surgery. An ischaemic threshold <60 per cent or ischaemia in ⩾3–5 segments is an indicator of high risk.

ADDITIONAL INFORMATION

A normal stress echo study is defined as showing normal wall motion at rest and with stress. Those patients with a normal exercise stress echo have an annual risk of cardiac death or nonfatal myocardial infarction of <1 per cent and are therefore regarded as being in a 'low-risk' group. The annual risk for those with a normal pharmacological stress echo is a little higher which is thought to reflect the fact that many of these patients are unable to exercise because of co-morbidities. Several factors indicate high risk, including extensive regional wall motion abnormalities (four to five segments) at rest or induced with stress, or the presence of a low ischaemic threshold (<60–70 per cent).

Stress protocols

Exercise stress

Exercise stress can be undertaken using either a treadmill or a bicycle: treadmill exercise limits the echo assessment to baseline and peak stress (i.e. immediately post exercise), whereas bicycle exercise means that images can be acquired during the test at different levels of exertion. 'Peak' stress images must all be acquired within 60 seconds of completing exercise, before the effects of exercise start to wear off and the patient enters the recovery phase.

For treadmill exercise a symptom-limited Bruce protocol is most commonly used, with the level of exercise increasing at 3-min intervals. For bicycle exercise, workload is usually increased in increments of 25W every 2–3min. Exercise usually continues (all else being equal) until the patient attains 85 per cent of their age-predicted heart rate (220 – patient's age in years).

Dobutamine stress

Dobutamine stress protocols begin with an IV infusion of dobutamine at 5μg/kg/min, increasing the infusion rate at 3-min intervals to 10, 20, 30 and 40μg/kg/min. If patients are failing to approach their target heart rate with the dobutamine infusion alone, IV atropine can also be administered in divided doses of 0.25mg every minute (up to a maximum of 1.0mg) to increase heart rate. Acquisition of images at low/intermediate levels of dobutamine stress as well as at peak stress allows for assessment of myocardial viability.

Vasodilator stress

Vasodilator stress usually causes a relatively small increase in heart rate together with a mild fall in blood pressure. It is less sensitive than exercise or dobutamine stress for detecting mild/moderate coronary disease, and so vasodilator stress should therefore be used only when exercise or dobutamine stress are contraindicated.

Dipyridamole stress is performed with an IV infusion of 0.56 mg/kg dipyridamole given over 4 min, followed by no infusion for 4 min. If no end points have been reached by this time, a further infusion of 0.28 mg/kg is given over 2 min, followed if necessary by IV atropine administered in divided doses of 0.25 mg every minute (up to a maximum of 1.0 mg) to increase heart rate. Baseline images are acquired prior to the infusion, and stress images are acquired after the first 4-min infusion and, if given, the second infusion (±atropine). Adverse effects of dipyridamole can be treated using 240 mg IV aminophylline.

Adenosine stress is performed with an IV infusion of 140 μg/kg/min adenosine given over 6 min. Baseline images are acquired prior to the infusion, and stress images are acquired 3 min into the infusion.

Stress echo and valvular disease

Aortic stenosis

Assessing the severity of aortic stenosis in patients with impaired LV function can be difficult. One measure of aortic stenosis severity is aortic valve area, calculated by the continuity equation (p. 155). In the presence of impaired LV function a reduced aortic valve area may be the result of aortic stenosis, but it can also result from reduced cardiac output failing to open the aortic valve cusps to their full extent during systole. Aortic valve gradient (velocity) does not help, as gradients underestimate the severity of aortic stenosis in the presence of impaired LV function.

It can therefore be difficult to assess whether a patient with 'low gradient, low flow aortic stenosis' has a significantly stenosed valve ('true' aortic stenosis) or whether the findings are primarily the result of reduced valve opening secondary to low cardiac output ('functional' aortic stenosis). 'Low gradient, low flow aortic stenosis' has been defined as an aortic valve orifice area $<1.0\ cm^2$ and a mean valve gradient <30 mmHg in a patient with a LV ejection fraction <40 per cent.

Dobutamine stress echo can be useful in this situation. To distinguish between 'true' and 'functional' aortic stenosis, dobutamine is initially infused at 5 μg/kg/min with increases, if necessary, at 5 min intervals to 10 μg/kg/min and 20 μg/kg/min. If there is true (fixed) aortic stenosis, the aortic valve area will remain essentially unchanged (usually remaining $<1.2\ cm^2$) but the mean valve gradient will increase (usually to a value >30 mmHg). If the 'stenosis' is functional, the valve area will increase relatively more, and the mean gradient relatively less, with the dobutamine infusion.

It is important to look for any regional wall motion abnormalities during such a study, which would indicate coexistent myocardial ischaemia, and also to assess the overall LV response to dobutamine. The presence of LV 'contractile reserve' is indicated by an increase in stroke volume with dobutamine stress, as shown by an increase in velocity time integral (VTI) of >20 per cent. Patients with contractile reserve have a better perioperative mortality than those without.

Mitral stenosis

In patients with mitral stenosis, stress echo can be helpful in those whose symptoms appear disproportionate to resting haemodynamic measurements, and also those who are asymptomatic but who appear to have severe stenosis. Doppler studies of the mitral and tricuspid valves can be performed during stress, and those who have exertional breathlessness with a mean mitral valve gradient >15 mmHg and a pulmonary artery systolic pressure >60 mmHg are likely to benefit from intervention.

After the stress echo study

Following the stress echo study, continue to monitor the patient carefully until they are asymptomatic and any ECG, echo or haemodynamic changes have returned to baseline. Patients should rest in the echo department for 30 min before going home, and they should be driven home by a companion. The results of the study should, where possible, be discussed with the patient before they leave. If the results are not immediately available, advise the patient how and when they will hear the results of the study.

You should begin your study report with the patient's demographic details and a summary of the indication for the study. Comment on the image quality and whether a contrast agent was used. Describe the stress protocol and the adequacy of the patient's response to it, noting in particular any symptoms (e.g. chest pain) and/or ECG changes, together with changes in heart rate and blood pressure. If an exercise protocol was used, include the exercise duration and peak heart rate attained; for a pharmacological protocol, include information on the drug(s) and doses administered. Review all the images and record the wall motion scores at each level of stress, summarizing them in your stress echo report in an easily understood visual format (as in Fig. 8.2). Finally, conclude your report with a summary of whether your findings are normal or indicate ischaemia, necrosis or viability (stunning or hibernation). If you have undertaken any valvular assessments as part of the study, include these details in your report too.

FURTHER READING

ACCF/ASE/ACEP/AHA/ASNC/SCAI/SCCT/SCMR. Appropriateness criteria for stress echocardiography. *Circulation* 2008; **117**: 1478–97.

Becher H, Chambers J, Fox K, *et al.* BSE procedure guidelines for the clinical application of stress echocardiography, recommendations for performance and interpretation of stress echocardiography. *Heart* 2004; **90**(suppl VI): vi23–30.

Chambers J. Low 'gradient', low flow aortic stenosis. *Heart* 2006; **92**: 554–8.

Das M, Pellikka P, Mahoney D, *et al.* Assessment of cardiac risk before nonvascular surgery: dobutamine stress echocardiography in 530 patients. *J Am Coll Cardiol* 2000; **35**: 1647–53.

Marwick PH. Stress echocardiography. *Heart* 2003; **89**: 113–18.

Pellikka PA, Nagueh SF, Elhendy AA, *et al.* American Society of Echocardiography recommendations for performance, interpretation, and application of stress echocardiography. *J Am Soc Echocardiogr* 2007; **20**: 1021–41.

Sicari R, Nihoyannopoulos P, Evangelista A, *et al.* Stress echocardiography expert consensus statement. *Eur J Echocardiogr* 2008; **9**: 415–37.

9 Advanced echo techniques

Contrast studies

There are two very different types of echo contrast study, using:

- agitated saline bubble contrast
- echo contrast agents.

Agitated saline bubble contrast

An agitated saline bubble contrast is simple to perform and is used primarily to detect a right-to-left shunt, most commonly a patent foramen ovale (PFO, p. 297). A suspension of tiny air bubbles is injected intravenously while an echo is performed. Normally the bubbles fill the right heart where they are clearly visible on echo (Fig. 9.1), but they are then filtered out as they pass through the lungs – no bubbles will therefore be seen in the left heart. If bubbles *are* seen within the left heart, this indicates that the agitated saline bubble contrast (and hence blood) is managing to cross directly from the right heart into the left via a right-to-left shunt, bypassing the lungs.

Normally the presence of an intracardiac shunt will allow blood to flow from left to right (high pressure to low pressure), but during a Valsalva manoeuvre the blood flow will momentarily reverse from right to left. To demonstrate a transient right-to-left shunt you can use 'agitated' saline:

- Draw up 8.5 mL of normal saline and 0.5 mL of air into a 10 mL Luer lock syringe.
- Using a 3-way tap, connect this to another (empty) 10 mL Luer lock syringe, and then attach this to an intravenous cannula sited in the patient's antecubital vein.

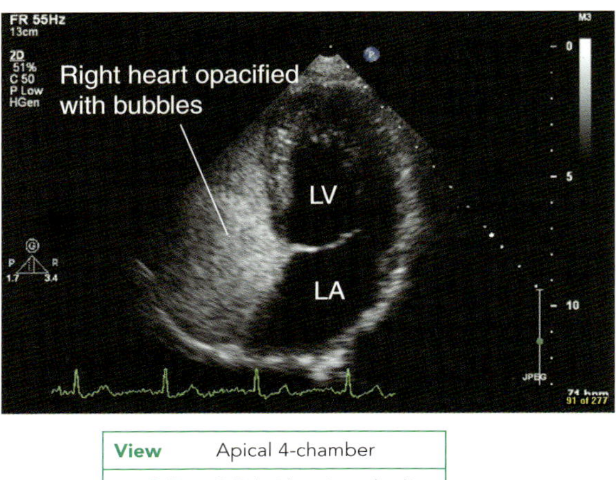

View	Apical 4-chamber
Modality	2-D (with agitated saline contrast)

Fig. 9.1 Agitated saline bubble contrast study (LA = left atrium; LV = left ventricle)

- Withdraw 1 mL of the patient's blood into the syringe containing the saline/air mixture.
- With the 3-way tap turned off to the patient, repeatedly squirt the saline/blood/air mixture back and forth between the two syringes for a few seconds until a suspension of tiny air bubbles is created in the mixture.
- Obtain a good apical 4-chamber view with your echo probe.
- With the patient performing a Valsalva manoeuvre, ensure you are recording the echo images and rapidly inject the 10 mL mixture. When the bubbles appear in the right atrium, ask the patient to release the Valsalva manoeuvre.
- Watch carefully for air bubbles crossing into the left atrium as the patient releases the Valsalva – some authorities regard the crossing of a single bubble as indicative of a shunt, others require three or more bubbles before making the diagnosis.

An agitated saline contrast study can be performed during transthoracic (TTE) or transoesophageal (TOE) echo. Although the image quality is better with TOE, patients usually perform a better Valsalva manoeuvre during TTE.

An additional use of agitated saline bubble contrast is to assist with echo guidance during pericardiocentesis. If there is doubt about whether the pericardiocentesis needle is in the pericardial cavity, a small amount of agitated saline can be injected through the pericardiocentesis needle. If the needle is in the right place, the bubbles will appear within the pericardial effusion. If the pericardiocentesis needle has inadvertently punctured the heart, the bubbles will be seen within one of the cardiac chambers instead.

Echo contrast agents

One of the limitations of TTE is image quality, which can be suboptimal in patients with poor echo windows. Good image quality is particularly important to obtain clear endocardial border definition for accurate left ventricular (LV) function assessment, for instance during stress echocardiography, and also to help identify LV masses and morphological abnormalities. The use of echo contrast agents is one way in which image quality can be enhanced.

As we have already seen, agitated saline bubble contrast does not normally pass through the lungs (unless a shunt is present) and so it is of little value in LV opacification. Echo contrast agents are different – they are specifically designed to pass though the lungs and reach the left heart. In order to achieve this, the bubbles within these echo contrast agents must be very small, usually measuring around 1–10μm in diameter. The exact composition of the bubbles varies between manufacturers, but they typically consist of a shell (e.g. lipid, phospholipid, human albumin) enclosing a cavity filled with gas (e.g. air, perfluoropropane, sulphur hexafluoride).

Echo contrast microbubbles are not just passive reflectors of ultrasound. Instead, when they are struck by an incident ultrasound beam, the microbubbles resonate, emitting an ultrasound signal of their own at higher harmonics than the incident beam. The use of appropriate settings on the echo machine (e.g. harmonic imaging, intermittent imaging) optimizes the detection of the 'resonant' signal generated by the microbubbles while at the same time suppressing the usual ultrasound signal returned from the surrounding tissues.

Echo contrast agent microbubbles are relatively 'fragile' and tend to be disrupted by the intensity of conventional ultrasound – the use of a low mechanical index (low-MI imaging) reduces this, although in some situations a higher MI can be used to deliberately disrupt the microbubbles (for example, to assess myocardial perfusion by disrupting the microbubbles in the myocardium with a brief high-MI pulse, and then observing how quickly the microbubbles are replenished).

Echo contrast agents include Definity® (known in Europe as Luminity®) and Optison®, both licensed by the United States Food and Drug Administration (FDA). Both are indicated for use in patients for LV opacification, endocardial border definition and Doppler.

Clinical applications

Echo contrast agents are useful in improving visualization of the LV, particularly in cases where image quality is suboptimal and two or more contiguous LV segments cannot be seen with conventional imaging. This improves the accuracy of LV volume and ejection fraction measurements, and is especially valuable in the assessment of regional wall motion during stress echo studies (Chapter 8).

Improved imaging of the LV endocardium can also help in the identification of morphological abnormalities including isolated ventricular non-compaction, apical hypertrophic cardiomyopathy, intracardiac masses such as tumours and thrombus, and LV aneurysm.

The enhanced LV imaging obtained with echo contrast agents can be particularly useful when performing portable studies in the intensive care unit, where the inability to position the patient optimally means that image quality is frequently suboptimal. Echo contrast agents can also improve spectral Doppler signals, aiding in the assessment of valvular disease and LV diastolic function.

Contraindications

For full details about the safe and appropriate use of echo contrast agents, refer to the relevant product datasheet. The following contraindications apply to Definity® and Optison®:

- known hypersensitivity to the products
- right-to-left, bidirectional or transient right-to-left cardiac shunts.

The agents are for intravenous use and must not be administered by the intra-arterial route.

High-risk patients with pulmonary hypertension or unstable cardiopulmonary conditions should be monitored during and for 30 min after administration (including vital signs, ECG and oxygen saturations). All other patients should be closely observed during and following administration. Resuscitation equipment and trained personnel must be available.

3-D echo

The cornerstone of most echo studies is 2-D imaging, in which the transducer images the heart by taking a 'slice' through a single plane. However, since the 1970s there has been interest in the potential for 3-D echo, in which sufficient data could be collected to construct a 3-D image which could then be manipulated to allow the operator to move back and forth 'through' the image to allow a view to be constructed in virtually any plane. Rapid developments in computer hardware and software together with advances in miniaturization during the 1990s made 3-D echo a practical possibility, and many departments now use 3-D echo as part of their imaging repertoire.

Early 3-D echo made use of offline processing of 2-D images to construct a 3-D image. More recently, matrix array transthoracic (and transoesophageal) transducers have become available that allow the acquisition of 3-D data ('volumetric scanning') in real time (Fig. 9.2). Matrix array transducers contain a grid of 2000–3000 elements that acquire a pyramid-shaped volume of data, with much of the initial 'number crunching' being performed by

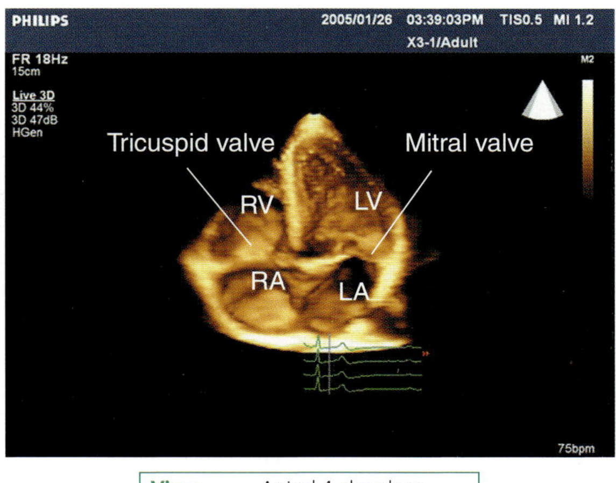

View	Apical 4-chamber
Modality	3D echo

Fig. 9.2 Three-dimensional (3-D) echo (LA = left atrium; LV = left ventricle; RA = right atrium; RV = right ventricle) (Figure reproduced with permission of Philips)

processors within the transducer (to reduce the amount of data that needs to be sent to the echo machine via the transducer cable, which could become unwieldy as a result). As well as creating greyscale 3-D images, 3-D echo can be combined with colour Doppler to allow 3-D reconstruction of regurgitant jets and shunts.

One clear advantage of 3-D over 2-D echo is in the measurement of LV volumes and mass. Using 2-D echo these parameters are calculated using a limited number of measurements, and the calculations are based on assumptions about LV geometry that may be misleading (Chapter 11). 3-D echo offers the capability to visualize the whole LV, making such measurements more accurate and more reproducible. 3-D echo is also not prone to the problem of foreshortening which can affect the reliability of 2-D measurements. As well as the LV, 3-D echo has also proven valuable in right ventricular assessment. Other uses for 3-D echo are listed in Table 9.1.

Table 9.1 Indications for 3-D echo

3-D echo offers advantages over 2-D echo in:

- calculation of ventricular volumes and mass
- assessment of valvular anatomy (especially mitral valve)
- calculation of valvular regurgitant volumes
- assessment of congenital heart disease
- assessment of left ventricular dyssynchrony
- planning surgery for structural heart disease

Disadvantages of 3-D echo are that it can be more time-consuming than 2-D echo and the equipment needed is more expensive. The image quality is not as good as 2-D echo, and patients need to be in a regular heart rhythm for a 3-D study.

Intravascular ultrasound

Intravascular ultrasound (IVUS) provides direct imaging of the coronary arteries, using a miniature ultrasound probe that can be passed down the coronary arteries via a catheter. IVUS probes use very high frequency ultrasound (typically 20–50 MHz) to image the wall of the artery, revealing not just the diameter of the lumen but also the characteristics of any atherosclerotic plaques (Fig. 9.3).

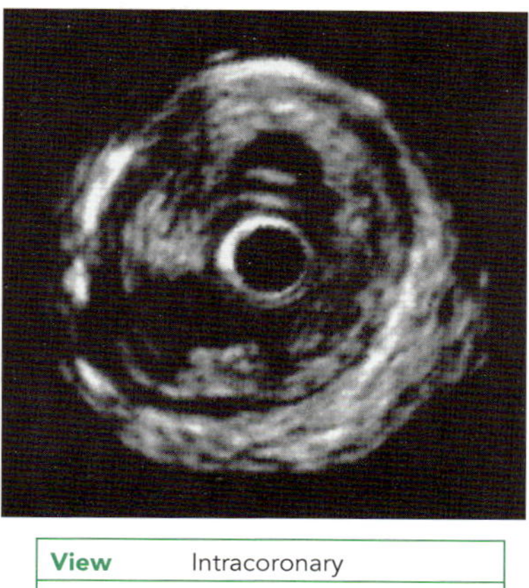

View	Intracoronary
Modality	Intravascular ultrasound

Fig. 9.3 Intravascular ultrasound of abnormal left circumflex coronary artery (Figure adapted with permission from the BMJ Publishing Group (*Heart* 2001; **85**: 567–70))

Coronary angiography (p. 107) commonly underestimates the severity of coronary atherosclerosis, particularly when the atheroma is diffusely distributed. IVUS plays an important role in clarifying the extent of coronary atheroma and can help identify obstructive disease that might be overlooked by angiography alone. IVUS has also provided an insight into the phenomenon of coronary artery remodelling, in which arterial diameter can increase as plaque accumulates, preserving the diameter of the lumen (so the vessel looks unobstructed on angiography) even though significant atheroma is present (as revealed by IVUS).

IVUS can also be helpful in guiding coronary artery stenting in percutaneous coronary intervention procedures. Performing an IVUS study immediately after stent deployment allows an assessment of how well-deployed the stent is, i.e. whether it is fully expanded and well-apposed to the walls of the artery.

Epicardial echo

The use of TOE during surgical procedures has grown over recent years, not only in the assessment of structural heart disease during cardiac surgery but also in monitoring cardiac performance more generally. However, not all patients can undergo such an intraoperative TOE examination and in these cases epicardial echo provides a useful alternative (Table 9.2).

Epicardial echo involves placing an echo probe directly on the surface of the heart while the heart is exposed during a sternotomy. The probe must of course be kept sterile, and so it is placed within a sterile sheath together with some acoustic gel. As there are no intervening structures during epicardial echo, an echo probe with a higher frequency than a normal transthoracic probe can be used and this will enhance image quality. Seven standard views are recommended by the American Society of Echocardiography and the Society of Cardiovascular Anesthesiologists (Table 9.3).

Table 9.2 Indications for epicardial echo

Epicardial ultrasound can be used as an alternative to intraoperative TOE in patients where:

- there are oesophageal abnormalities that contraindicate the passage of a TOE probe
- attempts to pass a TOE probe have been unsuccessful
- areas need to be inspected that cannot be clearly visualized with intraoperative TOE

TOE, transoesophageal echo.

Table 9.3 Epicardial echo views (and transthoracic echo (TTE) equivalents)

Epicardial echo view	Equivalent TTE view
Aortic valve short axis	Parasternal aortic valve short axis
Aortic valve long axis	Suprasternal aortic valve long axis
Left ventricular basal short axis	Modified parasternal mitral valve basal short axis
Left ventricular mid short axis	Parasternal mid-left ventricle short axis
Left ventricular long axis	Parasternal long axis
2-chamber	Modified parasternal long axis
Right ventricular outflow tract	Parasternal short axis

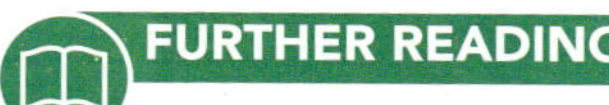

FURTHER READING

Hung J, Lang R, Flachskampf F, *et al.* 3D echocardiography: a review of the current status and future directions. *J Am Soc Echocardiogr* 2007; **20**: 213–33.

Mintz GS, Nissen SE, Anderson WD, *et al.* American College of Cardiology clinical expert consensus document on standards for acquisition, measurement and reporting of intravascular ultrasound studies (IVUS). *Eur J Echocardiogr* 2001; **2**: 299–313.

Mulvagh SL, Rakowski H, Vannan MA, *et al.* American Society of Echocardiography consensus statement on the clinical applications of ultrasonic contrast agents in echocardiography. *J Am Soc Echocardiogr* 2008; **21**: 1179–201.

Olszewski R, Timperley J, Cezary S, *et al.* 2007. The clinical applications of contrast echocardiography. *Eur J Echocardiogr* 2007; **8**: S13–23.

Reeves ST, Glas KE, Eltzschig H, *et al.* Guidelines for performing a comprehensive epicardial echocardiography examination: recommendations of the American Society of Echocardiography and the Society of Cardiovascular Anesthesiologists. *Anesth Analg* 2007; **105**: 2–28.

Schoenhagen P, Nissen S. Understanding coronary artery disease: tomographic imaging with intravascular ultrasound. *Heart* 2002; **88**: 91–6.

Sugeng L, Mor-Avi V, Lang RM. Three-dimensional echocardiography: coming of age. *Heart* 2008; **94**: 1123–5.

10 Alternative cardiac imaging techniques

Echo is not the only technique for obtaining diagnostic information about the heart. Several cardiac imaging techniques are available, some of which provide similar information to echo (e.g. assessment of left ventricular (LV) function with cardiac magnetic resonance imaging (MRI)) and some of which can provide additional information about the heart that echo alone cannot obtain (e.g. visualization of coronary stenoses with coronary angiography). Knowledge of these alternative imaging techniques can help you decide when another test might replace or supplement an echo study.

Nuclear cardiology

Nuclear cardiology uses radioactive isotopes, administered intravenously, to image the heart and to provide information about myocardial perfusion (myocardial perfusion imaging) and ventricular function (radionuclide ventriculography).

Uses of nuclear cardiology

Myocardial perfusion imaging uses a radiopharmaceutical (e.g. thallium-201 or a technetium-99m-labelled radiopharmaceutical) to assess myocardial blood flow, providing valuable information about coronary artery disease with a high degree of sensitivity and specificity (Fig. 10.1).

After the radiopharmaceutical has been administered intravenously, its distribution in the myocardium can be assessed using single photon emission computed tomography (SPECT) imaging. Imaging is performed at rest and again after stress (exercise or pharmacological), and comparison of

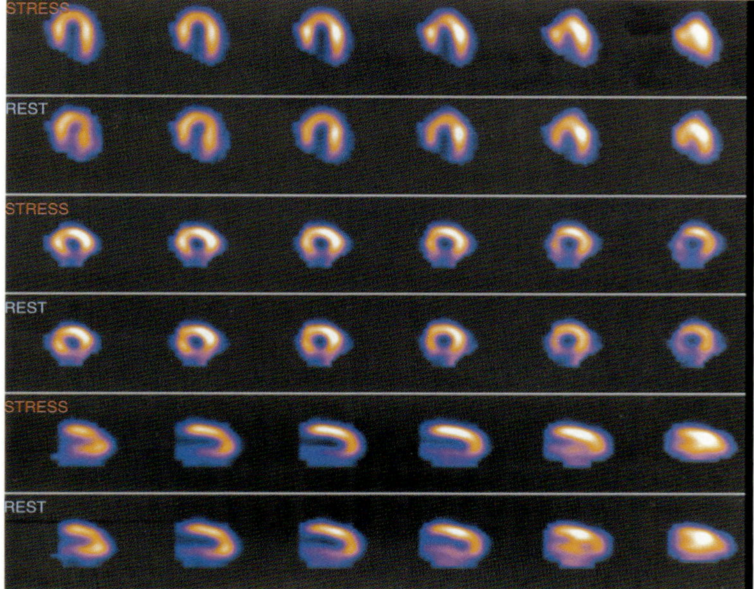

Fig. 10.1 Myocardial perfusion imaging (showing inferior wall defect)

the rest and stress images allows identification of areas of normal perfusion, reversible ischaemia (normal perfusion at rest but reduced perfusion after stress) and fixed ischaemia (reduced perfusion at rest and after stress). The use of ECG gating also allows myocardial function to be assessed with the calculation of a LV ejection fraction.

Radionuclide ventriculography gives an accurate assessment of ventricular function. It is most commonly performed using red blood cells labelled with technetium-99m which are administered intravenously. The count-rate of the radioactivity can be measured using a gamma camera over many cardiac cycles and, with the use of ECG gating, the average count rate at different stages of the cardiac cycle can be calculated. From this, an accurate measure of ejection fraction can be derived.

Disadvantages of nuclear cardiology

The principal drawback of nuclear cardiology is the patient's exposure to ionizing radiation. The typical effective radiation dose of a ^{99m}Tc dynamic cardiac scan is 6 mSv, equivalent to 2.7 years' exposure to natural background radiation. For a ^{201}Tl myocardial perfusion scan the typical dose is 18 mSv, equivalent to 8 years' background radiation (for comparison, the typical dose of a single chest X-ray is 0.02 mSv, or 3 days' background radiation). Further information on radiation doses and the lifetime additional risk of fatal cancer, can be found on the website of the Health Protection Agency (www.hpa.org.uk).

Cardiac magnetic resonance imaging

MRI is a highly versatile technique for cardiac imaging and provides both anatomical and functional information. Cardiac MRI is performed with a scanner containing a large superconducting magnet; radio waves are transmitted into the heart, aligning hydrogen nuclei, and as the nuclei subsequently 'relax' they emit radio waves of their own which can be detected by the scanner. The detected signal can then be used to reconstruct an image of the heart (Fig. 10.2).

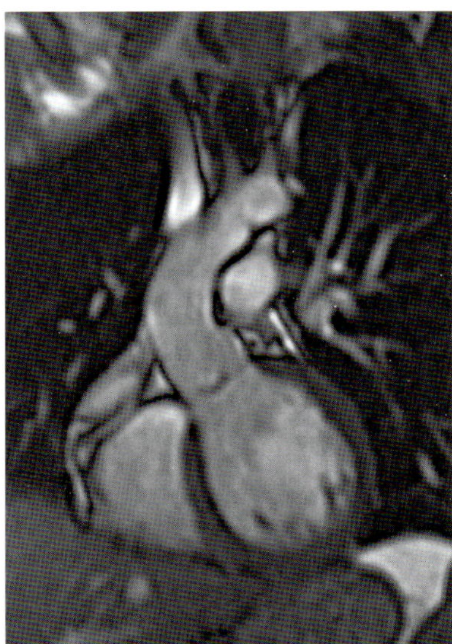

Fig. 10.2 Cardiac magnetic resonance imaging (MRI) scan

Uses of cardiac MRI

One of the great advantages of cardiac MRI over many other cardiac imaging techniques is the wide range of information that it can provide – as well as anatomical information (usually with excellent image quality) cardiac MRI can also measure blood flow velocities, making it suitable for the assessment of valvular abnormalities and shunts. Its uses include the assessment of:

- cardiac chamber dimensions and function
- valvular heart disease
- cardiomyopathies
- cardiac masses
- congenital heart disease
- pericardial disease
- aortic abnormalities.

Cardiac MRI does not have the spatial resolution to image the coronary arteries very well, but it can nevertheless aid in the assessment of coronary artery disease in a similar manner to a stress echo study (Chapter 8). A cardiac MRI scan can be combined with pharmacological stress, as for stress echo, to identify myocardial ischaemia, necrosis and viability. The use of a gadolinium-based contrast agent can provide valuable information on myocardial perfusion.

Disadvantages of cardiac MRI

Although cardiac MRI does not involve exposure to ionizing radiation, it does expose the patient to a powerful magnetic field and is therefore contraindicated in patients with certain types of metallic implant (e.g. pacemakers, implantable defibrillators and cerebrovascular aneurysm clips). Some patients with claustrophobia are unable to tolerate the enclosed conditions found in many MRI scanners. For certain cardiac MRI studies patients require an intravenous injection of a gadolinium-based contrast agent, and in patients with renal impairment this may pose a risk of nephrogenic systemic fibrosis.

Cardiac computed tomography

The development of multislice computed tomography (MSCT) has led to the increasing use of CT scanning to image the heart. MSCT scanners contain a gantry carrying an X-ray source and a number of detectors that rotates around the patient. Multiple image 'slices' are obtained as the patient is moved through the gantry during the scan, and an ECG is also recorded. The slices are then processed by the appropriate software, and the ECG data can be used to 'gate' the images so that the heart can be examined at different points in the cardiac cycle. Processing of the imaging data allows the heart to be viewed in any plane and from any angle, either as a 3-D volume rendered image or as cross-sectional slices (Fig. 10.3).

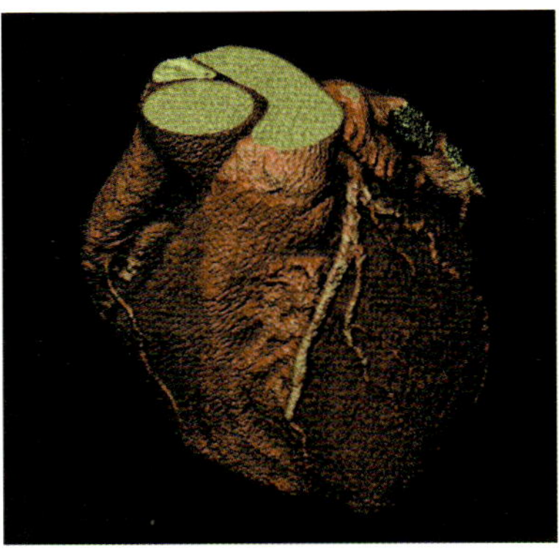

Fig. 10.3 Cardiac computed tomography (CT) (volume rendered image). Figure adapted with permission from the BMJ Publishing Group (*Heart* 2008; **94**: 781–92)

Modern MSCT scanners commonly have 16 or 64 slices, but models offering even more slices (256 and 320 slices) are becoming available. Cardiac CT scanning is very fast, as it typically takes no more than 15 s to acquire the images. However, some patient preparation is required, as cardiac studies require the injection of an intravascular contrast agent and many patients also require a beta-blocker to slow their heart rate. Examining and reporting the images usually takes 10–30 min, depending on the complexity of the case.

Uses of cardiac CT

The main use of MSCT is in assessment of the coronary arteries. A calcium score can be obtained, which reflects the amount of calcification present in the coronary arteries; this information can then be used to estimate the patient's risk of future cardiovascular events. The coronary arteries themselves can be imaged with the use of contrast (CT coronary angiography, CTCA), and any stenoses can be identified (although assessing the precise severity of stenoses is more difficult).

MSCT can also be used to image the cardiac chambers, allowing measurements to be made, and movie images show ventricular function. Cardiac masses can be examined, as can congenital abnormalities. Unfortunately cardiac CT does not provide information on blood flow, but it does allow valvular morphology to be assessed.

Disadvantages of cardiac CT

Cardiac CT involves exposure to ionizing radiation, and patients do need to have a relatively slow (and regular) pulse and must be able to hold their breath during the scan. For the assessment of the heart valves and chambers, echo is generally the preferred modality, but for coronary artery imaging (which cannot be performed with echo) cardiac CT offers a useful non-invasive alternative to cardiac catheterization.

Cardiac catheterization

Cardiac catheterization allows imaging of the coronary arteries and cardiac chambers (using a contrast agent) and also the measurement of intracardiac pressures and oxygen saturations. It is an invasive technique, requiring a catheter to be passed to the heart via a peripheral vessel.

In the case of a left heart study, the catheter is passed under local anaesthetic into the femoral or radial artery and then guided to the heart under fluoroscopic screening. Once the catheter in position, a contrast agent is injected to visualize the left and right coronary arteries in turn (coronary angiography, Fig. 10.4). Larger volumes of contrast can be used to visualize the LV and aorta. Intracardiac pressure measurements can be taken, and blood can be sampled from the tip of the catheter to assess oxygen saturation. For a right heart study the catheter is passed via the femoral vein and again allows intracardiac pressure and oxygen saturation measurements. Cardiac output can also be calculated.

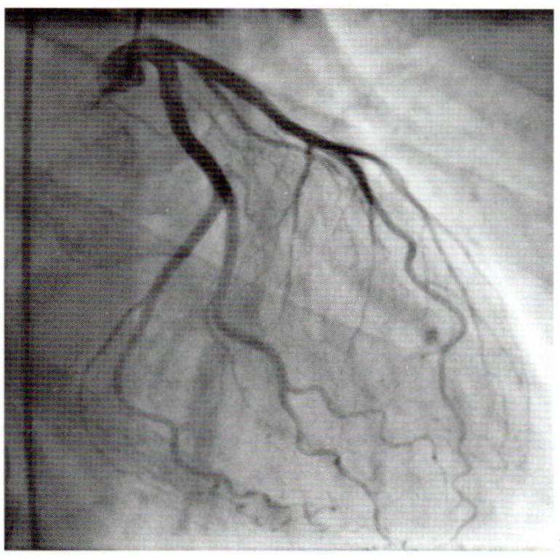

Fig. 10.4 Coronary angiogram (showing left coronary artery)

Uses of cardiac catheterization

Cardiac catheterisation is most commonly used to assess the coronary arteries in cases of suspected coronary artery disease. Although echo can provide information about myocardial ischaemia (e.g. regional LV wall motion abnormalities) it cannot visualize the coronary arteries themselves. Cardiac catheterization also has a role to play in supplementing the echo assessment of valvular, LV and congenital cardiac abnormalities.

Disadvantages of cardiac catheterization

Cardiac catheterization is an invasive procedure, carrying a risk of trauma to the vessels where catheters are inserted, and also carries a risk of arrhythmias, myocardial infarction, stroke and death. There is also exposure to radiation and an intravascular contrast agent.

FURTHER READING

Butler R, Gunning M, Nolan J. *Essential Cardiac Catheterization*. Hodder Arnold, London, 2007.

Pennell D. Cardiovascular magnetic resonance. *Heart* 2001; **85**: 581–9.

Roberts WT, Bax JJ, Davies LC. Cardiac CT and CT coronary angiography: technology and application. *Heart* 2008; **94**: 781–92.

Schwaiger M, Melin J. Cardiological applications of nuclear medicine. *Lancet* 1999; **354**: 661–6.

PART 3

Clinical Cases

11 The left heart and its function

Echo assessment of the left ventricle

In many echo departments, assessment of left ventricular (LV) function is the single commonest echo request. One reason for this is that symptoms and signs that can indicate heart failure are common and echo is a non-invasive, straightforward and relatively inexpensive technique for confirming whether LV dysfunction is present. This chapter will cover the assessment of LV dimensions and overall LV systolic and diastolic function (together with assessment of the left atrium (LA)). The assessment of regional systolic function, in the context of coronary artery disease, is discussed in Chapter 12.

The key challenge in using echo to assess the LV lies in summarizing the size and function of a complex 3-D structure using just a handful of parameters. Trying to represent the LV within a limited number of measurements is fraught with pitfalls, not least when using volumetric measures that rely on assumptions about the geometrical shape of the LV, which are not necessarily correct, particularly if the shape of the LV is distorted or abnormalities are limited just to one or two areas of the ventricular wall. The key is to use common sense – if there is a clear discrepancy between your 'eyeball' assessment of the LV and the figures coming out of your calculations, highlight this in your report.

A comprehensive echo evaluation of the LV should include assessment of:

- LV dimensions
  - LV shape
  - wall thickness
  - cavity size

- LV mass
- LV systolic function
  - global function
  - regional function (see Chapter 12)
- LV diastolic function
- LV outflow tract (LVOT) morphology (see Chapter 18, Hypertrophic cardiomyopathy)
- LV masses or thrombus (see Chapter 21).

Left ventricular dimensions

In measuring LV dimensions it is important not to 'miss the wood for the trees' – as LV measurements only provide a selective snapshot of the LV in the regions where the measurements are taken, you must ensure that your report also includes a description of any abnormalities that are not reflected in the figures alone. Take the time to 'eyeball' the LV as a whole in several views (at least part of the LV is visible is almost every standard view of the heart) and if the overall shape is abnormal, be sure to describe this (Fig. 11.1). A good example of this is the presence of an LV aneurysm, in which case describe its location and identify whether it is a true aneurysm or a pseudoaneurysm (Chapter 12), or the presence of a localised area of hypertrophy in hypertrophic cardiomyopathy.

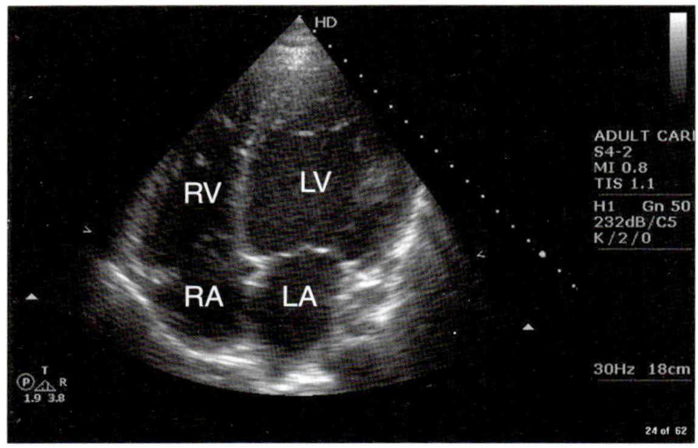

View	Apical 4-chamber
Modality	2-D

Fig. 11.1 Dilated left ventricle (LA = left atrium; LV = left ventricle; RA = right atrium; RV = right ventricle)

Linear LV measurements

Next, take some measurements of the LV wall and cavity dimensions in both systole and diastole. Linear LV measurements are traditionally made using M-mode echo (although comparable measurements can be obtained directly from a 2-D echo image if you prefer), in either the parasternal long axis or parasternal short axis view. M-mode has the advantage of high temporal resolution, which makes it easier to visualize motion of the endocardium. If you are using M-mode:

1. align the M-mode cursor so that it is perpendicular to the septal and posterior LV walls (i.e. at 90° to the long axis of the LV cavity) and lies at the tips of the mitral valve leaflets (Fig. 11.2)
2. obtain an M-mode trace and, when you are happy with it, freeze the trace on the screen
3. identify end-diastole and end-systole (see box) and the endocardial/ epicardial borders correctly.

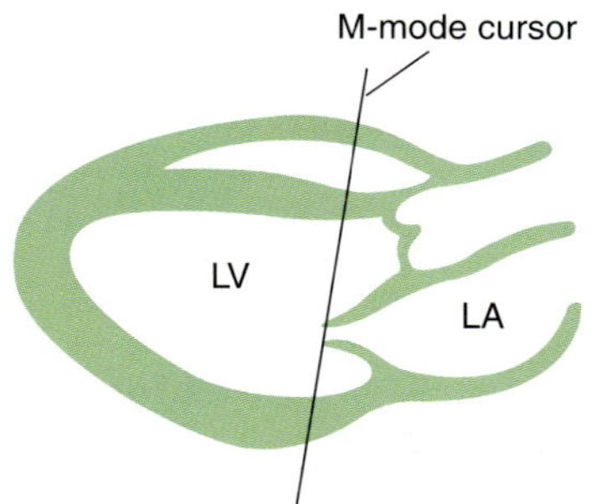

Fig. 11.2 Positioning of M-mode cursor for measurement of LV dimensions (LA = left atrium; LV = left ventricle)

END-DIASTOLE AND END-SYSTOLE

End-diastolic measurements are often taken at the onset of the QRS complex on the ECG trace. However, the American Society of Echocardiography (ASE) recommends that end-diastole is taken as the frame after mitral valve closure or the frame in the cardiac cycle in which the LV internal dimension is largest.

End-systolic measurements are often taken as the point when the LV internal dimension is at its narrowest, but the ASE also suggests using the frame preceding mitral valve opening as an alternative. The apical 2-chamber view does not show mitral valve opening very well, and so measurements taken in this view should not be based on the timing of mitral valve opening.

Starting at the right ventricular (RV) border of the interventricular septum (Fig. 11.3), use the callipers to measure the diastolic LV dimensions:

- IVSd (interventricular septal wall dimension – diastole)
- LVIDd (LV internal dimension – diastole)
- LVPWd (LV posterior wall dimension – diastole)

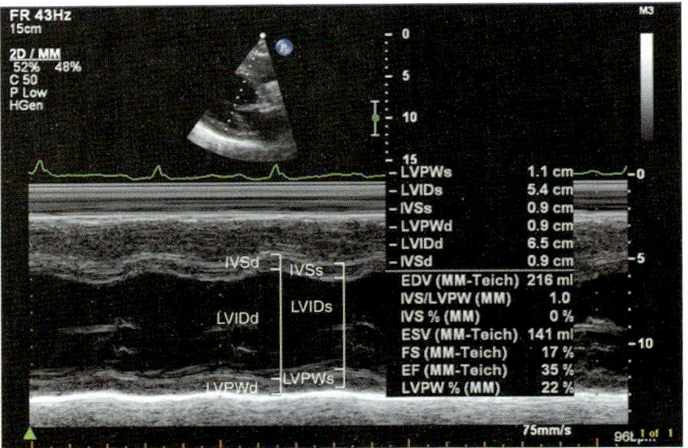

View	Parasternal long axis
Modality	M-mode

Fig. 11.3 M-mode in dilated cardiomyopathy (EDV = end-diastolic volume; EF = ejection fraction; ESV = end-systolic volume; FS = fractional shortening; IVS = interventricular septum; IVSd = interventricular septal wall dimension – diastole; IVSs = interventricular septal wall dimension – systole; LVIDd = left ventricular internal dimension – diastole; LVIDs = left ventricular internal dimension – systole; LVPW = left ventricular posterior wall; LVPWd = left ventricular posterior wall dimension – diastole; LVPWs = left ventricular posterior wall dimension – systole)

Then repeat the process for the systolic LV dimensions:

- IVSs (interventricular septal wall dimension – systole)
- LVIDs (left ventricular internal dimension – systole)
- LVPWs (left ventricular posterior wall dimension – systole)

In the past it has been recommended that such M-mode measurements be taken from leading edge to leading edge, but the improved resolution of contemporary echo machines means than measurements can instead be taken directly from the tissue–blood interface. The echo machine will display the measurements as you make them, and will often also display a number of calculated parameters (e.g. ejection fraction, fractional shortening) based on these measurements (Fig. 11.3).

It is a good idea to make several measurements on different cardiac cycles and obtain an average. It is also possible to adjust the LV internal dimensions for the patient's body surface area (BSA), measured in square metres. The Mosteller formula is commonly used to calculate BSA:

$$\text{BSA (m}^2\text{)} = \sqrt{\frac{\text{height (cm)} \times \text{weight (kg)}}{3600}}$$

Table 11.1 shows the reference ranges for men and women.

Table 11.1 Reference ranges for men and women

	Normal	Mild	Moderate	Severe
Men				
IVSd (cm)	0.6–1.2	1.3–1.5	1.6–1.9	≥2.0
LVIDd (cm)	4.2–5.9	6.0–6.3	6.4–6.8	≥6.9
LVIDd/BSA (cm/m^2)	2.2–3.1	3.2–3.4	3.5–3.6	≥3.7
LVPWd (cm)	0.6–1.2	1.3–1.5	1.6–1.9	≥2.0
Women				
IVSd (cm)	0.6–1.2	1.3–1.5	1.6–1.9	≥2.0
LVIDd (cm)	3.9–5.3	5.4–5.7	5.8–6.1	≥6.2
LVIDd/BSA (cm/m^2)	2.4–3.2	3.3–3.4	3.5–3.7	≥3.8
LVPWd (cm)	0.6–1.2	1.3–1.5	1.6–1.9	≥2.0

BSA = body surface area; IVSd = interventricular septal wall dimension – diastole; LVIDd = left ventricular internal dimension – diastole; LVPWd = left ventricular posterior wall dimension – diastole.

Reference ranges reproduced with permission of the British Society of Echocardiography and British Heart Foundation.

COMMON PITFALLS

Pitfalls in the assessment of LV dimensions include:

- *Failure to take measurements at the correct time points (end-systole or end-diastole)*
- *Failure to take measurements perpendicular to the long axis of the LV*
- *Failure to identify the endocardium correctly – be particularly careful to avoid mistaking chordae tendineae for the endocardium of the LV posterior wall*

Volumetric left ventricular measurements

Volumetric measurements are based upon the principle that LV volumes can be calculated from 2-D measurements of the LV as long as certain assumptions about the shape of the LV apply. The more distorted the LV (e.g. as a result of an aneurysm), the less reliable such volumetric measurements become.

Modified Simpson's rule method

Modified Simpson's rule method is the best (and most commonly used) way of calculating LV volumes. It is also known as the biplane method of discs, as it works on the principle that the LV cavity can be considered as a stack of elliptical discs of differing sizes from base to apex. If the volume of each disc is known (from its area and thickness), then the overall LV volume is equal to the volume of all the discs added together.

Echo machines automate much of the process and require the operator simply to measure the length of the LV (long axis) and to trace the outline of the LV endocardium in one (or preferably two) planes. To do this:

1. In the apical 4-chamber view obtain the best view you can of the LV, paying particular attention to clear endocardial border definition and avoidance of foreshortening.
2. Freeze a loop and find the end-diastolic image. Now trace the endocardial border from the mitral valve annulus all the way down to the apex and then back up to the annulus on the opposite side. Ignore any papillary muscle that may be visible. The machine will normally join up the start and finish points with a straight line across the mitral valve, to enclose the entire LV cavity within the traced area. The machine will then automatically split the traced area into a stack of discs (usually 20).
3. Measure the length of the LV long axis from the apex to the mid-point of the mitral valve. The machine will now use these measurements to calculate LV end-diastolic volume (LVEDV, Fig. 11.4).
4. Scroll to the end-systolic frame and repeat steps 2 and 3 to obtain the LV end-systolic volume (LVESV).
5. Although a measurement taken in just one plane will give you a value for LVEDV and LVESV, this does make the assumption that each of the discs is circular. Repeating the measurements in the apical 2-chamber view takes better account of the elliptical cross-section of the LV and any regional wall motion abnormalities.

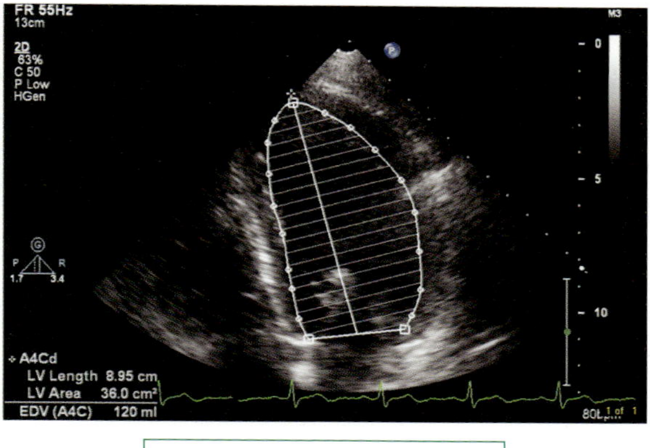

View	Apical 4-chamber
Modality	2-D

Fig. 11.4 Measurement of left ventricular (LV) volume using the modified Simpson's rule method (EDV = end-diastolic volume)

Area–length method

The area–length method can be useful for estimating LV volumes when the endocardium cannot be seen clearly enough to allow accurate tracing. However, it does make major assumptions (and simplifications) about the shape of the LV:

1. In the parasternal short axis view, mid-LV (papillary muscle) level, freeze a loop and find the end-diastolic frame. Perform planimetry by tracing the endocardial border to calculate the cross-sectional area of the LV cavity at this level in cm^2. Ignore the presence of the papillary muscles as you trace the endocardium.
2. In the apical 4-chamber view, in the end-diastolic frame, measure the length of the LV long axis from the apex to the mid-point of the mitral valve in cm.
3. The LVEDV, in mL, is given by:

$$\text{LVEDV} = \frac{5 \times \text{area} \times \text{length}}{6}$$

4. Scroll to the end-systolic frame and repeat steps 1 to 3 to obtain the LVESV.

Both LVEDV and LVESD can be adjusted for BSA ('LV volume index'). Table 11.2 shows the reference ranges for males and females.

Table 11.2 Left ventricle volumes – reference ranges

	Normal	Mild	Moderate	Severe
Men				
LVEDV (mL)	67–155	156–178	179–201	⩾202
LVESV (mL)	22–58	59–70	71–82	⩾83
LVEDV/BSA (mL/m^2)	35–75	76–86	87–96	⩾97
LVESV/BSA (mL/m^2)	12–30	31–36	37–42	⩾43
Women				
LVEDV (mL)	56–104	105–117	118–130	⩾131
LVESV (mL)	19–49	50–59	60–69	⩾70
LVEDV/BSA (mL/m^2)	35–75	76–86	87–96	⩾97
LVESV/BSA (mL/m^2)	12–30	31–36	37–42	⩾43

BSA = body surface area; LVEDV = left ventricular end-diastolic volume; LVESV = left ventricular end-systolic volume.
Reference ranges reproduced with permission of the British Society of Echocardiography and British Heart Foundation.

LV VOLUMES AND 3-D ECHO

3-D echo gets around many of the problems inherent in assessing LV volumes using 2-D echo. Because 3-D echo can visualize the whole LV, volume calculations do not require any assumptions to be made about LV geometry. The assessment of LV volumes (and mass) using 3-D echo has been well validated and shown to be more accurate (and reproducible) than 2-D techniques (Chapter 9).

Left ventricular mass

A normal LV mass is 96–200 g (men) and 66–150 g (women). LV mass increases with LV hypertrophy (LVH, Fig. 11.5), which can be a result of a primary cardiomyopathy (e.g. hypertrophic or infiltrative cardiomyopathy) or secondary to increased LV afterload (e.g. hypertension, aortic stenosis). The echo assessment of LVH includes:

- description of the overall appearance of the LV (concentric versus asymmetrical hypertrophy)
- measurement of LV dimensions
- calculation of LV mass
- assessment of LV function (systolic and diastolic)
- a search for underlying causes, such as aortic stenosis or aortic coarctation.

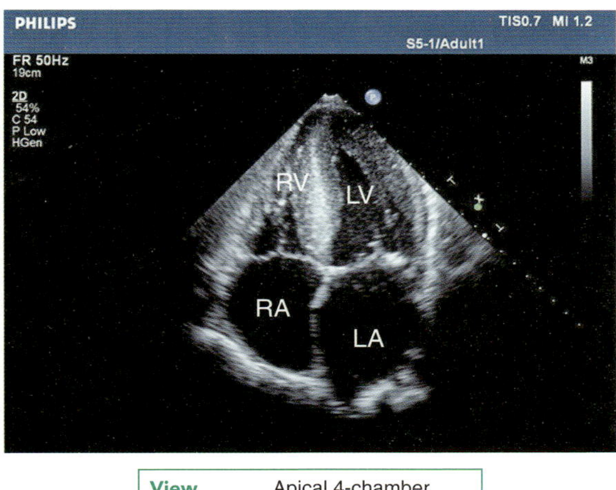

View	Apical 4-chamber
Modality	2-D

Fig. 11.5 Severe left ventricular hypertrophy (with dilated atria) (LA = left atrium; LV = left ventricle; RA = right atrium; RV = right ventricle) (Figure reproduced with permission of Philips)

LV mass using linear measurements

As described earlier under 'Linear LV measurements', use M-mode (or 2-D) echo to obtain the following measurements (in cm) at end-diastole:

- IVSd
- LVIDd
- LVPWd.

LV mass, in grams, can then be calculated using the following formula:

$$\text{LV mass} = \{0.8 \times [1.04 \times ((\text{LVIDd} + \text{LVPWd} + \text{IVSd})^3 - (\text{LVIDd})^3)]\} + 0.6$$

LV mass using volumetric measurements

Volumetric calculations of LV mass are based on measuring the LV cavity volume, as outlined above, and subtracting this from the total volume of the LV (enclosed within the epicardium). This subtraction leaves the 'shell' volume, i.e. the volume occupied by the ventricular myocardium. The LV mass then equals this 'shell' volume multiplied by the myocardial density (1.05 g/mL). There are several ways of going about this.

The **area–length formula** is based on the method used to calculate LVEDV, outlined earlier under 'Volumetric LV measurements':

1. In the parasternal short axis view, mid-LV (papillary muscle) level, freeze a loop and find the end-diastolic frame. Perform planimetry by tracing the endocardial border to calculate the endocardial cross-sectional area (A_2) of the LV at this level in cm^2. Ignore the presence of the papillary muscles as you trace the endocardium.
2. In the same view, perform planimetry by tracing the *epicardial* border to calculate the epicardial cross-sectional area (A_1) of the LV in cm^2.
3. Calculate the mean wall thickness (t) in cm using the formula:

$$t = \sqrt{\frac{A_1}{\pi}} - \sqrt{\frac{A_2}{\pi}}$$

4. In the apical 4-chamber view, in the end-diastolic frame, measure the length (L) of the LV long axis from the apex to the mid-point of the mitral valve in cm.
5. LV mass, in grams, is given by the following formula:

$$\text{LV mass} = 1.05 \times \{[(5/6) \times A_1 \times (L + t)] - [(5/6) \times A_2 \times L]\}$$

The **truncated ellipsoid formula** is based on similar measurements but is more complex. Here the length of the LV long axis (L), as measured from the apical 4-chamber view, is split in two by the short axis plane in which the planimetry of the LV cross-sectional areas was performed. The distance from the apex to the short axis plane is denoted by 'a', and from this plane to the mitral annulus plane by 'd', both measured in cm. There is also a further variable, 'b', which is the short axis radius given by:

$$b = \sqrt{\frac{A_2}{\pi}}$$

LV mass, in grams, is given by the following formula:

$$\text{LV mass} = 1.05 \times \pi \left\{ (b+t)^2 \left[\left\{ \frac{2}{3}(a+t) + d - \frac{d^3}{3(a+t)^2} \right\} - b^2 \left\{ \frac{2}{3}a + d - \frac{d^3}{3a^2} \right\} \right] \right\}$$

You can also use a technique based on the **modified Simpson's rule method**; however, this method is very dependent on being able to obtain clear definition of both endocardial and epicardial borders. To calculate LV mass:

1. Using the apical 4- and 2-chamber views calculate LVEDV (i.e. the cavity volume) as described earlier.
2. Now repeat the process, but this time use planimetry to trace the epicardial border of the LV, to obtain the total LV volume.
3. The myocardial volume is the total LV volume minus the LVEDV. Multiply this by the myocardial density (1.05 g/mL) to calculate LV mass.
4. LV mass can be adjusted for BSA ('LV mass index').

Table 11.3 shows the reference ranges for males and females.

Table 11.3 Left ventricle mass – reference ranges

	Normal	Mild	Moderate	Severe
Men				
LV mass (g)	96–200	201–227	228–254	>254
LV mass/BSA (g/m^2)	50–102	103–116	117–130	>130
Women				
LV mass (g)	66–150	151–171	172–182	>182
LV mass/BSA (g/m^2)	44–88	89–100	101–112	>112

BSA = body surface area; LV = left ventricle.
Reference ranges reproduced with permission of the British Society of Echocardiography and British Heart Foundation.

COMMON PITFALLS

Pitfalls in the assessment of LV mass include:

Linear measurements:

- Small measurement errors can become greatly magnified because of the cubing of LV dimensions in the linear LV mass formula
- Linear measurements should not be used in cases with distorted LV geometry (e.g. isolated areas of hypertrophy)

Volumetric measurements

- Failure to trace the endocardium or epicardium accurately.

Left ventricular systolic function

The assessment of left ventricular systolic function forms a cornerstone of any echo study and is an essential part of the management of patients with suspected systolic heart failure, which is a common condition with considerable morbidity and mortality.

Heart failure

Heart failure affects 1–2 per cent of the population and is particularly common in the elderly, affecting over 10 per cent of those aged over 85 years. Heart failure is regarded as a clinical syndrome in which patients have the symptoms and signs of heart failure (Table 11.4) together with objective evidence of a structural or functional cardiac abnormality at rest. Heart failure can be classified as:

- systolic and/or diastolic
- acute or chronic
- left- and/or right-sided
- high output (e.g. thyrotoxicosis) or low output.

There are many causes of systolic heart failure, including:

- coronary artery disease
- hypertension
- valvular disease
- viral myocarditis
- cardiomyopathy (Chapter 18)
- cardiotoxic drugs e.g. anthracyclines
- alcohol.

Table 11.4 Clinical features of heart failure

Symptoms	Signs
May be asymptomatic Breathlessness Fatigue Ankle swelling	Tachycardia, gallop rhythm Tachypnoea Elevated jugular venous pressure Cardiomegaly Pulmonary congestion/oedema Peripheral oedema Ascites Hepatomegaly

Echo assessment of LV systolic function

As the assessment of LV function is based on many of the linear and/or volumetric measurements already discussed in this chapter, the same pitfalls apply. The calculations assume that the LV has a regular geometrical shape and that the function of each segment of the LV is the same. It is therefore important to be aware of the limitations of each of the following methods and to use them judiciously. Indeed, some centres do not quantify LV function at all and have a policy of simply providing an 'eyeball' assessment of overall function, grading LV function as 'normal' or 'mildly/moderately/severely impaired' rather than putting a figure on it. Nonetheless, quantitative assessment can be useful and remains widely used. The key point is to use common sense – if there is a clear discrepancy between how LV function appears to you and the figures coming out of your calculations, highlight this in your report.

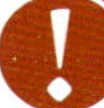

COMMON PITFALLS

Pitfalls in the assessment of LV systolic function include:

- Failure to take accurate measurements of chamber dimensions
- Using measures that do not take full account of abnormal LV morphology or regional wall motion abnormalities
- For Doppler-related measures, such as stroke volume, failure to align the ultrasound beam with the direction of blood flow
- Attempting to measure dP/dt when there is insufficient mitral regurgitation to obtain a clear continuous wave (CW) trace

Fractional shortening

Fractional shortening (FS) is a measure of the percentage change in LV dimensions between diastole and systole. A normal FS lies in the range 25–43 per cent. FS is calculated from the LVIDd and LVIDs:

$$FS = \frac{LVIDd - LVIDs}{LVIDd} \times 100\%$$

Ejection fraction

Ejection fraction (EF) is the most widely quoted measure of LV systolic performance, and expresses (as a percentage) the proportion of blood pumped out of the LV with each heartbeat. A normal EF is ⩾55 per cent. EF is calculated from the LVEDV and LVESV:

$$EF = \frac{LVEDV - LVESV}{LVEDV} \times 100\%$$

It is also possible to calculate EF using linear rather than volumetric measurements (i.e. based upon M-mode measurements alone), using the formula:

$$EF = \frac{LVIDd^3 - LVIDs^3}{LVIDd^3} \times 100\%$$

However, this method takes no account of variations in regional wall motion and is highly prone to inaccuracies. EF is often automatically calculated by an echo machine as soon as the linear measurements of LVIDd and LVIDs have been entered by the sonographer (Fig. 11.3), but rather than accepting this value you should, where possible, go on to assess EF using volumetric measurements.

EF AND TRASTUZUMAB (HERCEPTIN)

Accurate measurement of EF is always desirable, but there are situations in which it can be crucial. One of these is in the monitoring of patients with breast cancer receiving trastuzumab (Herceptin), a drug that can affect LV function. It is recommended by the National Institute for Health and Clinical Excellence that cardiac function should be assessed prior to starting treatment, and that treatment should not be offered to those with an EF ⩽ 55 per cent. Patients on treatment should have a cardiac functional assessment every 3 months and if the EF drops by 10 percentage (ejection) points or more from baseline and to below 50 per cent then treatment should be suspended. The British Society of Echocardiography stresses the importance of measuring EF accurately in these patients, using the modified Simpson's rule method (or 3-D echo) and with the availability of LV contrast as appropriate, and that echo departments should have recent audit data to demonstrate that they can reproducibly measure EF to the requirements of these guidelines.

Table 11.5 shows the reference ranges for LV fractional shortening and ejection fraction. There are several other techniques for the quantification of LV systolic function and these are discussed below.

Table 11.5 Left ventricular (LV) systolic function – reference ranges

	Normal	Mild	Moderate	Severe
LV fractional shortening (%)	25–43	20–24	15–19	<15
LV ejection fraction (%)	$\geqslant 55$	45–54	36–44	$\leqslant 35$

Reference ranges reproduced with permission of the British Society of Echocardiography and British Heart Foundation.

Stroke distance

Stroke distance (SD) is the average distance travelled by the blood during each heartbeat. In the apical 5-chamber view, use pulsed-wave (PW) Doppler to measure the velocity time integral (VTI) of outflow in the LVOT to give VTI_{LVOT} (in cm). Place the sample volume at the level of the aortic valve annulus, just proximal to the cusps. SD equals the VTI_{LVOT}. A normal SD is in the range 18–22 cm.

Stroke volume

Stroke volume is the quantity of blood ejected into the aorta by the LV with each heartbeat. It can be measured as follows:

1. In the parasternal long axis view, measure the diameter of the LVOT in cm at the level of the aortic valve annulus, just proximal to the cusps (Fig. 11.6), and use this to calculate the cross-sectional area (CSA) of the LVOT in cm^2:

$$CSA_{LVOT} = 0.785 \times (\text{LVOT diameter})^2$$

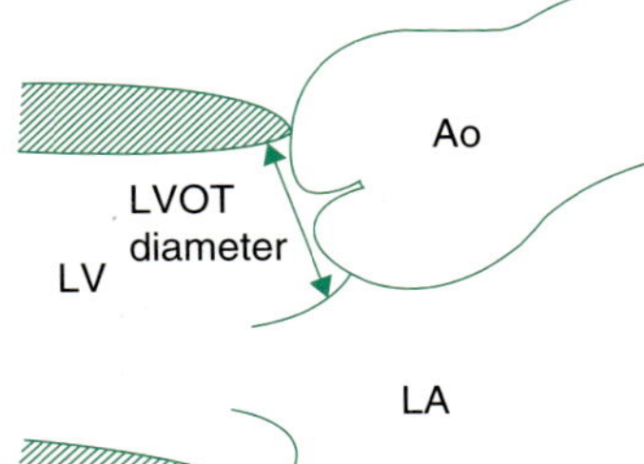

Fig. 11.6 Measurement of LVOT diameter (Ao = aorta; LA = left atrium; LV = left ventricle; LVOT = left ventricular outflow tract)

2. In the apical 5-chamber view, use PW Doppler to measure the VTI of outflow in the LVOT. Place the sample volume at the level of the aortic valve annulus, at the same point where the LVOT diameter was measured (Fig. 11.7) and obtain a PW trace of flow in the LVOT to measure VTI_{LVOT} (in cm) (Fig. 11.8).

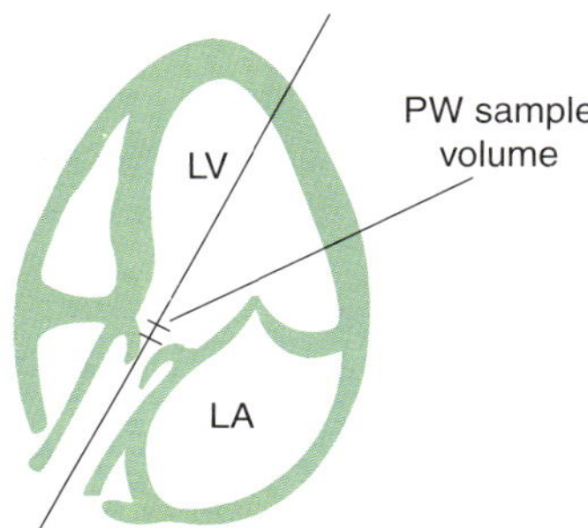

Fig. 11.7 Positioning of sample volume for pulsed-wave (PW) Doppler of left ventricular outflow tract velocity time integral (VTI) (LA = left atrium; LV = left ventricle)

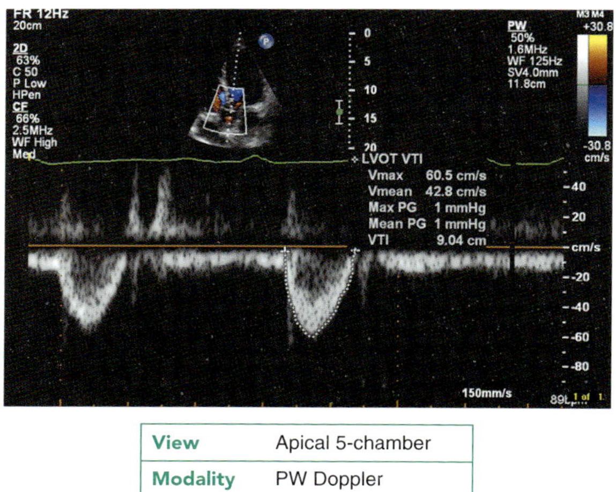

View	Apical 5-chamber
Modality	PW Doppler

Fig. 11.8 Pulsed-wave (PW) Doppler of left ventricular outflow tract (LVOT) (PG = pressure gradient; V_{max} = peak velocity; V_{mean} = mean velocity; VTI = velocity time integral)

3. The LV stroke volume (SV), in mL/beat, can then be calculated from:

$$SV = CSA_{LVOT} \times VTI_{LVOT}$$

A normal SV lies in the range 60–100 mL/beat. The calculation of SV depends on a good alignment of the Doppler interrogation angle with the direction of flow, and upon the assumption that flow in the LVOT is laminar and the LVOT cross-section is circular. It is essential to measure the LVOT diameter as accurately as possible. SV can, in principle, be measured anywhere in the heart where a cross-sectional area and VTI can be measured, but in practical terms measurement at the LVOT is relatively straightforward.

Stroke volume index

Stroke volume index (SVI) is SV adjusted for BSA, measured in mL/beat/m^2:

$$SVI = \frac{SV}{BSA}$$

Cardiac output

Cardiac output (CO) can be calculated from the SV and the heart rate (HR, in beats/min). A normal cardiac output is 4–8 L/min:

$$CO = \frac{SV \times HR}{1000}$$

Cardiac index

Cardiac index (CI) is CO adjusted for BSA, measured in L/min/m^2:

$$CI = \frac{CO}{BSA}$$

Rate of ventricular pressure rise (dP/dt)

With normal LV systolic function, the rate of rise in ventricular pressure (dP/dt) during systole is rapid. If systolic function is impaired, dP/dt starts to fall. The measurement of dP/dt requires the presence of mitral regurgitation:

1. In the apical 4-chamber view, use CW Doppler to obtain a spectral trace of mitral regurgitation, ensuring careful alignment of the ultra-sound beam with the regurgitant jet. Set the sweep speed as high as possible to 'spread out' the trace and make it easier to mark the relevant timepoints.
2. Using the trace, mark the points where the regurgitant jet velocity reaches 1 m/s and also 3 m/s. Measure the time interval (dt) between these two points in seconds (Fig. 11.9).
3. At 1 m/s the pressure gradient driving the regurgitant jet is 4 mmHg (Bernoulli equation), and at 3 m/s the gradient is 36 mmHg, giving a change in pressure gradients (dP) between the two velocities of 32 mmHg.

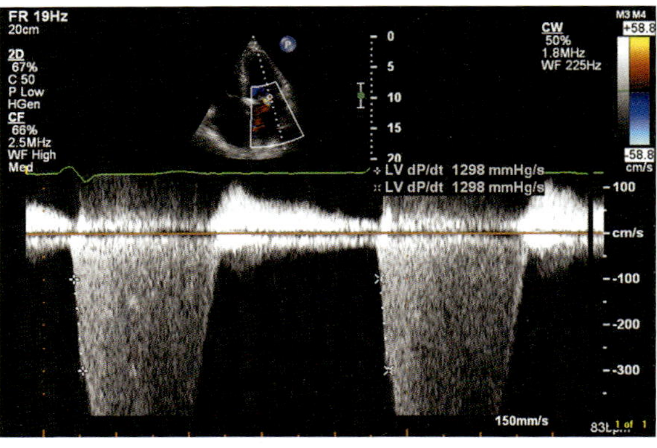

View	Apical 4-chamber
Modality	CW Doppler

Fig. 11.9 Measurement of the rate of rise in ventricular pressure (dP/dt) (CW = continuous wave; LV = left ventricle)

4. dP/dt is therefore calculated, in mmHg/s, by dividing the measured time interval (dt) into 32. The longer the duration of dt, and the smaller the value for dP/dt, the worse the LV systolic function. A normal LV will have a dP/dt > 1200 mmHg/s (and a dt < 0.027 s), whereas a severely impaired LV usually has a dP/dt < 800 mmHg/s (and a dt > 0.04 s).

dP/dt should not be used if there is *acute* mitral regurgitation, or if there is significant aortic stenosis or hypertension.

SAMPLE REPORT

LV wall thickness is normal. The LV is moderately dilated (LVIDd 6.6 cm, LVEDV 190 mL). LV systolic function is moderately impaired and the impairment is global with no specific regional wall motion abnormalities. Fractional shortening 17 per cent, ejection fraction 38 per cent using modified Simpson's rule method. The stroke volume is 40 mL/beat with a cardiac output of 3 L/min. The mitral valve leaflets are structurally normal but the annulus is dilated and there is moderate functional mitral regurgitation, with a dP/dt of 986 mmHg/s. The findings indicate moderately impaired LV systolic function.

Management of impaired LV systolic function

Patients with LV systolic dysfunction are treated with diuretics to relieve symptoms and any contributing factors (e.g. hypertension, valvular disease, myocardial ischaemia) should be treated as appropriate. Both morbidity and mortality are improved by the use of angiotensin-converting enzyme (ACE) inhibitors (or angiotensin receptor blockers) and beta-blockers (e.g. bisoprolol, carvedilol). In some patients there is also a role for aldosterone antagonists (e.g. spironolactone) and digoxin.

Patients with moderate to severe heart failure despite optimal medical treatment, a LVEF ≤ 35 per cent and broad QRS complexes on the ECG (QRS duration ≥ 120 ms) may gain a reduction in symptoms and in mortality with the implantation of a biventricular pacemaker (cardiac resynchronization therapy, CRT – see box). Those at high risk of ventricular arrhythmias may benefit from an implantable cardioverter defibrillator (ICD).

CARDIAC RESYNCHRONIZATION THERAPY

Echo can help in patient selection for CRT by demonstrating impaired synchrony in contraction both between LV and RV (interventricular dyssynchrony) and between different walls within the LV (intraventricular dyssynchrony). Many different measures are available, often using advanced techniques such as tissue Doppler imaging (TDI) and 3-D echo.

Interventricular dyssynchrony can be assessed by measuring the time from the start of the QRS complex on the ECG to the start of aortic and pulmonary flow (as measured using PW Doppler in the apical 5-chamber and parasternal short axis views, respectively). If the difference between the onset of aortic and pulmonary flow is ≥40 ms, significant dyssynchrony is present.

Intraventricular dyssynchrony can be assessed by measuring the time from the start of the QRS complex on the ECG to the peak of LV septal and posterior wall contraction (as measured using M-mode in the parasternal long axis view). If the difference in peak contraction between the two walls is ≥130 ms, significant dyssynchrony is present.

Left ventricular diastolic function

The diagnosis and management of diastolic heart failure has always been somewhat controversial because it is harder to characterize, and the treatment strategies are less well studied than for systolic heart failure. Clinically, a diagnosis of diastolic heart failure is usually considered when a patient has symptoms and/or signs of heart failure (as for systolic heart failure) but their LV systolic function is normal or near-normal (EF > 50 per cent).

Diastolic heart failure is also known as 'heart failure with preserved ejection fraction' (HFPEF), distinguishing it from systolic heart failure ('heart failure with reduced ejection fraction', HFREF). There is however evidence that diastolic dysfunction is also present in patients with systolic dysfunction, so some authorities regard the distinction between systolic and diastolic failure as false and argue that systolic and diastolic dysfunction are part of a single spectrum, and that diastolic dysfunction is often a precursor to systolic dysfunction. It certainly seems that there is significant overlap between systolic and diastolic dysfunction and they should not be regarded as mutually exclusive entities.

HEART FAILURE WITH PRESERVED EF

Many authorities argue that LV diastolic dysfunction can be present regardless of whether systolic function is normal or not. However, if you wish to specifically diagnose heart failure with preserved EF, you need to confirm that systolic function is indeed virtually normal. The European Society of Cardiology criteria for 'normal or mildly abnormal LV function' are:

- LV ejection fraction > 50 per cent
- LV end-diastolic volume index < 97 mL/m^2
- LV end-systolic volume index < 49 mL/m^2.

Causes of impaired LV diastolic function

Diastolic dysfunction is thought to reflect 'stiffness' or impaired relaxation of the LV, and so occurs in conditions where the LV becomes less compliant:

- ageing
- hypertension
- LVH
- myocardial ischaemia
- aortic stenosis
- infiltrative cardiomyopathies.

Impairment of LV relaxation increases LV end-diastolic pressure and this consequently impacts on the pulmonary circulation, leading to pulmonary congestion and breathlessness.

Echo assessment of LV diastolic function

Any assessment of LV diastolic function should also include a full assessment of LV dimensions, mass and systolic function as outlined earlier in this chapter. Remember to look for features indicative of the underlying aetiology of diastolic dysfunction (e.g. aortic stenosis, ischaemic heart disease). LA size should also be assessed, as outlined on page 137. LA dilatation indicates elevated LA pressure.

Many methods are available to characterize LV diastolic function on echo, but the most widely used are:

- LV inflow
- pulmonary venous flow
- TDI of the mitral annulus.

LV inflow

To assess LV inflow, perform PW Doppler in the apical 4-chamber view with the sample volume placed at the tips of the mitral valve leaflets (Fig. 11.10). Obtain a PW Doppler trace (Fig. 11.11) and measure:

- Peak E wave velocity
- Peak A wave velocity
- E:A ratio
- E wave deceleration time (DT)
- isovolumic relaxation time (IVRT).

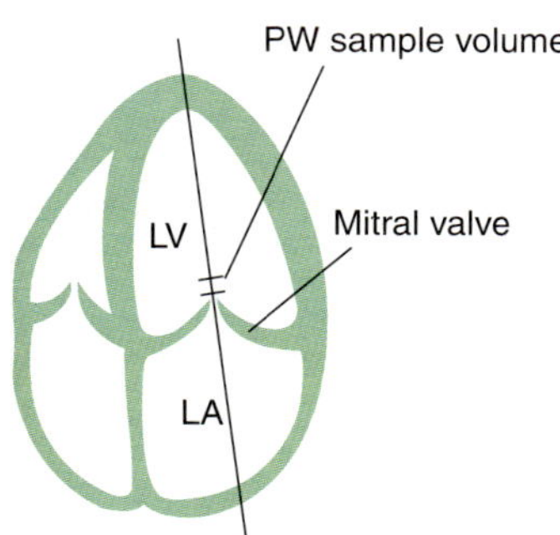

Fig. 11.10 Positioning of sample volume for pulsed-wave (PW) Doppler of mitral valve inflow (LA = left atrium; LV = left ventricle)

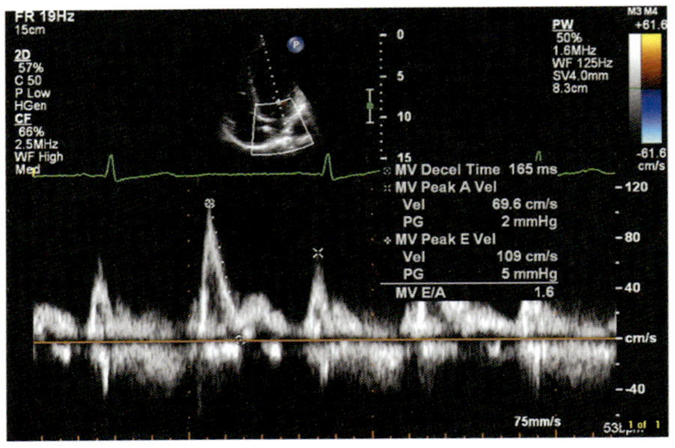

View	Apical 4-chamber
Modality	PW Doppler

Fig. 11.11 Pulsed-wave (PW) Doppler of mitral valve (MV) inflow (PG = pressure gradient; Vel = velocity)

E:A ratio is simply the ratio between peak E and A wave velocities:

$$\text{E:A ratio} = \frac{\text{Peak E wave velocity}}{\text{Peak A wave velocity}}$$

The E wave is normally taller than the A wave, and the E:A ratio normally lies in the range 1–2.

E wave deceleration time is the time period between the peak of the E wave and the end of the E wave (measured by extrapolating the E wave deceleration slope down to the baseline), and is normally 150–200 ms.

IVRT is the time period between aortic valve closure and mitral valve opening, during which LV pressure falls but there is no change in LV volume. There are various methods of measuring IVRT. The simplest is to tilt the probe, obtain a 5-chamber view and adjust the PW Doppler sample volume to lie between the mitral and aortic valves (so that both the mitral inflow and aortic outflow traces are seen on the same PW Doppler trace). Freeze the trace and measure the time period between the end of the aortic outflow trace and the start of the mitral inflow trace – this is the IVRT, and is normally 50–100 ms.

Pulmonary venous flow

To assess pulmonary venous flow, perform PW Doppler in the apical 4-chamber view with the sample volume placed inside one of the pulmonary veins (the right upper pulmonary vein is usually easiest to locate, Fig. 11.12).

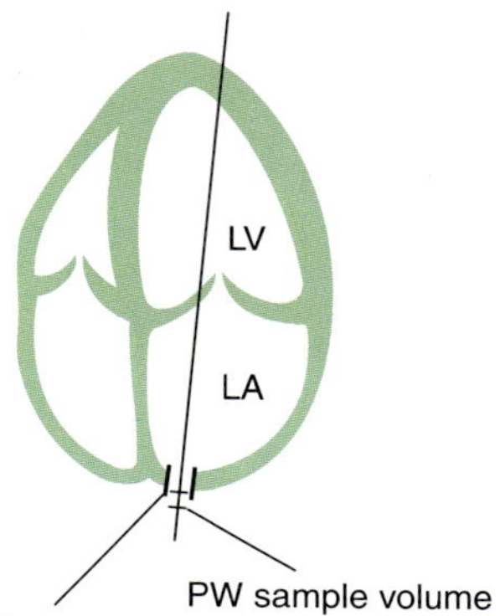

Fig. 11.12 Positioning of sample volume for pulsed-wave Doppler of pulmonary venous flow (LA = left atrium; LV = left ventricle)

Pulmonary vein flow normally consists of three components: the S wave represents forward flow into the left atrium during ventricular systole, and the smaller D wave represents forward flow during ventricular diastole. If the patient is in sinus rhythm, the S and D waves are followed by an 'a' wave, representing flow reversal in the pulmonary vein during atrial systole.

Obtain a PW Doppler trace (Fig. 11.13) and measure:

- peak systolic ('S' wave) velocity (PV_S)
- peak diastolic ('D' wave) velocity (PV_D)
- peak atrial reversal ('a' wave) velocity (PV_a)
- duration of atrial reversal (a_{dur}).

Normally $PV_S > PV_D$ and $PV_a < 0.35$ m/s. The duration of atrial reversal (a_{dur}) measured in the pulmonary vein is normally < 20 ms longer than the duration of the A wave (A_{dur}) measured on LV inflow.

TDI of the mitral annulus

TDI of the mitral annulus is undertaken in the apical 4-chamber view, placing the sample volume (which should be small, usually 2–3 mm) in the myocardium of the septum and then the lateral wall. The optimal location is

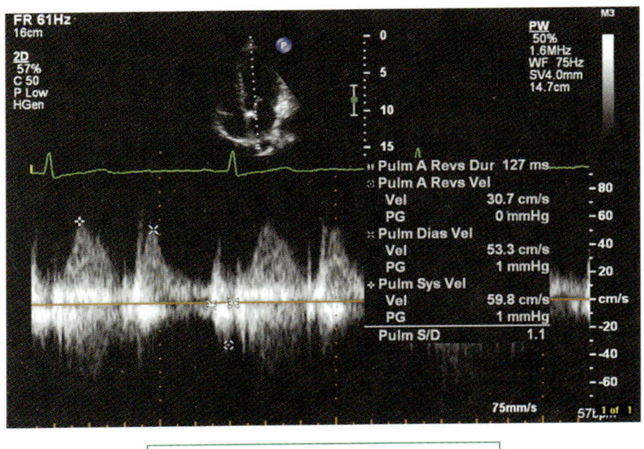

View	Apical 4-chamber
Modality	PW Doppler

Fig. 11.13 Pulsed-wave (PW) Doppler of pulmonary venous flow (Dur = duration; PG = pressure gradient; Revs = reversal; S/D = S (systolic) wave/D (diastolic) wave; Vel = velocity)

1 cm below the mitral annulus (Fig. 11.14). In each location a tissue Doppler recording should be made (Fig. 11.15) using a low gain setting and an aliasing velocity 15–20 cm/s.

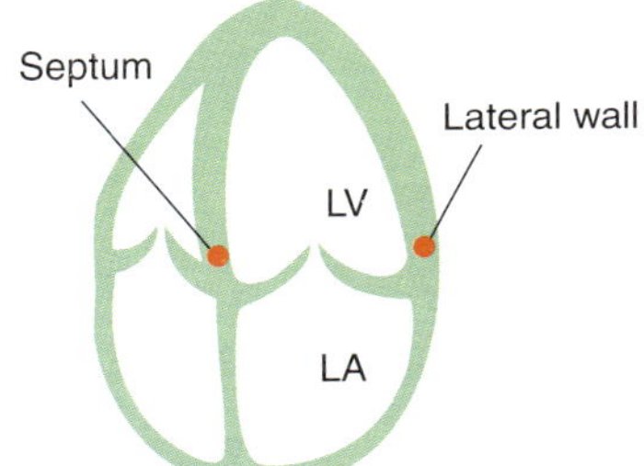

Fig. 11.14 Positioning of sample volume for tissue Doppler imaging (TDI) of the mitral annulus (LA = left atrium; LV = left ventricle)

The mitral annular tissue Doppler recording shows an *early myocardial velocity* (E_m or E') which corresponds to early diastolic relaxation, the myocardium moving away from the transducer. This is followed by a further movement away from the transducer, corresponding to *atrial contraction* (A_m or A'). Normally $E_m > A_m$ with a ratio between the two velocities in the range 1–2. If there is diastolic dysfunction, the E_m:A_m ratio reverses. The ratio between the peak LV inflow E wave velocity and E_m should also be

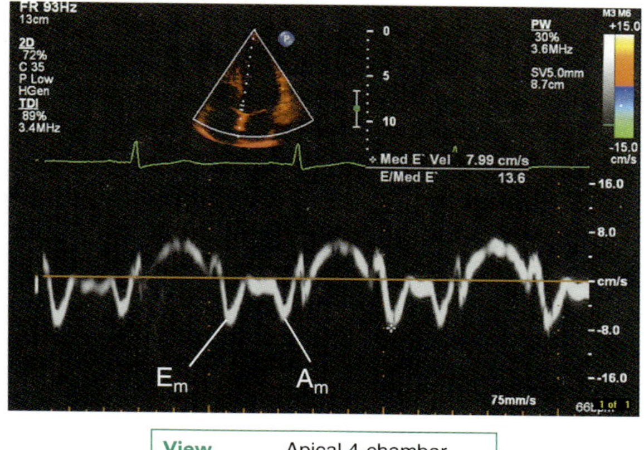

View	Apical 4-chamber
Modality	PW Tissue Doppler

Fig. 11.15 Pulsed-wave (PW) trace of mitral annulus (septal wall) obtained with tissue Doppler imaging (TDI) (Med E′ Vel = medial early myocardial velocity)

calculated; this ratio reflects LA pressure. Normal E/E_m ratios are <8 at the septum and <10 at the lateral wall.

Interpretation of results

The assessment of LV diastolic function should combine each of the measures discussed above (Fig. 11.16). Using these measures, LV diastolic function can be classified as:

- normal
- mildly impaired (abnormal relaxation)
- moderately impaired (pseudonormal)
- severely impaired (restrictive filling).

Mild impairment of diastolic function causes a reversal of the usual E:A ratio and a lengthening of IVRT and E wave DT. As diastolic function worsens further, the E:A ratio returns to normal ('pseudonormalization'). For this reason, E:A ratio should not be used as the only measure of diastolic function.

Although the E:A ratio pseudonormalizes with moderate dysfunction, pulmonary venous Doppler shows a reversal of the normal ratio between PV_S and PV_D, such that $PV_S < PV_D$. There is also an increase in PV_a (≥0.35 m/s) and also in $a_{dur}–A_{dur}$, which becomes ≥20 ms (normally it is <20 ms).

Mitral annular tissue Doppler shows a reversal of the normal E_m:A_m ratio with mild diastolic dysfunction, the degree of reversal increasing in magnitude as the diastolic dysfunction becomes increasingly severe.

SAMPLE REPORT

The LA is moderately dilated (volume 70 mL). There is moderate concentric LV hypertrophy. LV systolic function is normal (LVEF 64 per cent, LVEDV index 82 mL/m^2). There is significant reversal of the LV inflow E:A ratio (2.2) with shortening of IVRT (42 ms) and DT (138 ms). Pulmonary vein Doppler shows marked reversal of the PV_S:PV_D ratio, with a PV_a of 0.41 m/s and a_{dur}–A_{dur} of 25 ms. Mitral annular tissue Doppler shows marked reversal of the E_m:A_m ratio and a septal E:E_m ratio of 18. These findings indicate severely impaired LV diastolic function.

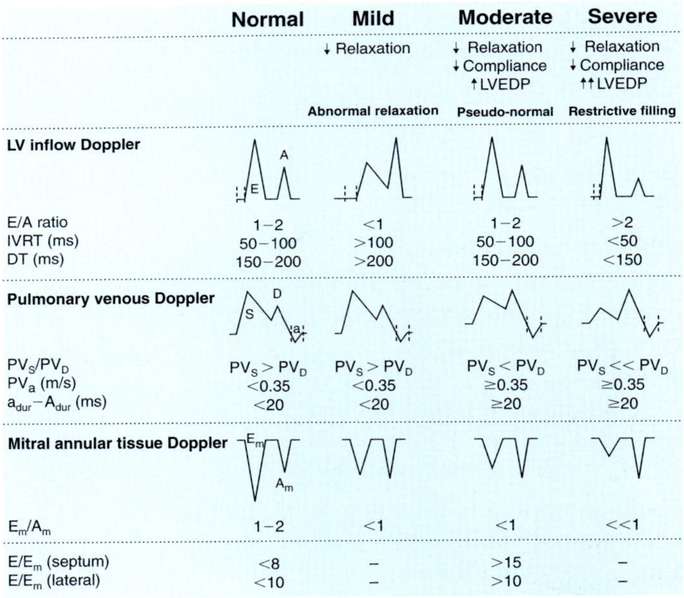

	Normal	Mild	Moderate	Severe
		↓ Relaxation	↓ Relaxation ↓ Compliance ↑ LVEDP	↓ Relaxation ↓ Compliance ↑↑ LVEDP
		Abnormal relaxation	**Pseudo-normal**	**Restrictive filling**
LV inflow Doppler	E A			
E/A ratio	1–2	<1	1–2	>2
IVRT (ms)	50–100	>100	50–100	<50
DT (ms)	150–200	>200	150–200	<150
Pulmonary venous Doppler	S D a			
PV_S/PV_D	$PV_S > PV_D$	$PV_S > PV_D$	$PV_S < PV_D$	$PV_S << PV_D$
PV_a (m/s)	<0.35	<0.35	≥0.35	≥0.35
$a_{dur}-A_{dur}$ (ms)	<20	<20	≥20	≥20
Mitral annular tissue Doppler	E_m A_m			
E_m/A_m	1–2	<1	<1	<<1
E/E_m (septum)	<8	–	>15	–
E/E_m (lateral)	<10	–	>10	–

Fig. 11.16 Classification of left ventricular (LV) diastolic dysfunction (A = peak A-wave velocity; A_m = atrial contraction; a_{dur} = duration of atrial reversal; DT = deceleration time; E = peak E-wave velocity; E_m = early myocardial velocity on tissue Doppler imaging of mitral annulus (also known as E'); IVRT = isovolumic relaxation time; LVEDP = left ventricular end-diastolic pressure; PV_a = peak atrial reversal ('a' wave) velocity; PV_D = peak diastolic ('D' wave) velocity; PV_S = peak systolic ('S' wave) velocity (Adapted with permission of the British Society of Echocardiography and British Heart Foundation)

Management of impaired LV diastolic function

Patients with LV diastolic dysfunction are treated with diuretics to relieve fluid congestion and any contributing factors (e.g. hypertension, myocardial ischaemia) should be treated as appropriate. The value of ACE inhibitors or angiotensin receptor blockers remains unclear.

Echo assessment of the left atrium

The left atrium (LA) can be seen in several views:

- left parasternal window
  - parasternal long axis view
  - parasternal short axis view (aortic valve level)
- apical window
  - apical 4-chamber view
  - apical 2-chamber view
  - apical 3-chamber (long axis) view
- subcostal window
  - subcostal long axis view.

An echo evaluation of the LA should include assessment of:

- LA morphology and dimensions
- presence of any LA masses (e.g. tumour, thrombus)
- presence of spontaneous echo contrast.

LA masses and spontaneous echo contrast are discussed in Chapter 21.

Left atrial dimensions

LA dilatation (Fig. 11.17) can result from:

- mitral valve disease
- dilated cardiomyopathy
- restrictive cardiomyopathy
- LV diastolic dysfunction
- atrial fibrillation.

LA diameter is measured at end-systole in the parasternal long axis view, using either 2-D or M-mode imaging (Fig. 11.18).

LA volume is measured using the modified Simpson's rule method:

1. In the apical 4-chamber view obtain the best view you can of the LA, paying particular attention to avoidance of foreshortening.

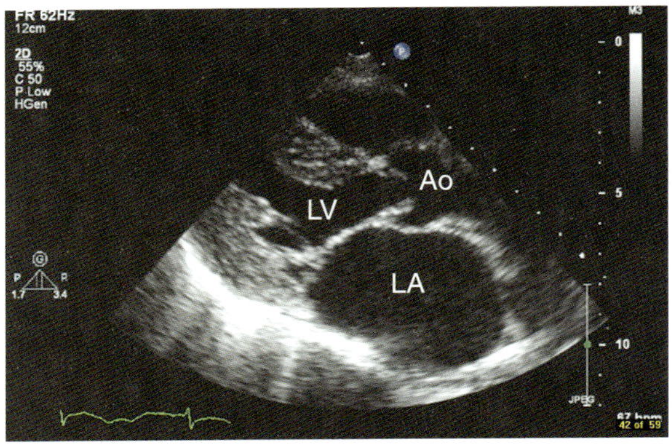

View	Parasternal long axis
Modality	2-D

Fig. 11.17 Dilated left atrium (LA) (with left ventricular (LV) hypertrophy) (Ao = aorta)

COR TRIATRIATUM

Cor triatriatum is a rare congenital abnormality in which the LA is partitioned into two chambers by a membrane, best seen in the apical 4-chamber view. The membrane contains one or more perforations allowing blood to flow between the two chambers, but nonetheless there is a degree of obstruction to LV inflow which can be assessed using PW Doppler. Cor triatriatum dexter is the name given to this condition when it occurs in the right atrium.

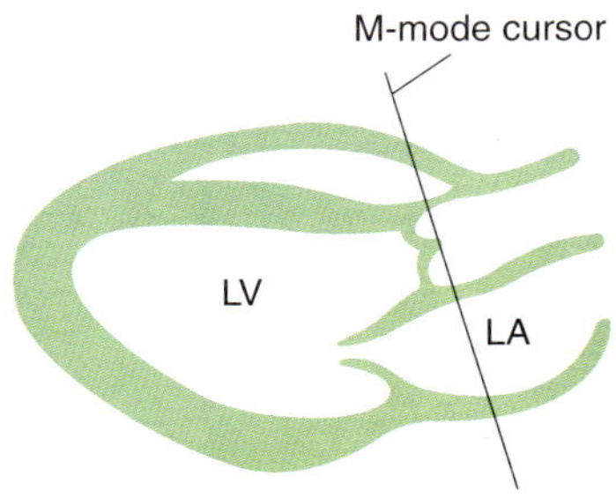

Fig. 11.18 Positioning of M-mode cursor for measurement of left atrial (LA) diameter (LV = left ventricle)

2. Freeze a loop and find the end-systolic image. Now trace the endocardial border around the LA to obtain an area measurement. Ignore any pulmonary veins that may be visible.
3. Measure the length of the LA long axis from the mid-point of the mitral annulus to the superior border (back wall) of the LA.
4. Repeat the measurements in the apical 2-chamber view.
5. If the echo machine does not calculate LA volume for you, it can be calculated from:

$$\text{LA volume} = \frac{0.85 \times \text{LA area (4-chamber)} \times \text{LA area (2-chamber)}}{\text{LA length}}$$

Reference values for LA dimensions are given in Table 11.6.

Table 11.6 Left atrial (LA) dimensions – reference ranges

	Normal	Mild	Moderate	Severe
Men				
LA diameter (cm)	3.0–4.0	4.1–4.6	4.7–5.2	⩾5.3
LA volume (mL)	18–58	59–68	69–78	⩾79
LA diameter/BSA (cm/m^2)	1.5–2.3	2.4–2.6	2.7–2.9	⩾3.0
LA volume/BSA (mL/m^2)	16–28	29–33	34–39	⩾40
Women				
LA diameter (cm)	2.7–3.8	3.9–4.2	4.3–4.6	⩾4.7
LA volume (mL)	22–52	53–62	63–72	⩾73
LA diameter/BSA (cm/m^2)	1.5–2.3	2.4–2.6	2.7–2.9	⩾3.0
LA volume/BSA (mL/m^2)	16–28	29–33	34–39	⩾40

BSA = body surface area.
Reference ranges reproduced with permission of the British Society of Echocardiography and British Heart Foundation.

FURTHER READING

Dickstein K, Cohen-Solal A, Filippatos G, *et al.* ESC Guidelines for the diagnosis and treatment of acute and chronic heart failure. *Eur Heart J* 2008; **29**: 2388–442.

Lang RM, Bierig M, Devereux RB, *et al.* Recommendations for chamber quantification: a report from the American Society of Echocardiography's Guidelines and Standards Committee and the Chamber Quantification Writing Group, developed in conjunction with the European Association of

Echocardiography, a branch of the European Society of Cardiology. *J Am Soc Echocardiogr* 2005; **18**: 1440–63.

Paulus WJ, Tschöpe C, Sanderson JE, *et al*. How to diagnose diastolic heart failure: a consensus statement on the diagnosis of heart failure with normal left ventricular ejection fraction by the Heart Failure and Echocardiography Associations of the European Society of Cardiology. *Eur Heart J* 2007; **28**: 2539–50.

Senior R, Ashrafian H. Screening for isolated diastolic dysfunction – a bridge too far? *Eur J Echocardiogr* 2005; **6**: 79–82.

Senior R, Bhatia VK. *British Society of Echocardiography Distance Learning Module 13: Evaluation of Systolic Function of the Left Ventricle*. Accessible from the BSE website (www.bsecho.org).

12 Coronary artery disease and regional left ventricular function

Chapter 11 looked at the global assessment of left ventricular (LV) dimensions and function. However, abnormalities of LV function can affect one or more specific areas of the LV wall and then the LV is said to show a regional wall motion abnormality (RWMA). RWMA is the result of coronary artery disease affecting the function of the myocardium, either because the blood supply to a particular area of myocardium has become reduced (ischaemia) or blocked altogether, causing death (necrosis) of the myocytes. The identification of RWMA by echo can therefore reveal a great deal about the status of the coronary circulation.

The coronary arteries

Normal coronary artery anatomy

As discussed in Chapter 2, the coronary circulation normally arises as two separate vessels from the sinuses of Valsalva – the left coronary artery (LCA) from the left sinus, and the right coronary artery (RCA) from the right sinus (Fig. 2.5, p. 12). The initial portion of the LCA is the left main stem which soon divides into the left anterior descending (LAD) and circumflex (Cx) arteries. The LAD runs down the anterior interventricular groove and the Cx runs in the left atrioventricular groove. The RCA runs in the right atrioventricular groove, and in most people gives rise to the posterior descending artery which runs down the posterior interventricular groove.

All the arteries supply branches to the myocardium in their respective territories, and as there is some anatomical variation from one person to the next, there can be a little variability in which vessel is responsible for supplying blood to each territory. Nonetheless, each vessel's territory is fairly well defined and so wall motion abnormalities in a particular region give an indication of the coronary vessel(s) likely to be involved.

Regional left ventricular function

The LV is conventionally split into 16 or 17 different regions or 'segments'. In the 16-segment model the LV is sliced longitudinally into thirds (basal, mid-cavity and apical). The basal and mid-cavity slices each contain six segments and the apical slice contains four segments. The American Heart Association's 17-segment model contains all these segments plus one more – an apical 'cap' (Fig. 12.1). The 16-segment model remains popular for echo purposes, but if you are going to compare echo findings with other modalities (e.g. nuclear cardiology) then it is better to use the more widely

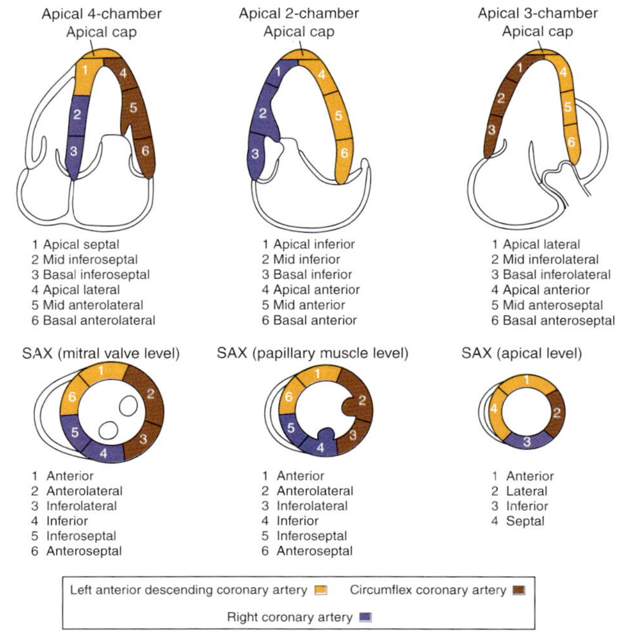

Fig. 12.1 The 17-segment model of LV segmentation (SAX = short axis)

applicable 17-segment model. Whichever model you choose, ensure that your nomenclature is consistent.

In the 17-segment model, the six segments in each of the basal and mid-cavity slices are termed anterior, anteroseptal, inferoseptal, inferior, inferolateral (sometimes also called posterior) and anterolateral. The boundaries of the septum are defined by the attachment of the right ventricle (RV), and each of the six circumferential segments occupies 60° in the short axis view. As the LV narrows towards the apex, there are just four apical segments, termed anterior, septal, inferior and lateral. The apical cap is at the very tip of the ventricle, where there is no LV cavity.

Each segment is assigned to one of the coronary arteries (LAD, Cx or RCA), as indicated by the colour-coding in Fig. 12.1, although there can be some overlap depending on each individual's coronary anatomy. Normal wall motion during systole is indicated by an endocardial excursion >5 mm and by wall thickening >50 per cent. Each segment should be inspected in turn, where possible in two separate views, and scored according to its motion:

- X = unable to interpret (suboptimal image quality)
- 1 = normokinetic
- 2 = hypokinetic
- 3 = akinetic
- 4 = dyskinetic
- 5 = aneurysmal.

Myocardial ischaemia and infarction

Myocardial ischaemia results from the development of an atherosclerotic plaque in one or more coronary arteries, limiting the flow of blood to the myocardium downstream. This normally does not cause symptoms until the lumen is obstructed by ⩾70 per cent, at which point the patient develops exertional chest discomfort and/or breathlessness. The chest discomfort is typically central in location and heavy or tight in character, and may radiate into the neck and jaw and down one or both arms. The symptoms are rapidly relieved with rest and/or nitrates.

An acute coronary syndrome occurs when an atherosclerotic plaque ruptures, exposing the lipid-rich core to the bloodstream. This leads to the rapid formation of a thrombus which acutely obstructs flow down the coronary artery. If this leads to necrosis of a portion of myocardium, cardiac markers (e.g. troponins, creatine kinase) will be released into the circulation, and the detection of these markers is one of the key diagnostic features of a myocardial infarction. Unstable symptoms without a rise in cardiac markers is termed unstable angina.

Echo assessment of myocardial ischaemia and infarction

Areas of myocardial ischaemia and infarction typically lead to hypokinetic, akinetic, dyskinetic or aneurysmal myocardial segments. By assessing wall motion in each of the LV segments a comprehensive picture of LV regional wall motion can be compiled and likely abnormalities in the supplying coronary arteries identified. The assessment of regional LV function should also include an assessment of LV dimensions, morphology and global LV systolic and diastolic function (see Chapter 11).

Myocardial ischaemia is frequently assessed by stress echo (see Chapter 8), in which any changes in wall motion are assessed in response to exercise or pharmacological stress. In the classical ischaemic response, the myocardium is normokinetic at rest but its wall motion worsens on stress.

Stress echo can also have an important role following **myocardial infarction**, identifying areas where the myocardium is still viable. Areas of myocardial necrosis are typically akinetic or hypokinetic at rest and remain unchanged with stress. However, sometimes improvement in wall motion is seen with stress, indicating that the myocardium is still viable but is stunned or hibernating. Stunned myocardium is likely to improve spontaneously with time, whereas hibernating myocardium will usually only improve with coronary revascularization.

Echo can help in the differential diagnosis of acute chest pain, which includes not just acute coronary syndromes but also conditions such as aortic dissection (p. 274) and pulmonary embolism. Echo is also important in the diagnosis of many of the complications of myocardial infarction, discussed later in this chapter.

Management of myocardial ischaemia and infarction

Myocardial ischaemia

Stable angina is managed with drugs to relieve symptoms and to reduce the risk of coronary thrombosis. Symptomatic relief can be obtained with glyceryl trinitrate used as required, and with one or more regular anti-ischaemic agents (beta-blockers, calcium channel blockers, nitrates, nicorandil or ivabradine). Cardioprotective drugs include aspirin, statins and angiotensin-converting enzyme (ACE) inhibitors.

Unstable angina is also managed with cardioprotective and anti-ischaemic drugs, but with the addition of antithrombotic agents such as heparin and glycoprotein IIb/IIIa antagonists.

Coronary revascularization has an important role in patients with troublesome symptoms or a high risk of coronary events. Revascularization can be achieved with percutaneous coronary intervention (PCI) or coronary artery bypass grafting (CABG).

Myocardial infarction

Myocardial infarctions are subgrouped and managed according to the accompanying ECG changes: the presence of ST segment elevation defines an ST elevation myocardial infarction (STEMI) in which urgent restoration of coronary blood flow, with primary PCI or thrombolysis, is required. Other ECG changes (ST segment depression, T wave inversion) are seen in a non-STEMI (NSTEMI), in which the mainstay of therapy is aggressive treatment with antiplatelet and antithrombotic drugs and reduction in myocardial oxygen demand, followed by coronary angiography and coronary revascularization (as guided by symptoms and risk stratification).

As for stable angina, patients who have had a myocardial infarction should receive appropriate cardioprotective drugs including aspirin, beta-blockers, statins and ACE inhibitors.

Complications of myocardial infarction

Left ventricular aneurysm

Aneurysmal dilatation of the LV can occur in areas where the infarcted myocardium has become weakened and thinned. Patients may have clinical features of impaired LV function and persistent ST segment elevation on the ECG.

Echo assessment

Identify the region of the LV affected with reference to the usual segmental nomenclature. Look for the characteristic dyskinetic wall motion within the aneurysmal segment. In contrast with pseudoaneurysms (see below), 'true' aneurysms have a wide 'neck', which is at least half the diameter of the aneurysm itself (Fig. 12.2), and are lined by myocardium rather than pericardium.

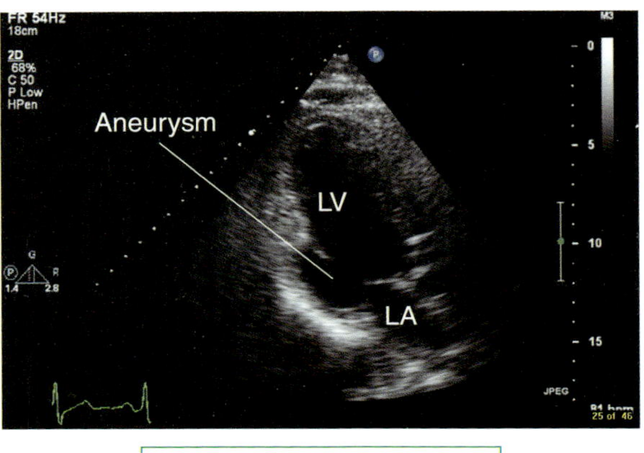

View	Apical 3-chamber
Modality	2-D

Fig. 12.2 Left ventricular (LV) inferolateral (posterior) wall aneurysm (LA = left atrium)

Look for evidence of mural thrombus, which can form as a consequence of impaired wall motion. Undertake a full assessment of LV systolic and diastolic function.

Mural thrombus

Mural thrombus can occur where stasis of blood occurs, for example within an LV aneurysm or on an akinetic segment (Fig. 21.3, p. 289). The assessment of intracardiac thrombus is described on page 287.

Papillary muscle rupture

Acute mitral regurgitation can occur following myocardial infarction as a result of papillary muscle dysfunction or rupture. Papillary muscle dysfunction most commonly occurs in inferior myocardial infarction; where rupture occurs, it is often due to rupture of the posteromedial papillary muscle (which has a single blood supply, usually from the RCA or Cx artery) rather than the anterolateral papillary muscle (which has a dual blood supply). Patients may present with acute pulmonary oedema, cardiogenic shock and a new systolic murmur. Urgent surgical intervention is required.

Echo assessment

Use 2-D imaging to assess the structure of the mitral valve leaflets, annulus, papillary muscles and chordae. In cases of papillary muscle rupture, look for evidence of a flail mitral leaflet with an attached piece of papillary muscle, and its chordal attachments, prolapsing into the left atrium (LA) during systole.

Use Doppler assessment to examine the nature and extent of mitral regurgitation, as outlined in Chapter 14. Assess LV dimensions and function, and LA dimensions (in acute severe mitral regurgitation the LA will not have had time to dilate).

Be alert to alternative diagnoses – haemodynamic decompensation with a new systolic murmur can also occur in post-infarction ventricular septal defect (VSD; described below).

Post-infarction ventricular septal defect

Rupture of the interventricular septum, due to a focal area of myocardial necrosis, causes an acquired VSD. There is usually a sudden deterioration in the patient's condition and a new harsh systolic murmur. It is associated with a high mortality and requires urgent surgical intervention.

Echo assessment

Assess the interventricular septum using 2-D and colour Doppler to identify the location and size of the VSD – some post-infarction VSDs are small and can be challenging to find. Do not forget that post-infarction VSDs can be multiple, so check to see if there is more than one jet on colour Doppler. Doppler imaging will show a left-to-right shunt, with a high-velocity jet. Assess LV and RV dimensions and function.

Ventricular rupture and cardiac tamponade

Rupture of the ventricular free wall is usually a devastating complication, causing rapid haemorrhage into the pericardium and fatal cardiac tamponade in around 75 per cent of cases. However, sometimes the ventricular rupture can be contained by adhesions or thrombosis, causing a more stable (but nonetheless still extremely dangerous) situation which can, if time permits, be repaired surgically.

A chronic ventricular rupture is known as a pseudoaneurysm. The distinction between a 'true' aneurysm and a pseudoaneurysm is that the wall of a true aneurysm is composed of myocardium, but with a pseudoaneurysm the myocardium has been breached and the pseudoaneurysm is lined by pericardium.

Echo assessment

Look for evidence of a pericardial effusion with associated thrombus in the pericardial space, and for evidence of flow between the ventricle and the pericardium on colour Doppler. Assess the location and dimensions of the rupture and the pericardial effusion, and look for features of cardiac tamponade. A pericardial effusion alone is common after myocardial infarction and does not, in itself, necessarily indicate a ventricular rupture.

A pseudoaneurysm is well demarcated from the surrounding myocardium and has a narrow 'neck', which is less than half the diameter of the aneurysm itself. Thrombus may be present within the aneurysm.

DRESSLER'S SYNDROME

A pericardial effusion may be seen following a myocardial infarction and should be assessed as outlined in Chapter 19. Pericardial effusion occurring 2–10 weeks after the myocardial infarction is likely to be due to Dressler's syndrome, a form of pericarditis also known as postmyocardial infarction syndrome. Patients may present with pleuritic chest pain, fever and a pericardial friction rub. Dressler's syndrome is thought to be an autoimmune response, caused by the release of myocardial antigens, and is also seen in some patients after cardiac surgery (post-pericardiotomy syndrome).

FURTHER READING

Bassand JP, Hamm CW, Ardissino D, *et al*. Guidelines for the diagnosis and treatment of non-ST-segment elevation acute coronary syndromes. *Eur Heart J* 2007; **28**: 1598–660.

Cerqueira MD, Weissman NJ, Dilsizian V, *et al*. Standardized myocardial segmentation and nomenclature for tomographic imaging of the heart. *Circulation* 2002; **105**: 539–42.

Lang RM, Bierig M, Devereux RB, *et al*. Recommendations for chamber quantification: a report from the American Society of Echocardiography's Guidelines and Standards Committee and the Chamber Quantification Writing Group, developed in conjunction with the European Association of Echocardiography, a branch of the European Society of Cardiology. *J Am Soc Echocardiogr* 2005; **18**: 1440–63.

Van de Werf F, Bax J, Betriu A, *et al*. Management of acute myocardial infarction in patients presenting with persistent ST-segment elevation. *Eur Heart J* 2008; **29**: 2909–45.

13 The aortic valve

Echo views of the aortic valve

The aortic valve is usually assessed in the:

- left parasternal window
  - parasternal long axis view
  - parasternal short axis view (aortic valve level)
- apical window
  - apical 5-chamber view.

The **parasternal long axis view** (Fig. 6.2, p. 56) bisects the aortic valve, showing the right coronary cusp anterior to the non-coronary cusp. 2-D imaging shows the structure of the aortic valve and allows an assessment of cusp mobility. An M-mode study of the valve, at the level of the cusp tips, shows the cusps opening at the start of systole (Fig. 13.1). The aortic root as a whole moves anteriorly during systole, being pushed forwards by the expanding left atrium (LA) as it fills during diastole. Conditions that enhance LA filling, such as mitral regurgitation, exaggerate this anterior motion of the aortic root. The aortic valve cusps close at the end of systole to make a single thin closure line. This M-mode pattern of normal aortic valve cusp motion is described as 'box-shaped'. While in this view, use colour Doppler to assess valvular flow.

The **parasternal short axis view** (**aortic valve level**) shows the valve 'face on' and all three cusps can be seen together with the surrounding cardiac structures (Fig. 6.5, p. 60). Colour Doppler shows the location and extent of any valvular regurgitation.

The **apical 5-chamber view** allows further 2-D inspection of the valve (Fig. 6.9, p. 64) and a colour Doppler assessment of any regurgitant flow.

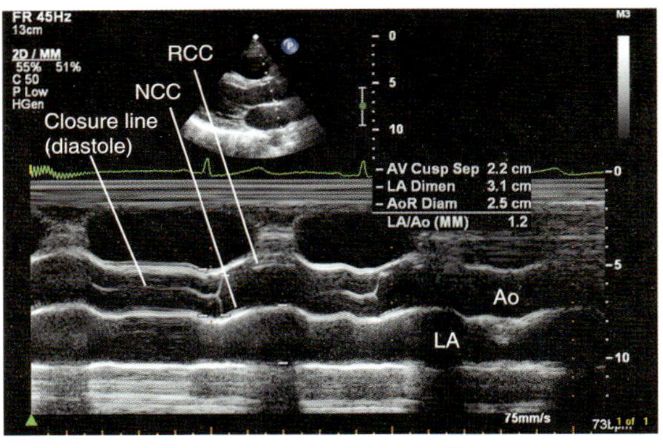

View	Parasternal long axis
Modality	M-mode

Fig. 13.1 M-mode of normal aortic valve (Ao = aorta; LA = left atrium; NCC = non-coronary cusp; RCC = right coronary cusp)

In this view a good alignment of continuous wave (CW) Doppler with the valve can usually be obtained, allowing an assessment of forward (and any regurgitant) flow. The normal aortic valve has a peak forward flow velocity <1.7 m/s and a valve area >2.0 cm^2.

Additional information can also be obtained from the:

- right parasternal window
- apical 3-chamber (long axis) view
- subcostal window
  - subcostal short axis view
- suprasternal window
  - aorta view.

The **right parasternal window** provides an additional view from which the aortic valve can be interrogated using CW Doppler (e.g. using a standalone pencil probe). The **apical 3-chamber (long axis) view** is similar in many ways to the parasternal long axis view, but offers the advantage of a suitable angle for CW Doppler assessment (Fig. 6.11, p. 66). The **subcostal short axis view** is seldom used but can visualize the aortic valve in short axis when good views cannot be obtained from the standard locations. The **suprasternal window (aorta view)** allows Doppler assessment of flow in the descending thoracic aorta, which is useful in aortic regurgitation.

Aortic stenosis

Aortic stenosis is the obstruction of blood flow from the left ventricle (LV) due to a narrowing of the aortic valve, or an obstruction just below or above the level of the valve.

Causes of aortic stenosis

Calcific degeneration of the aortic valve is one of the commonest causes of aortic stenosis. This is characterized by progressive fibrosis and calcification of the aortic valve, beginning at the base of the cusps. The early stage of this process is often referred to as 'aortic sclerosis', but this term is somewhat misleading – it implies a benign process, but in fact aortic sclerosis is often a prelude to the development of significant stenosis later on.

Bicuspid aortic valve (p. 303) is also a common cause of aortic stenosis in the West, and is thought to be responsible for around half of cases of severe aortic stenosis in adults. The stenotic process is similar to that seen in calcific degeneration, but occurs at a younger age. Fibrosis typically starts in a patient's teens, with gradual calcification in their thirties onwards. Patients who require surgery for stenosis of a bicuspid aortic valve do so on average 5 years earlier than those with calcific degeneration of a tricuspid aortic valve.

Rheumatic aortic stenosis is less common than rheumatic mitral stenosis, and the two often coexist in the same patient. There is fusion of the commissures of the aortic valve cusps and the cusps themselves become fibrotic and eventually calcified.

Sub- and supravalvular obstruction cause a form of aortic stenosis in which the valve itself is unaffected but the obstruction lies below or above the valve. Subvalvular aortic stenosis results from a fixed obstruction in the LV outflow tract (LVOT), usually a fibromuscular ridge or membrane, and may be associated with other congenital heart defects in up to half of cases. In supravalvular aortic stenosis there is a fixed obstruction in the ascending aorta, just above the sinuses of Valsalva, due to a diffuse narrowing or a discrete membrane.

Clinical features of aortic stenosis

The clinical features of aortic stenosis are summarized in Table 13.1. Many cases of aortic stenosis are detected incidentally, either because of a systolic murmur heard during a routine examination or as an incidental finding during an echocardiogram for other indications. The appearance of symptoms has significant implications for the patient's outlook: those with angina as a result of aortic stenosis have an average life expectancy of 5 years, those with exertional syncope 3 years, and those with heart failure just 1 year.

Table 13.1 Clinical features of aortic stenosis

Symptoms	Signs
Often asymptomatic	Slow-rising pulse
Angina	Low systolic blood pressure and narrow pulse pressure
Exertional dizziness and syncope	Sustained apex beat (as a result of left ventricular hypertrophy)
Breathlessness	Soft aortic component to second heart sound (A_2)
	Ejection click
	Ejection systolic murmur
	Signs of heart failure in advanced cases

Echo assessment of aortic stenosis

2-D and M-mode

Use 2-D and M-mode echo to assess the structure of the valve (Fig. 13.2):

- Is it a tricuspid aortic valve, or is it bicuspid (or pseudobicuspid), unicuspid or quadricuspid? If there is cusp fusion, describe which cusps are involved.
- Is there any thickening or calcification of the cusps? Is this diffuse or focal? If focal, which area of each cusp is affected?
- Is cusp mobility normal or reduced? How much is it reduced?
- Is there any doming of the cusps?
- Is there any evidence of sub- or supravalvular stenosis?

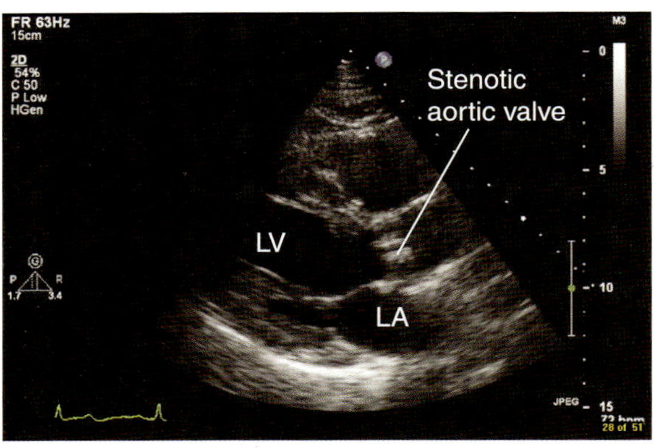

View	Parasternal long axis
Modality	2-D

Fig. 13.2 Moderate aortic stenosis (LV = left ventricle; LA = left atrium)

SUB- OR SUPRAVALVULAR AORTIC STENOSIS

Always be alert to this possibility if the transaortic pressure gradient is unexpectedly high in the presence of an aortic valve that does not look stenosed. If you suspect sub- or supravalvular stenosis, use pulsed-wave (PW) Doppler to assess blood flow at different levels above and below the valve to detect where the main flow acceleration occurs. Use 2-D echo to look carefully for a discrete membrane causing obstruction above or below the valve.

Colour Doppler

Colour Doppler imaging will show an increase in flow velocity and/or turbulent flow downstream of the stenosis.

CW and PW Doppler

Use CW Doppler to obtain a trace of forward flow through the aortic valve (Fig. 13.3). You should obtain traces from the apex and from at least one other position, such as the suprasternal or right parasternal position, and recordings should be made with both an imaging probe and a standalone 'pencil' probe. Ignore traces obtained from ectopic beats (and the beat following an ectopic).

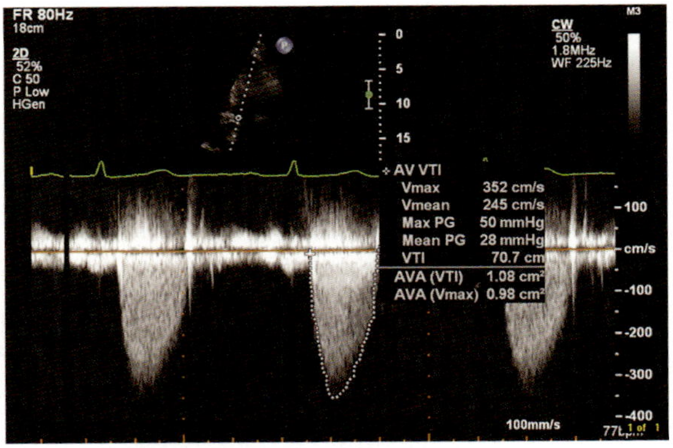

View	Apical 5-chamber
Modality	CW Doppler

Fig. 13.3 Doppler assessment of valve gradient in moderate aortic stenosis (AVA = aortic valve area; PG = pressure gradient; V_{max} = peak velocity; V_{mean} = mean velocity; VTI = velocity time integral)

The CW Doppler trace will give peak transaortic velocity (V_{max}), which relates to peak transaortic pressure gradient (ΔP_{max}) via the simplified Bernoulli equation:

$$\Delta P_{max} = 4 \times V_{max}^2$$

If peak velocity in the LVOT is >1.0 m/s, the full Bernoulli equation should be used for greater accuracy:

$$\Delta P_{max} = 4 \times (V_2^2 - V_1^2)$$

where V_2 is the peak transaortic velocity, assessed by CW Doppler, and V_1 is the peak LVOT velocity, assessed by PW Doppler.

PEAK-TO-PEAK AND INSTANTANEOUS GRADIENTS

Transaortic gradient can also be assessed during cardiac catheterization, by measuring the fall in systolic pressure on withdrawing a catheter across the aortic valve. The gradient measured in this way is a **peak-to-peak** gradient – it is the difference between the peak pressure in the LV and the peak pressure in the aorta (which do not occur simultaneously – see Fig. 2.6, p. 13). In contrast, the gradient measured by echo Doppler is an **instantaneous** gradient – it measures the maximum *instantaneous* pressure difference between the two chambers. Instantaneous gradients are greater than peak-to-peak gradients, and so peak transaortic gradients measured by echo will be higher than gradients measured by cardiac catheterization.

The mean transaortic pressure gradient (ΔP_{mean}) can be obtained by tracing the Doppler envelope, from which the echo machine can calculate a mean value by averaging the instantaneous gradients throughout the trace. Alternatively, ΔP_{mean} can be estimated from the ΔP_{max} using the equation:

$$\Delta P_{mean} = \frac{\Delta P_{max}}{1.45} + 2\text{mmHg}$$

Conditions that increase stroke volume (e.g. aortic regurgitation, pregnancy) increase transaortic flow during systole and can therefore lead to an *overestimation* of transaortic pressure gradients. Conversely, transaortic pressure gradients are *underestimated* in the presence of impaired LV function. These problems can, to some extent, be compensated for by using the continuity equation to measure aortic valve effective orifice area (EOA_{AV}). To do this:

1. Measure the diameter of the LVOT in the parasternal long axis view, and then use this to calculate the cross-sectional area (CSA) of the LVOT:

$$CSA_{LVOT} = 0.785 \times (\text{LVOT diameter})^2$$

2. Now measure the velocity time integral (VTI) of flow in the LVOT (using PW Doppler) and across the aortic valve (using CW Doppler) to give VTI_{LVOT} and VTI_{AV}, respectively.
3. Use the continuity equation to calculate aortic valve EOA as follows:

$$EOA_{AV} = \frac{CSA_{LVOT} \times VTI_{LVOT}}{VTI_{AV}}$$

COMMON PITFALLS

Pitfalls in the echo assessment of aortic stenosis include:

- A poor Doppler signal outline, which may lead the sonographer to 'miss' the true peak of the Doppler velocity signal.
- Failure to align the Doppler beam with the flow through the aortic valve, which leads to an underestimation of transaortic peak velocity (the extent of error increases rapidly with misalignment of more than 20°).
- Accidentally mistaking a mitral regurgitation trace for an aortic stenosis trace (particularly when using a pencil probe), and thus making measurements from the wrong valve.
- Overestimation of the severity of stenosis because of coexistent aortic regurgitation.
- Underestimation of the severity of aortic stenosis because of coexistent mitral stenosis or impairment of LV function.
- Inappropriate use of the continuity equation (it cannot be used if there are serial stenoses, i.e. sub/supravalvular stenoses, or if the LVOT is not circular, as in hypertrophic obstructive cardiomyopathy or subvalvular stenosis).

If you measured the LVOT diameter in centimetres, this will give you an EOA_{AV} in cm^2. Some versions of the continuity equation use the ratio of peak velocities in the LVOT and across the aortic valve instead of using VTIs – however, although the results are often very similar, they are not identical and it is better to use VTI for the calculation.

You will find more information on the assessment of aortic stenosis in the setting of impaired LV function in Chapter 8, 'The stress echo study'.

Associated features

If aortic stenosis is present you should:

- assess any coexistent aortic regurgitation
- assess any coexistent disease affecting the other valves (as patients undergoing aortic valve surgery may also require any other valvular abnormalities to be corrected at the same time)
- assess LV dimensions and function. Obstruction to LV outflow by the aortic valve raises LV pressure, leading to LV hypertrophy and subsequently dilatation and impaired function
- assess aortic root morphology and dimensions (aortic root dilatation is a common finding in aortic stenosis)
- if the aortic valve is bicuspid, check for the presence of coarctation of the aorta (bicuspid aortic valve and coarctation of the aorta are sometimes associated).

Severity of aortic stenosis

Severity of aortic stenosis can be quantified by (Table 13.2):

- V_{max}
- P_{max}
- P_{mean}
- EOA.

Table 13.2 Indicators of aortic stenosis severity

	Mild	Moderate	Severe
Aortic V_{max} (m/s)	1.7–2.9	3.0–4.0	>4.0
Aortic P_{max} (mmHg)	<36	36–64	>64
Aortic P_{mean} (mmHg)	<25	25–40	>40
Aortic valve EOA (cm^2)	1.5–2.0	1.0–1.4	<1.0

EOA, effective orifice area; P_{max} = peak pressure; P_{mean} = mean pressure; V_{max} = peak velocity. Reference ranges reproduced with permission of the British Society of Echocardiography and British Heart Foundation.

SAMPLE REPORT

The aortic valve is tricuspid and heavily calcified with severely reduced cusp mobility. There is doming of the cusps during systole. The transaortic peak velocity is 5.2 m/s (peak gradient 92 mmHg, mean gradient 65 mmHg) and the aortic valve effective orifice area is 0.6 cm^2. There is no associated aortic regurgitation and the mitral valve is normal. There is moderate concentric left ventricular hypertrophy with good systolic function. The aortic root is dilated, measuring 4.2 cm at the level of the sinuses of Valsalva. The findings are consistent with severe aortic stenosis.

Management of aortic stenosis

Echo surveillance

Patients with aortic stenosis should be advised to report symptoms immediately. Asymptomatic patients with an aortic V_{max} of >4 m/s should be reassessed every 6 months, and if V_{max} increases by >0.3 m/s per year, surgery should be considered. Annual reassessment is advised for those with lesser degrees of stenosis.

Drug therapy

There is no specific drug therapy to reverse aortic stenosis, although there has been research interest in the potential of statin therapy to slow the progression of the disease.

Surgery

Surgical replacement of the valve is the definitive treatment for aortic stenosis. Biological prosthetic valves are generally preferred for older patients or those who wish to avoid the need for long-term anticoagulation, while mechanical prosthetic valves are preferred for younger patients. Surgery is indicated for severe symptomatic aortic stenosis. Asymptomatic patients should be considered for surgery if they have LV systolic dysfunction, or if they develop symptoms (or a fall in blood pressure or complex ventricular arrhythmias) on exercise testing. Replacement of a moderate or severely stenosed aortic valve is usually advisable if patients are due to undergo heart surgery for another reason, such as bypass grafting or mitral valve surgery.

Balloon valvuloplasty can be used as a bridge to valve replacement in unstable patients, or for patients who need urgent non-cardiac surgery. Transcatheter aortic valve implantation (TAVI, page 232) is a new technique for aortic valve replacement in patients who cannot undergo conventional valve surgery.

Aortic regurgitation

Aortic regurgitation is the flow of blood from the aorta back through the aortic valve during diastole. It can result from a problem with the aortic valve itself or from a problem with the aortic root affecting an otherwise normal valve.

Causes of aortic regurgitation

Valvular causes include:

- bicuspid aortic valve, causing incomplete closure of the valve
- calcific degeneration of the aortic valve
- rheumatic aortic valve disease
- infective endocarditis
- connective tissue diseases (e.g. rheumatoid arthritis, systemic lupus erythematosus).

Aortic root causes result from dilatation and/or distortion of the aortic root. These include:

- hypertension
- Marfan syndrome
- Ehlers–Danlos syndrome
- osteogenesis imperfecta
- aortic dissection
- sinus of Valsalva aneurysm
- cystic medial necrosis
- syphilitic aortitis
- Behçet disease.

Some conditions, such as ankylosing spondylitis, can affect both the aortic valve and the aortic root.

Clinical features of aortic regurgitation

The clinical features of aortic regurgitation are summarized in Table 13.3. Chronic aortic regurgitation places a volume overload on the LV, which, with time, dilates and becomes increasingly impaired, at which point the patient may develop symptoms and signs of heart failure. The disease process can therefore be insidious, although once heart failure does develop patients often decline rapidly. Infective endocarditis and aortic dissection can cause acute aortic regurgitation, in which the patient can have clinically severe regurgitation but the usual markers of severity (such as LV dilatation) have not had time to develop.

Table 13.3 Clinical features of aortic regurgitation

Symptoms	Signs
May be asymptomatic Symptoms of heart failure: breathlessness, orthopnoea, paroxysmal nocturnal dyspnoea Symptoms may also indicate the aetiology (e.g. fever in infective endocarditis)	Collapsing pulse Low diastolic blood pressure and wide pulse pressure Displaced apex beat (as a result of left ventricular dilatation) Early diastolic murmur Signs of heart failure in advanced cases

Echo assessment of aortic regurgitation

2-D and M-mode

Use 2-D and M-mode echo to assess the structure of both the aortic valve and the aortic root:

- Is it a normal tricuspid aortic valve, or is it bicuspid (or pseudobicuspid), unicuspid or quadricuspid? Are the valve cusps thickened or calcified?
- Are there any features of aortic stenosis (which may coexist with regurgitation)?
- Is there any prolapse? Which cusps are affected?
- Are there any features of infective endocarditis (vegetations, aortic root abscess)?
- Is there dilatation of the aortic root and/or any indication of dissection?

Use M-mode to interrogate the *mitral* valve. The diastolic jet of aortic regurgitation may hit the anterior mitral valve leaflet, causing fluttering of the leaflet, which can be seen on M-mode echo (Fig. 13.4). This pushes the anterior leaflet backwards during diastole, causing premature closure of the mitral valve and thereby partly obstructing the normal flow of blood through the mitral valve orifice. This can cause a diastolic murmur, called an Austin Flint murmur. These effects on the mitral valve are an indicator of severe aortic regurgitation.

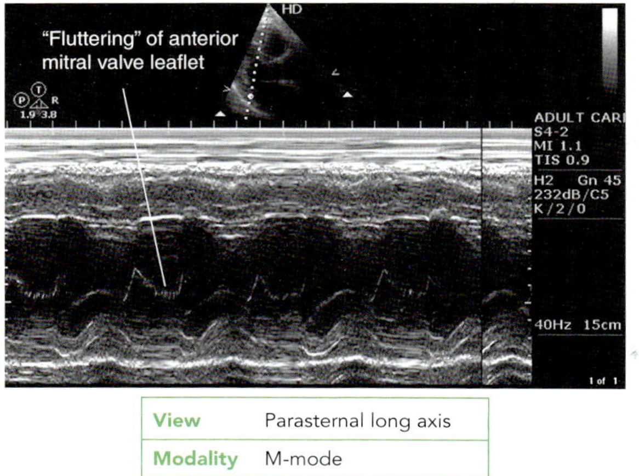

View	Parasternal long axis
Modality	M-mode

Fig. 13.4 Aortic regurgitation causing 'fluttering' of anterior mitral valve leaflet

The LV also requires careful assessment. M-mode and 2-D imaging will show LV dimensions and function. In chronic aortic regurgitation, volume overload leads to progressive LV dilatation but with hyperkinetic wall motion, particularly of the posterior wall and septum.

Colour Doppler

Use colour Doppler to examine the jet of aortic regurgitation (Fig. 13.5). How far the jet extends back into the LV is an unreliable indicator of severity, but assessing the width of the jet (in the parasternal long axis view) in relation to the diameter of the LVOT is a useful guide to severity (see below). The measurements should be taken just below (within 1 cm of the level of) the aortic valve. Colour M-mode imaging in the parasternal long axis view, with the cursor placed just below the aortic valve, can be a useful way to measure the width of the jet and of the LVOT.

Measure the width of the vena contracta (VC) – the narrowest region of colour flow at the level of the aortic valve – in the parasternal long axis view. This also helps gauge severity. VC cannot be reliably measured if there is more than one regurgitant jet, or if the shape of the jet is irregular. If the jet

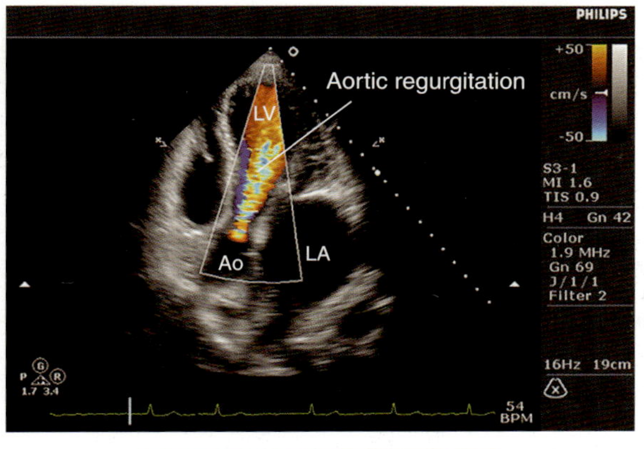

View	Apical 5-chamber
Modality	Colour Doppler

Fig. 13.5 Aortic regurgitation (Ao = aorta; LA = left atrium; LV = left ventricle) (Figure reproduced with permission of Philips)

is eccentric, the measurement of VC should be made perpendicular to the direction of the jet rather than to the orientation of the LVOT.

CW and PW Doppler

Record the CW Doppler trace in the apical 5-chamber view, with the probe carefully aligned with the direction of the regurgitant jet (Fig. 13.6). An inverted trace can also be obtained from the suprasternal view. The CW Doppler trace is faint in mild aortic regurgitation, and denser in moderate or severe regurgitation. The pressure half-time of the diastolic deceleration slope, which equates to the rate of deceleration of the regurgitant jet, is a guide to severity, particularly in acute regurgitation.

PW Doppler can be used to map the extent of the regurgitant jet in the LV, by positioning the sample volume at various points in the LV (in the apical 5-chamber view) and checking for regurgitant flow, although this is not a good indicator of severity. PW Doppler can also be used to look for diastolic flow reversal in the upper descending aorta, using a suprasternal view and placing the sample volume in the descending aorta (just beyond the origin of the left subclavian artery). It is normal to have a brief reversal of aortic flow in diastole, but flow reversal throughout the whole of diastole (pandiastolic) indicates moderate or severe aortic regurgitation. Obtain a VTI of the diastolic flow reversal – severe regurgitation is indicated by a VTI > 15 cm.

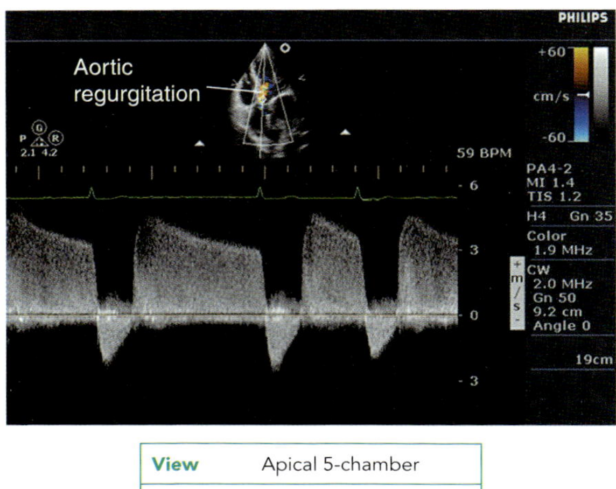

View	Apical 5-chamber
Modality	CW Doppler

Fig. 13.6 Aortic regurgitation (Figure reproduced with permission of Philips)

Regurgitant volume

The volume of blood entering the LV via the mitral valve during diastole should normally equal the volume of blood leaving it via the LVOT (stroke volume). In the presence of aortic regurgitation, LVOT outflow will be greater than mitral valve inflow as the systolic LVOT outflow will consist of the blood that has entered via the mitral valve plus the blood that entered the ventricle via aortic regurgitation during diastole. The difference between LVOT outflow and mitral valve inflow gives the regurgitant volume.

Although simple in principle, measurement of regurgitant volume is difficult in practice. First, the measurement is not valid if there is significant mitral regurgitation. Second, any error in measurement of mitral valve orifice area or LVOT diameter can have a large impact on the result. If you wish to measure regurgitant fraction, you can do so as follows:

1. In the apical 4-chamber view, measure the diameter of the mitral annulus in cm, and then use this to calculate the CSA of the mitral valve in cm^2. This calculation makes the assumption that the mitral orifice is circular:

$$CSA_{MV} = 0.785 \times (\text{mitral annulus diameter})^2$$

2. In the apical 4-chamber view, measure the VTI of mitral valve inflow (using PW Doppler) to give VTI_{MV}, in cm. It is generally easiest to place

the sample volume at the valve tips (some place it at the level of the mitral valve annulus).

3. The stroke volume of the mitral valve (SV_{MV}), in mL/beat, can then be calculated from:

$$SV_{MV} = CSA_{MV} \times VTI_{MV}$$

4. In the parasternal long axis view, measure the diameter of the LVOT in cm, and then use this to calculate the cross-sectional area (CSA) of the LVOT in cm^2:

$$CSA_{LVOT} = 0.785 \times (\text{LVOT diameter})^2$$

5. In the apical 5-chamber view, measure the VTI of LVOT outflow (using PW Doppler) to give VTI_{LVOT}, in cm.
6. The stroke volume of the LVOT (SV_{LVOT}), in mL/beat, can then be calculated from:

$$SV_{LVOT} = CSA_{LVOT} \times VTI_{LVOT}$$

7. Aortic regurgitant volume (RV) can be calculated from:

$$RV = SV_{LVOT} - SV_{MV}$$

8. Aortic regurgitant fraction (RF) can be calculated from:

$$RF = \frac{RV}{SV_{MV}} \; (\times 100 \text{ to express as a percentage})$$

Once you have calculated the aortic RV, you can also calculate the regurgitant orifice area (ROA). This is the average size of the orifice in the aortic valve, in cm^2, through which the regurgitation occurs during diastole, and equals the aortic RV (in mL) divided by the VTI of the aortic regurgitation Doppler trace (VTI_{AR}), measured in cm using CW Doppler:

$$ROA = \frac{RV}{VTI_{AR}}$$

Proximal isovelocity surface area (PISA) assessment

The use of PISA in the assessment of aortic regurgitation is not as common as it is for mitral regurgitation, as it is technically more challenging to obtain suitable images and the technique has not been so well studied in relation to the aortic valve.

COMMON PITFALLS

Pitfalls in the echo assessment of aortic regurgitation include:

- An eccentric jet usually leads to underestimation of severity.
- Measuring the width of the regurgitant jet on colour Doppler too far below the aortic valve, where it tends to spread out, overestimates severity.

Associated features

If aortic regurgitation is present you should:

- assess any coexistent aortic stenosis
- assess any coexistent disease affecting the other valves (as patients undergoing aortic valve surgery may also require any other valvular abnormalities to be corrected at the same time)
- assess LV dimensions and function
- assess aortic root morphology and dimensions
- if the aortic valve is bicuspid, check for the presence of coarctation of the aorta (bicuspid aortic valve and coarctation of the aorta are sometimes associated).

Severity of aortic regurgitation

Severity of aortic regurgitation can be assessed by (Table 13.4):

- VC width
- ratio of jet width to LVOT width
- jet pressure half-time
- VTI of diastolic flow reversal in upper descending aorta
- RV
- RF
- ROA.

The ratio of jet width to LVOT width is commonly used to quantify severity, but can be misleading in jets that are eccentric or have a diffuse origin. In such cases it is generally better to use visual assessment to grade the ratio in terms of small, intermediate or large, and to use this as a gross guide to severity, than to stick slavishly to percentages. The VC width is a more reliable indicator of severity.

The pressure half-time of the diastolic deceleration slope shortens with increasing severity, as the rate of fall in aortic pressure is greater in severe

Table 13.4 Indicators of aortic regurgitation severity

	Mild	Moderate	Severe
Colour Doppler			
Vena contracta width (cm)	<0.3	–	>0.6
Ratio of jet width to LVOT width (%)	<25	–	⩾65
CW Doppler			
Pressure half-time (ms)	>500	–	<250
PW Doppler			
VTI diastolic flow reversal in upper descending aorta (cm)	–	–	15
Multimodality			
Regurgitant volume (mL/beat)	<30	30–59	⩾60
Regurgitant fraction (%)	<30	30–49	⩾50
Regurgitant orifice area (cm^2)	<0.10	0.10–0.29	⩾0.30

CW = continuous wave; LVOT = left ventricular outflow tract; PW = pulsed-wave; VTI = velocity time integral. Reference ranges reproduced with permission of the British Society of Echocardiography and British Heart Foundation.

regurgitation, but the half-time can also be affected by changes in LV compliance and the use of vasodilators.

SAMPLE REPORT

The aortic valve is tricuspid with cusps that are rheumatic in appearance. There is a dense central jet of aortic regurgitation with a vena contracta width of 0.7 cm and a ratio of jet width to LVOT width of 76 per cent. The pressure half-time of the regurgitant jet is 220 ms. The calculated aortic regurgitant volume is 78 mL/beat (regurgitant fraction 62 per cent) with a regurgitant orifice area of 0.38 cm^2. There is holodiastolic flow reversal in the upper descending aorta (VTI 21 cm). The LV is non-dilated and there is good LV systolic function. The aortic root is mildly dilated, measuring 4.1 cm at the level of the sinuses of Valsalva. The findings are consistent with severe aortic regurgitation.

Management of aortic regurgitation

Echo surveillance

- Patients with mild–moderate aortic regurgitation should be seen annually and have an echo every 2 years.

- Patients with severe regurgitation and normal LV function should be reviewed every 6 months, or annually if stable and not close to needing surgery.
- Patients with a dilated aortic root (especially those with Marfan syndrome or bicuspid aortic valve) should have an annual echo, or even more frequently if the aorta is enlarging.

Drug therapy

Patients who develop LV impairment should be treated with appropriate heart failure medication and hypertension should be well controlled. The 'pre-emptive' use of vasodilators in patients with normal LV function is unproven, but beta-blockers have a role to play in those with Marfan syndrome.

Surgery

Aortic valve surgery is indicated for symptomatic acute aortic regurgitation and in chronic aortic regurgitation when severe and symptomatic. In asymptomatic patients with severe aortic regurgitation, surgery is indicated for:

- LV impairment (ejection fraction ≤50 per cent)
- LV dilatation (end-diastolic diameter >7.0 cm or end-systolic diameter >5.0 cm)
- Patients needing heart surgery for other reasons (e.g. coronary artery bypass graft).

Regardless of aortic regurgitation severity, surgery is indicated for patients with aortic root disease and an aortic root diameter measuring:

- ≥4.5 cm in Marfan syndrome
- ≥5.0 cm with a bicuspid aortic valve
- ≥5.5 cm for other patients.

Surgery may involve aortic valve replacement or repair (where the valve is suitable), together with aortic root grafting where appropriate.

FURTHER READING

Chambers J. *British Society of Echocardiography Distance Learning Module 3: Echocardiographic Assessment of Aortic Stenosis*. Accessible from the BSE website (www.bsecho.org).

Maurer G. Aortic regurgitation. *Heart* 2006; **92**: 994–1000.

Ramaraj R, Sorrell VL. Degenerative aortic stenosis. *BMJ* 2008; **336**: 550–5.

The Task Force on the Management of Valvular Heart Disease of the European Society of Cardiology. Guidelines on the management of valvular heart disease. *Eur Heart J* 2007; **28**: 230–68.

Ward C. Clinical significance of the bicuspid aortic valve. *Heart* 2000; **83**: 81–5.

Zoghbi WA, Enriquez-Sarano M, Foster E, *et al*. American Society of Echocardiography: recommendations for evaluation of the severity of native valvular regurgitation with two-dimensional and Doppler echocardiography. *J Am Soc Echocardiogr* 2003; **16**: 777–802.

14 The mitral valve

Echo views of the mitral valve

The mitral valve is usually assessed in the:

- left parasternal window
  - parasternal long axis view
  - parasternal short axis view (mitral valve and papillary muscle levels)
- apical window
  - apical 4-chamber view
  - apical 2-chamber view
  - apical 3-chamber (long axis) view.

The **parasternal long axis view** (Fig. 6.2, p. 56) bisects the mitral valve, showing the anterior and posterior leaflets in the plane of the A2 and P2 scallops. 2-D imaging shows the structure of the mitral valve and allows an assessment of leaflet mobility. An M-mode study of the valve, at the level of the leaflet tips, shows the tips open widely in early diastole as blood flows from the left atrium (LA) into the left ventricle (LV), and the point at which the anterior leaflet tip reaches its most anterior position is called the E point (Fig. 14.1). The leaflets then move back together in mid-diastole before separating once again towards the end of diastole, as a result of the extra surge of blood through the valve that accompanies atrial systole. The maximum excursion of the anterior leaflet during this phase is called the A point. The anterior leaflet then follows a straight downward line to its closure point at the onset of systole. Once you have completed the M-mode recording, use colour Doppler to assess valvular flow.

The **parasternal short axis view** (**mitral valve level**) shows the valve 'face on' and all three scallops of both leaflets can be seen together with both

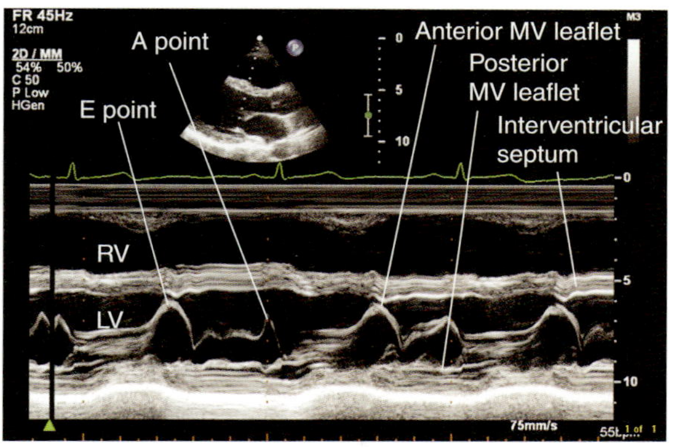

View	Parasternal long axis
Modality	M-mode

Fig. 14.1 M-mode of normal mitral valve (LV = left ventricle; MV = mitral valve; RV= right ventricle)

mitral commissures (Figs 6.6 (p. 61) and 14.2). The area of the valve orifice can be measured with planimetry in this view – a normal mitral valve has an orifice area of 4.0–6.0 cm^2. Colour Doppler shows the location and extent of any valvular regurgitation. Angling the probe down to the **papillary muscle level** (Fig. 6.7, p. 61) shows both papillary muscles. Sometimes there can be three papillary muscles if one of them happens to be bifid.

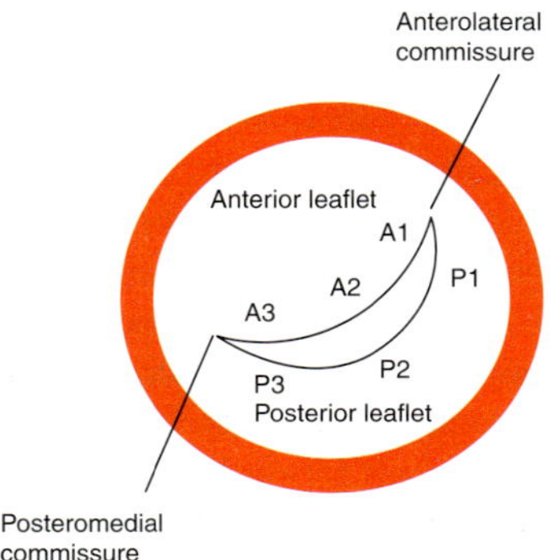

Fig. 14.2 Mitral valve scallops, as seen in the parasternal short axis view.

The **apical 4-chamber view** (Fig. 6.8, p. 63) shows the anterior mitral leaflet (A2 and A3 scallops) adjacent to the interventricular septum and the posterior leaflet (P1) adjacent to the lateral wall, together with the anterolateral papillary muscle and its chordae. The **apical 2-chamber view** (Fig. 6.10, p. 65) shows the anterior mitral leaflet in a 'bicommisural view', with the P1 and P3 scallops of the posterior leaflet on either side and the A2 scallop of the anterior leaflet in the middle. The **apical 3-chamber view** (Fig. 6.11, p. 66) is similar to the parasternal long axis view, showing the A2 and P2 scallops.

In each of the apical views inspect the valve structure with 2-D echo and assess flow with colour Doppler. The apical views permit a good alignment of continuous wave (CW) and pulsed-wave (PW) Doppler with the valve to assess forward (and any regurgitant) flow. Forward flow across a normal mitral valve has a pressure half-time of 40–70 ms. Additional information can also be obtained from the:

- subcostal window
  - subcostal long axis view
  - subcostal short axis view.

The **subcostal long axis view** provides an additional view from which the mitral valve can be examined. The **subcostal short axis view** is seldom used to examine the mitral valve, but with appropriate angulation of the probe it can be visualized.

Mitral stenosis

Mitral stenosis is the obstruction of diastolic blood flow from the LA to the LV due to a narrowing of the mitral valve. This is almost always due to rheumatic mitral valve disease, as a consequence of rheumatic fever earlier in life.

Causes of mitral stenosis

Rheumatic valve disease can affect any of the heart valves (or several in combination), but most commonly affects the mitral valve. The characteristic feature is fusion of the mitral leaflets along their edges, starting from the mitral commissures, restricting their ability to open. The leaflet edges become thickened, although there can be thickening and/or calcification elsewhere too. As the main body of each leaflet usually remains relatively pliable, the leaflets are seen to 'dome' during diastole, with the rising LA pressure causing the leaflet body to bow forwards towards the ventricle. This gives the leaflets what is described as a 'hockey stick' appearance. Rheumatic mitral stenosis also affects the chordae, causing fibrosis, shortening and calcification of the subvalvular apparatus.

Other causes of mitral stenosis are rare. These include congenital mitral stenosis, mitral annular calcification, systemic lupus erythematosus, rheumatoid arthritis, carcinoid syndrome and infective endocarditis. Beware of conditions that can cause obstruction of the mitral valve orifice and mimic mitral stenosis, such as left atrial myxoma, infective endocarditis with a large vegetation, ball thrombus or cor triatriatum.

MITRAL ANNULAR CALCIFICATION

Mitral annular calcification is relatively common in older patients (but can also be seen in younger patients with renal failure) and most commonly occurs in the posterior part of the mitral annulus, at the attachment point of the posterior leaflet, although rarely it can extend right round the annulus in severe cases. It is thought to be an indicator of cardiovascular risk and a marker of coronary artery disease. If annular calcification is massive, it can extend into the mitral leaflets and cause mitral stenosis. Unlike rheumatic mitral stenosis, mitral annular calcification does not affect the leaflet tips or cause fusion of the commissures.

Clinical features of mitral stenosis

The clinical features of mitral stenosis are summarized in Table 14.1. Most patients are female, and most will have other coexistent valve disease. Rheumatic mitral stenosis usually presents 20–40 years after an episode of rheumatic fever and is now relatively uncommon in developed countries. The onset of mitral stenosis tends to be gradual and so the symptoms can build up insidiously over a long period, but a new event (such as pregnancy or the onset of atrial fibrillation (AF)) can suddenly cause the symptoms to deteriorate. Patients usually remain asymptomatic until the mitral valve orifice area falls below 2.0 cm^2, at which point LA pressure starts to

Table 14.1 Clinical features of mitral stenosis

Symptoms	Signs
Often gradual onset	Atrial fibrillation is common
Breathlessness	Malar flush ('mitral facies')
Cough	Tapping apex beat (palpable first heart sound)
Peripheral oedema	Loud first heart sound
Haemoptysis	Loud pulmonary component to second heart sound (P_2) if pulmonary hypertension present
Peripheral emboli	Opening snap
	Low pitched mid-diastolic murmur (with presystolic accentuation if in sinus rhythm)

increase. As LA pressure rises, the LA starts to dilate. Pulmonary artery pressure also begins to rise and pulmonary hypertension develops. Once a patient becomes symptomatic, if left untreated the 10-year survival is around 50–60 per cent.

Echo assessment of mitral stenosis

2-D and M-mode

Use 2-D and M-mode echo to assess the structure of the valve and the subvalvular apparatus. Be sure to describe the appearance of the mitral leaflets, mitral annulus, chordae tendineae and papillary muscles:

- Do the mitral valve leaflets appear normal? Is there evidence of rheumatic valve disease (Fig. 14.3)?
- Does the mitral annulus appear normal? Is there annular calcification, and is this mild, moderate or severe?
- Is there any thickening of the leaflets? Is this mild, moderate or severe? Are both leaflets affected, and does this affect the tip or body of each leaflet?
- Is there any calcification of the leaflets? Is this focal or diffuse? Does the calcification affect either or both of the commissures?
- Is there fusion of one or both of the commissures?
- Are the chordae tendineae normal? Is there any chordal thickening, shortening or calcification? Does this affect the chordae to the anterior or posterior leaflet?

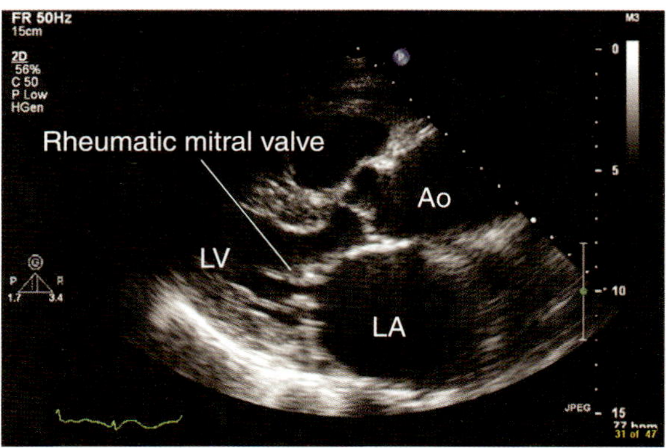

View	Parasternal long axis
Modality	2-D

Fig. 14.3 Rheumatic mitral valve (Ao = aorta; LA = left atrium; LV = left ventricle)

- Are the papillary muscles normal? Is there any calcification or fibrosis?
- Is mitral leaflet mobility normal or reduced? How much is it reduced (mild, moderate or severe)? Is there any doming during diastole?

In the parasternal short axis view (mitral valve level), if the image quality is good enough, perform planimetry to measure the mitral orifice area. Remember that a stenosed mitral valve, when open, is funnel shaped, so be careful to ensure that you are measuring the 'funnel' at its narrowest point, i.e. the level of the leaflet tips. If you angle the probe too far upwards (towards the LA) you will overestimate the orifice area. Once you've recorded a loop at the level of the tips, scroll the images back and forth until you find the one that shows the orifice at its widest point in the cardiac cycle. Take your measurement from this image, tracing around the inner edge of the leaflets – the echo machine will calculate the orifice area for you. Using M-mode in mitral stenosis, assess:

- Are the leaflet tips thickened?
- Is there reduced excursion of the mitral leaflets during diastole?
- Is there evidence of commissural fusion (shown by the posterior leaflet moving upwards, in the same direction as the anterior leaflet, as it opens during diastole, rather than downwards as a mirror image of the anterior leaflet)?

Colour Doppler

Use colour Doppler to look for any coexistent mitral regurgitation. The colour jet can also help in obtaining correct alignment of the probe for CW and PW Doppler recordings.

CW and PW Doppler

Use CW Doppler to obtain a trace of forward flow through the mitral valve (Fig. 14.4) from an apical 4-chamber view. Ignore traces obtained from ectopic beats (and the beat following an ectopic), and if the patient is in AF (as is often the case) you should average measurements taken from several beats.

From the trace, measure the **pressure half-time** of the mitral valve inflow by measuring the downward slope of the E wave (delineated by the '+' markers in Fig. 14.4, giving a pressure half-time of 223 ms). Pressure half-time is a measure of the rate of fall in pressure across the valve – specifically, the time taken for the transmitral pressure gradient to fall to half of its initial peak value. The narrower the valve, the longer it takes for the pressure gradient to fall and hence the longer the pressure half-time. An echo Doppler trace displays flow velocity rather than pressure, and the mathematical relationship between

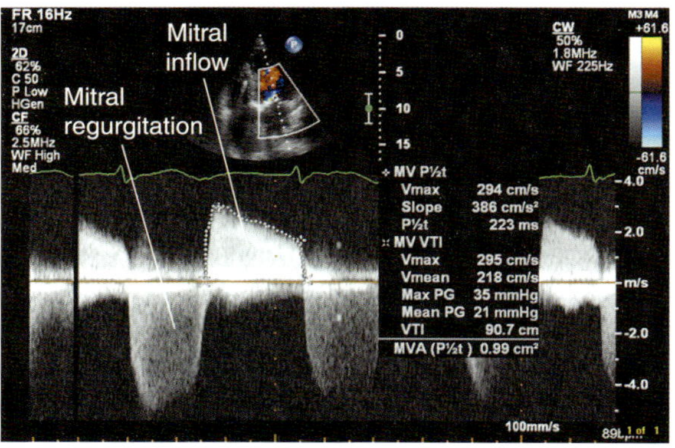

View	Apical 4-chamber
Modality	CW Doppler

Fig. 14.4 Severe mitral stenosis (and coexistent mitral regurgitation) (MV = mitral valve; MVA = mitral valve area; P1⁄2t = pressure half-time; PG = pressure gradient; V_{max} = peak velocity; V_{mean} = mean velocity; VTI = velocity time integral)

pressure and flow velocity means that a fall in pressure gradient to 0.5 of its original value equates to a fall in flow velocity to 0.7 of its original value.

Studies have shown that a mitral valve area of 1 cm^2 has a pressure half-time of approximately 220 ms, and that the relationship between pressure half-time and valve area is linear. It is therefore possible to estimate mitral valve area from pressure half-time using the equation:

$$\text{Mitral valve area} = \frac{220}{\text{pressure half-time}}$$

where mitral valve area is measured in cm and pressure half-time in ms. In Fig. 14.4, the pressure half-time of 223 ms gives a valve area of:

$$\text{Mitral valve area} = \frac{220}{223}$$

$$\text{Mitral valve area} = 0.99\ \text{cm}^2$$

This calculated valve area can be compared with the measured area you obtained from planimetry. Although pressure half-time is not affected by the presence of mitral regurgitation, it is influenced by conditions that alter compliance in the LA or LV, such as an atrial septal defect (ASD) or significant aortic regurgitation, which will shorten pressure half-time (and thus overestimate mitral valve area). Pressure half-time is also influenced by the acute haemodynamic changes that occur following mitral valvuloplasty (see p. 231).

Next, measure the **mean mitral pressure drop** by tracing the VTI of the mitral inflow (delineated by the 'X' markers in Fig. 14.4, giving a mean pressure gradient of 21 mmHg). Unlike pressure half-time, the mean pressure gradient is dependent not only on stenosis severity but also upon flow across the valve – conditions that increase transmitral flow (such as exercise or, as in the example in Figure 14.4, coexistent mitral regurgitation) will also increase the gradient.

Continuity equation

Mitral valve area can also be calculated using the continuity equation. This calculation relies on the volume of blood entering the LV via the mitral valve orifice during diastole (transmitral stroke volume) being equal to the volume of blood leaving the LV via the LV outflow tract (LVOT) during systole. This calculation cannot therefore be used in the presence of significant mitral or aortic regurgitation.

1. In the parasternal long axis view, measure the diameter of the LVOT in cm, and then use this to calculate the cross-sectional area (CSA) of the LVOT in cm^2:

$$CSA_{LVOT} = 0.785 \times (\text{LVOT diameter})^2$$

2. In the apical 5-chamber view, measure the velocity time integral (VTI) of LVOT outflow (using PW Doppler) to give VTI_{LVOT}, in cm.
3. The stroke volume of the LVOT (SV_{LVOT}), in mL/beat, can then be calculated from:

$$SV_{LVOT} = CSA_{LVOT} \times VTI_{LVOT}$$

4. This will be equal to the transmitral stoke volume (SV_{MV}):

$$SV_{MV} = SV_{LVOT}$$

5. In the apical 4-chamber view, measure the VTI of mitral valve inflow (using PW Doppler) to give VTI_{MV}, in cm.
6. Mitral valve area (MVA), in cm^2, can be calculated from:

$$MVA = \frac{SV_{MV}}{VTI_{MV}}$$

COMMON PITFALLS

Pitfalls in the echo assessment of mitral stenosis include:

- Inaccurate planimetry of the mitral orifice because of suboptimal 2-D image quality or heavy calcification of the mitral leaflet edges.
- Failure to planimeter the mitral leaflets at their tips, leading to an overestimation of orifice area.
- Failure to align the Doppler beam with flow through the valve during CW Doppler interrogation.
- Inaccurate measurement of pressure half-time due to a poor quality mitral inflow trace.
- Failing to recognize that conditions affecting LV compliance (e.g. coexistent aortic regurgitation, LV hypertrophy, recent valvuloplasty) will affect pressure half-time, as will the presence of an ASD.
- Failure to average several readings when patients are in AF.

Associated features

If mitral stenosis is present you should:

- assess any coexistent mitral regurgitation
- assess any coexistent disease affecting the other valves (as patients undergoing mitral valve surgery may also require any other valvular abnormalities to be corrected at the same time)
- assess LA size – the LA dilates in mitral stenosis
- look for evidence of blood stasis in the LA, as evidenced by spontaneous echo contrast or the presence of a thrombus
- assess LV dimensions and function. Systolic function is usually normal in mitral stenosis unless other pathology is present, but mitral stenosis impairs diastolic function
- assess the right heart for evidence of pulmonary hypertension, and comment on right atrial and ventricular size.

Severity of mitral stenosis

Severity of mitral stenosis can be quantified by:

- pressure half-time
- mean pressure drop
- valve area.

Table 14.2 summarizes the echo indicators of mitral stenosis severity. You should always state the method(s) you have used to measure mitral valve area in your report.

Table 14.2 Indicators of mitral stenosis severity

	Mild	Moderate	Severe
Pressure half-time (ms)	71–139	140–219	>219
Mean pressure drop (mmHg)	<5.0	5–10	>10
Valve area (cm^2)	1.6–2.0	1.0–1.5	<1.0

Reference ranges reproduced with permission of the British Society of Echocardiography and British Heart Foundation.

Indirect indicators that point towards more severe mitral stenosis include:

- LA dilatation
- pulmonary hypertension.

SAMPLE REPORT

The mitral valve is rheumatic in appearance, with fusion of the leaflets at both commissures and moderate thickening of both leaflet tips and the chordae tendineae. There is no calcification and the mitral annulus and papillary muscles appear normal. Mitral leaflet mobility is severely reduced, with doming during diastole. The mitral valve area measures 0.86 cm^2 by planimetry. The pressure half-time is 245 ms, giving a calculated valve area of 0.9 cm^2. The mean transmitral pressure drop is 14 mmHg. There is mild associated mitral regurgitation. The left atrium is severely dilated at 5.6 cm, and there is spontaneous echo contrast (the patient is also noted to be in atrial fibrillation). Left ventricular dimensions are normal with good systolic function. There is mild tricuspid regurgitation with an elevated pulmonary artery systolic pressure of 56 mmHg. The findings are consistent with severe mitral stenosis potentially suitable for balloon mitral valvuloplasty.

Management of mitral stenosis

Echo surveillance

Patients with asymptomatic but significant mitral stenosis should be advised to report symptoms immediately and should have annual clinical and echo evaluations.

Drug therapy

There is no specific drug therapy to reverse mitral stenosis, but diuretics are useful in treating breathlessness. Anticoagulation is important in those in AF and with thrombus in the LA.

Surgery

Patients with symptomatic severe mitral stenosis symptoms should be considered for intervention. If the valve is suitable this usually takes the form of percutaneous balloon mitral valvuloplasty (PBMV, p. 231). If unsuitable for this technique, surgical intervention can be offered.

Mitral regurgitation

Mitral regurgitation is the flow of blood from the LV back through the mitral valve during systole. Mitral regurgitation can result from dysfunction of any part of the mitral valve apparatus: the leaflets, annulus, papillary muscles or chordae tendineae. Different pathologies tend to affect different parts of the valve apparatus, and sometimes more than one part is affected.

Causes of mitral regurgitation

A trace amount of mitral regurgitation, in the absence of any structural heart disease, is a common finding in normal individuals. More significant mitral regurgitation can be the result of:

- myxomatous degeneration/mitral valve prolapse (MVP)
- rheumatic valve disease
- infective endocarditis
- ischaemic heart disease (papillary muscle dysfunction/rupture)
- mitral annular dilatation ('functional' mitral regurgitation, secondary to LV dilatation).

MVP is the single commonest cause of mitral regurgitation in the developed world, and as well as being a result of degenerative valve disease, it can also occur in collagen disorders such as Ehlers–Danlos syndrome or Marfan syndrome (Chapter 23), or papillary muscle dysfunction/rupture.

Mitral regurgitation in ischaemic heart disease can be intermittent, only occurring when an episode of myocardial ischaemia affects a papillary muscle, or it may be permanent following a myocardial infarction. It is characterized by 'tethering' of the valve during systole, causing failure of leaflet apposition. Myocardial infarction can also lead to rupture of a papillary muscle, leading to flailing of the affected leaflet segments (the attached portion of ruptured muscle can usually be seen swinging between atrium and ventricle on its chordal attachments), often with disastrous clinical consequences for the patient.

Rare causes of mitral regurgitation include:

- congenital (e.g. cleft mitral valve, which may be associated with a primum ASD)
- systemic lupus erythematosus
- osteogenesis imperfecta
- mitral annular calcification.

Clinical features of mitral regurgitation

The clinical features of mitral regurgitation are summarized in Table 14.3. Chronic mitral regurgitation places a volume overload on the LV, which, with time, dilates and becomes increasingly impaired, leading to an increase in LA pressure, at which point the patient develops symptoms. Pulmonary hypertension can ensue. Infective endocarditis and papillary muscle or chordal rupture can cause acute mitral regurgitation, in which the abrupt volume overload increases LV filling pressure and can lead to acute pulmonary oedema.

Table 14.3 Clinical features of mitral regurgitation (MR)

Symptoms	Signs
May be asymptomatic Symptoms of heart failure: breathlessness; orthopnoea; paroxysmal nocturnal dyspnoea; fatigue Symptoms may be insidious (chronic MR) or abrupt (acute MR) Symptoms may also indicate the aetiology (e.g. myocardial infarction, infective endocarditis)	Atrial fibrillation may be present Displaced apex beat (as a result of left ventricular dilatation) Pansystolic murmur, heard at apex and radiating to axilla Mid-late systolic click followed by late systolic murmur (mitral valve prolapse) Signs of heart failure in advanced (or acute) cases

Echo assessment of mitral regurgitation

2-D and M-mode

Use 2-D and M-mode echo to assess the structure of the valve and the subvalvular apparatus. Be sure to describe the appearance of the mitral leaflets, mitral annulus, chordae tendineae and papillary muscles:

- Do the mitral valve leaflets appear normal? Is there evidence of rheumatic valve disease, or of myxomatous degeneration?

- Does the mitral annulus appear normal? Is the annulus dilated? Is there annular calcification, and is this mild, moderate or severe?
- Is there any thickening of the leaflets? Is this mild, moderate or severe? Are both leaflets affected, and does this affect the tip or body of each leaflet?
- Is there any calcification of the leaflets? Is this focal or diffuse? Does the calcification affect either or both of the commissures?
- Are the chordae tendineae normal? Is there any chordal elongation or rupture? Does this affect the chordae to the anterior or posterior leaflet?
- Are the papillary muscles normal? Is there any rupture or partial rupture?
- Is mitral leaflet mobility normal? Is there any leaflet prolapse (see box)?
- Are there any vegetations? Where are they located? Are they mobile and/or pedunculated? What are their dimensions?
- Is there any evidence of an abscess or a mass? Where is it located? What are its dimensions?

MITRAL VALVE PROLAPSE

MVP should be diagnosed when:

- any part of either leaflet moves >2 mm behind the plane of the mitral annulus in the parasternal long axis view

or

- the coaptation point of the leaflets moves behind the annular plane in the apical 4-chamber view.

The population prevalence of MVP is around 2 per cent. As well as mitral regurgitation, MVP has also been associated with autonomic dysfunction (Barlow's syndrome) with symptoms including palpitations and syncope. In describing MVP, comment on:

- the leaflet scallops that are affected
- whether the prolapse is mild/moderate/severe
- the extent of any mitral regurgitation, and the direction of the regurgitant jet.

A **flail leaflet** usually results from rupture of a chordae tendineae or papillary muscle, and should be distinguished from MVP. The tip of a flail leaflet will point upwards into the atrium, whereas the tip of a prolapsing leaflet continues to point downwards towards the ventricle.

Using M-mode in mitral regurgitation, assess:

- Are the leaflet tips thickened?
- Is there evidence of MVP?

Colour Doppler

Use colour Doppler to examine the jet of mitral regurgitation in the parasternal (Fig. 14.5) and apical views. Describe:

- how far the regurgitant jet extends back into the LA – trace the area of the jet and of the LA
- the position of the jet in relation to the mitral leaflets (e.g. central jet, or evidence of regurgitation through a leaflet perforation)
- the direction of travel of the regurgitant jet (Fig. 14.6) within the atrium (central, anteriorly directed, posteriorly directed) and whether it impinges on the atrial wall or flows retrogradely up a pulmonary vein. Eccentric jets are usually directed *away from* the abnormal leaflet (e.g. anterior leaflet prolapse gives rise to a posteriorly directed jet).

Central jets can appear more severe than they really are on colour Doppler because of entrainment – blood cells along the sides of the jet are drawn along with the regurgitant blood. Conversely, eccentric jets that impinge on the LA wall can appear less severe than they are, because they cannot entrain blood cells on the side of the jet that hits the wall.

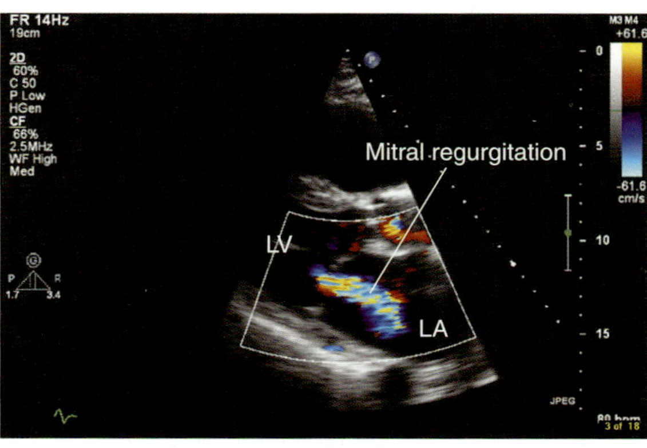

View	Parasternal long axis
Modality	Colour Doppler

Fig. 14.5 Mitral regurgitation (LA = left atrium; LV = left ventricle)

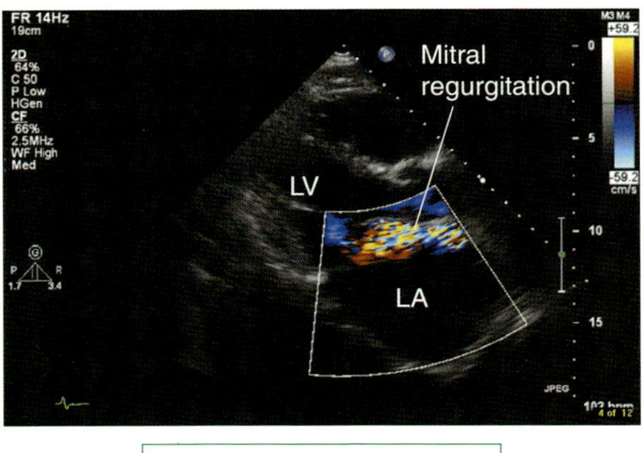

View	Parasternal long axis
Modality	Colour Doppler

Fig. 14.6 Mitral valve prolapse with eccentric (anterior) jet of mitral regurgitation (LA = left atrium; LV = left ventricle)

Measure the width of the vena contracta (VC) – the narrowest region of colour flow at the level of the mitral valve – in the parasternal long axis or apical 4-chamber or 3-chamber view. This helps gauge severity even if the jet is eccentric, but it cannot be used to assess the severity of multiple regurgitant jets. VC should *not* be measured in the apical 2-chamber view, as this runs parallel to the mitral orifice and the VC will appear wider than it is.

It is important to use appropriate (and consistent) colour gain settings for these assessments to avoid under/overestimating severity. For measurement of jet area and VC width, a Nyquist limit setting of 50–60 cm/s is usually appropriate.

CW and PW Doppler

Record the CW Doppler trace in the apical 4-chamber view, with the probe carefully aligned with the direction of the regurgitant jet (Fig. 14.7). The CW Doppler trace is faint in mild mitral regurgitation, and denser in moderate or severe regurgitation. The velocity of the regurgitant jet is usually high (e.g. 5 m/s) and, in chronic mitral regurgitation, remains high throughout systole. By contrast, in acute mitral regurgitation the jet velocity starts to fall towards the end of systole, as the pressure gradient between the ventricle and the LA equalizes more rapidly than it does in chronic mitral regurgitation. The LA (and LV) is usually non-dilated in acute regurgitation as it has not had time to dilate.

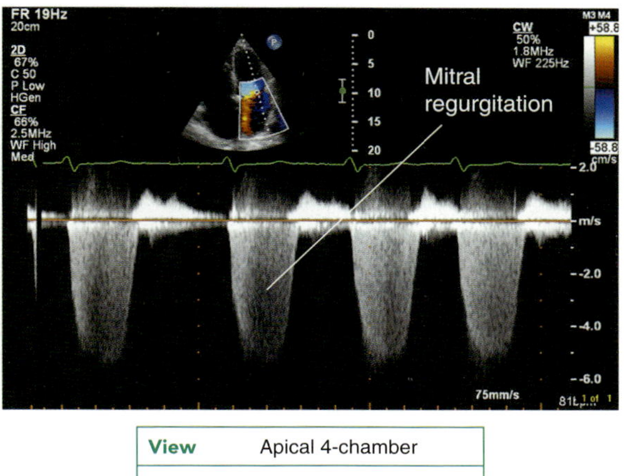

View	Apical 4-chamber
Modality	CW Doppler

Fig. 14.7 Mitral regurgitation

PW Doppler can be used to obtain a VTI of mitral valve inflow and LVOT outflow (which are necessary for calculation of regurgitant volume, see below). PW Doppler can also be used to assess flow, where possible, in the pulmonary veins. The pulmonary veins are reasonably easy to assess with transoesophageal echo, but somewhat harder with transthoracic echo. It is however usually possible to locate one or other of the right pulmonary veins in the corner of the LA, adjacent to the interatrial septum, in the apical 4-chamber view. Place the PW Doppler sample volume 1 cm into the pulmonary vein and obtain a recording (Fig. 14.8). Normally the systolic (S) wave is larger than the diastolic (D) wave: if the D wave is larger, then there is blunting of forward flow in the pulmonary vein; if the S wave is inverted, there is systolic flow reversal (indicative of severe mitral regurgitation).

Regurgitant volume

The volume of blood entering the LV via the mitral valve during diastole should normally equal the volume of blood leaving the LV via the LVOT (stroke volume) in systole. In the presence of mitral regurgitation, LVOT outflow will be less than mitral valve inflow as the LVOT outflow will be missing the regurgitant volume of blood that has re-entered the LA. The difference between mitral valve inflow and LVOT outflow gives the regurgitant volume.

As with any assessment of valvular regurgitant volume, any error in measurement of mitral valve orifice area or LVOT diameter can have a large

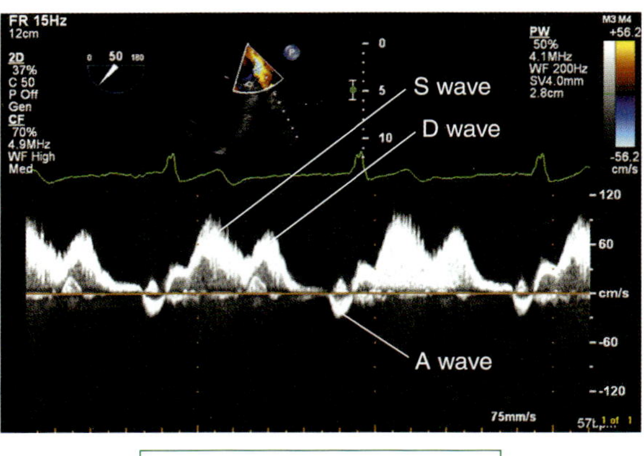

View	Transoesophageal echo – left upper pulmonary vein view
Modality	PW Doppler

Fig. 14.8 Normal pulmonary vein flow (transoesophageal echo)

impact on the result. Calculation of regurgitant volume is not appropriate if there is significant coexistent aortic regurgitation.

To measure mitral valve regurgitant volume:

1. In the apical 4-chamber view, measure the diameter of the mitral annulus in cm, and then use this to calculate the CSA of the mitral valve in cm^2. This calculation makes the assumption that the mitral orifice is circular:

$$CSA_{MV} = 0.785 \times (\text{mitral annulus diameter})^2$$

2. In the apical 4-chamber view, measure the VTI of mitral valve inflow (using PW Doppler) to give VTI_{MV}, in cm. It is generally easiest to place the sample volume at the valve tips (some place it at the level of the mitral valve annulus).
3. The stroke volume of the mitral valve (SV_{MV}), in mL/beat, can then be calculated from:

$$SV_{MV} = CSA_{MV} \times VTI_{MV}$$

4. In the parasternal long axis view, measure the diameter of the LVOT in cm, and then use this to calculate the CSA of the LVOT in cm^2:

$$CSA_{LVOT} = 0.785 \times (\text{LVOT diameter})^2$$

5. In the apical 5-chamber view, measure the VTI of LVOT outflow (using PW Doppler) to give VTI_{LVOT}, in cm.
6. The stroke volume of the LVOT (SV_{LVOT}), in mL/beat, can then be calculated from:

$$SV_{LVOT} = CSA_{LVOT} \times VTI_{LVOT}$$

7. Mitral regurgitant volume (RV) can be calculated from:

$$RV = SV_{MV} - SV_{LVOT}$$

8. Mitral regurgitant fraction (RF) can be calculated from:

$$RF = \frac{RV}{SV_{MV}} \text{ (}\times 100 \text{ to express as a percentage)}$$

Once you have calculated the mitral RV, you can also calculate the regurgitant orifice area (ROA). This is the average size of the orifice in the mitral valve, in cm^2, through which the regurgitation occurs during systole, and equals the mitral RV (in mL) divided by the VTI of the mitral regurgitation Doppler trace (VTI_{MR}), measured in cm using CW Doppler:

$$ROA = \frac{RV}{VTI_{MR}}$$

Proximal isovelocity surface area (PISA) assessment

The use of PISA has been well validated in the assessment of mitral regurgitation. The principle behind PISA is that blood flowing towards a circular orifice converges to form a series of hemispheric shells, each of which gets smaller and faster as it approaches the orifice. If the aliasing velocity (Nyquist limit) of the echo machine is adjusted it can be made to match the velocity of blood flow in the 'shells' – there will be a blue–red interface at the point in the series of shells where aliasing occurs, and at that position the velocity of blood flow equals the aliasing velocity you have selected (Fig. 14.9). Knowing the velocity of blood flow at that point, and calculating the surface area of the relevant hemisphere, you can calculate regurgitant flow rate:

1. Using colour Doppler in the apical 4-chamber view, narrow down the sector width and minimize the depth before zooming in on the location of the regurgitant jet through the mitral valve. Adjust the aliasing velocity by adjusting the zero point on the colour flow scale until you see

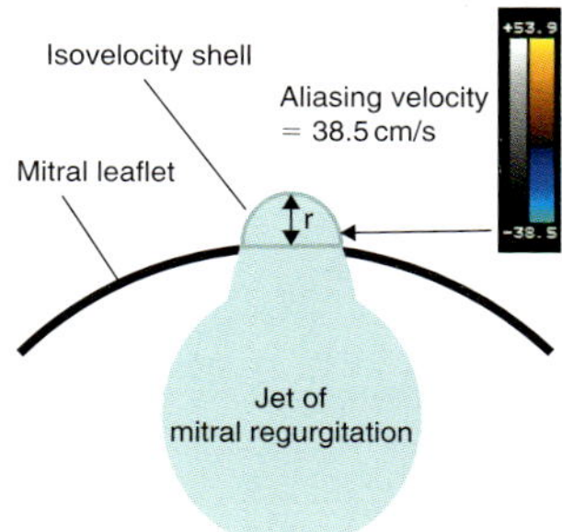

Fig. 14.9 The proximal isovelocity surface area (PISA) method uses the surface area of a hemispheric 'shell' of uniform velocity and the aliasing velocity to calculate regurgitant flow rate (r = shell radius)

a clear hemisphere of converging blood flow on the ventricular side of the valve, usually at a setting of 20–40 cm/s. There should be a clear interface between red- and blue-coloured flow, and the velocity of blood flow at this point equals the aliasing velocity (in cm/s).

2. Measure the radius (r) of this hemisphere by taking a measurement from the edge of the hemisphere (i.e. the red–blue interface) to the centre of the valve orifice. Use this to calculate PISA, the surface area of this hemisphere, in cm^2:

$$\text{PISA} = 2\pi r^2$$

3. The regurgitant flow rate, in mL/s, can be calculated from:

$$\text{Regurgitant flow rate} = \text{PISA} \times \text{aliasing velocity}$$

4. Next, use CW Doppler to measure the maximum velocity of the mitral regurgitant jet (V_{MR}) in cm/s. Use this to calculate regurgitant orifice area (ROA) in cm^2:

$$\text{ROA} = \frac{\text{Regurgitant flow rate}}{V_{MR}}$$

The PISA technique should not be used if a clear symmetrical hemisphere cannot be obtained or if the jet of mitral regurgitation is eccentric.

Associated features

If mitral regurgitation is present you should:

- assess any coexistent mitral stenosis
- assess any coexistent disease affecting the other valves (as patients undergoing mitral valve surgery may also require any other valvular abnormalities to be corrected at the same time)

COMMON PITFALLS

Pitfalls in the echo assessment of mitral regurgitation include:

- Measuring regurgitant jet area or VC width on colour Doppler with inappropriate colour gain settings.
- Underestimating the severity of eccentric jets on colour Doppler.
- Failure to align the Doppler beam with regurgitant flow during CW Doppler interrogation.
- Inaccurate measurement of mitral valve orifice area or LVOT diameter when calculating RV.
- Trying to calculate RV when there is coexistent aortic regurgitation.
- Using the PISA method to assess eccentric jets.
- Failure to average several readings when the patient is in AF.

- assess LA size – the LA dilates in chronic mitral regurgitation
- assess LV dimensions and function
- assess the right heart for evidence of pulmonary hypertension, and comment on right atrial and ventricular size.

Severity of mitral regurgitation

Severity of mitral regurgitation can be assessed by:

- jet area
- ratio of jet area to left atrial area
- VC width
- PISA radius
- RV
- RF
- ROA.

Table 14.4 summarizes the echo indicators of mitral regurgitation severity.

Indirect indicators that point towards more severe mitral regurgitation include:

- LA dilatation
- LV dilatation/dysfunction
- pulmonary vein systolic flow reversal
- pulmonary hypertension.

Table 14.4 Indicators of mitral regurgitation severity

	Mild	Moderate	Severe
Colour Doppler			
Jet area (cm^2, at Nyquist 50–60 cm/s)	<4	–	>10
Ratio of jet area to left atrial area (%)	<20	–	>40
Vena contracta width (cm)	<0.3	–	⩾0.7
PISA radius (cm, at Nyquist 40 cm/s)	<0.4	–	>1.0
Multimodality			
Regurgitant volume (mL/beat)	<30	30–59	⩾60
Regurgitant fraction (%)	<30	30–49	⩾50
Effective regurgitant orifice area (cm^2)	<0.20	0.20–0.39	⩾0.40

Reference ranges reproduced with permission of the British Society of Echocardiography and British Heart Foundation.

SAMPLE REPORT

There is myxomatous degeneration of the mitral valve leaflets. The chordae tendineae and papillary muscles appear normal. There is an extensive central jet of mitral regurgitation (jet area 11 cm^2 occupying 52 per cent of left atrial area) causing systolic flow reversal in the right upper pulmonary vein. The vena contracta width is 0.9 cm and the PISA radius is 1.2 cm. The regurgitant volume is 74 mL/beat (regurgitant fraction 57 per cent) with an effective orifice area of 0.45 cm^2. The left ventricle is mildly dilated with mildly impaired systolic function (ejection fraction 48 per cent). The pulmonary artery systolic pressure is 38 mmHg. The findings indicate severe mitral regurgitation secondary to myxomatous degeneration.

Management of mitral regurgitation

Echo surveillance

- Asymptomatic patients with moderate mitral regurgitation (and normal LV function) should be seen annually and have an echo every 2 years.
- Asymptomatic patients with severe mitral regurgitation (and normal LV function) should be seen every 6 months and have an echo every year.

Drug therapy and surgery

In patients with mitral regurgitation and heart failure, standard heart failure treatment (e.g. angiotensin-converting enzyme (ACE) inhibitors and beta-blockers) should be considered as usual. For those with preserved

LV function, there is no role for the routine use of drugs. Those with AF should be treated with anticoagulation.

Where patients require mitral valve surgery, valve repair is, where feasible, generally considered superior to valve replacement. For patients with severe symptomatic mitral regurgitation secondary to disease of the mitral leaflets, surgery should be considered if the LV ejection fraction (LVEF) is >30 per cent and the LV end-systolic diameter (LVESD) <5.5 cm. Those with severe LV dysfunction (LVEF <30 per cent and/or LVESD >5.5 cm) should first undergo optimization of medical therapy, with surgery considered if this fails and the likelihood of a durable repair is thought to be good.

In asymptomatic patients, mitral valve surgery should be considered if there is evidence of any of the following:

- AF
- LV dysfunction (LVEF <60 per cent and/or LVESD >4.5 cm)
- Pulmonary hypertension (resting pulmonary artery systolic pressure >50 mmHg).

MITRAL REGURGITATION AND 3-D ECHO

3-D echo is proving to be extremely useful in assessing mitral valve disease and in planning surgery. It offers more accurate visualisation and measurement of valve orifice area in mitral stenosis, and better assessment of the geometry of the mitral valve apparatus in assessing the cause of mitral regurgitation. Combining 3-D echo with colour Doppler is helpful in determining the origin and direction of regurgitant jets.

Ischaemic mitral regurgitation

Rupture of a papillary muscle following acute myocardial infarction requires urgent stabilization (intra-aortic balloon pump and vasodilators) followed by urgent surgery. In chronic ischaemic mitral regurgitation, it is generally agreed that severe regurgitation should be corrected at the time of coronary artery bypass surgery. In moderate ischaemic regurgitation the management strategies are more controversial.

Functional mitral regurgitation

Drug therapy is the mainstay of treatment in functional mitral regurgitation secondary to cardiomyopathy, although mitral valve surgery (in combination with LV reconstruction) may be considered in those with severe functional regurgitation and severely impaired LV function.

FURTHER READING

Grayburn PA. How to measure severity of mitral regurgitation. *Heart* 2008; **94**: 376–83.

Khattar R. *British Society of Echocardiography Distance Learning Module 7: Mitral Stenosis*. Accessible from the BSE website (www.bsecho.org).

Otto CM. Timing of surgery in mitral regurgitation. *Heart* 2003; **89**: 100–5.

Prendergast BD, Shaw TRD, Iung B, *et al*. Contemporary criteria for the selection of patients for percutaneous balloon mitral valvuloplasty. *Heart* 2002; **87**: 401–4.

The Task Force on the Management of Valvular Heart Disease of the European Society of Cardiology. Guidelines on the management of valvular heart disease. *Eur Heart J* 2007; **28**: 230–68.

Wilkins GT, Weyman AE, Abascal VM, *et al*. Percutaneous balloon dilatation of the mitral valve: an analysis of echocardiographic variables related to outcome and the mechanism of dilatation. *Br Heart J* 1988; **60**: 299–308.

Zoghbi WA, Enriquez-Sarano M, Foster E, *et al*. 2003. American Society of Echocardiography: Recommendations for evaluation of the severity of native valvular regurgitation with two-dimensional and Doppler echocardiography. *J Am Soc Echocardiogr* 2003; **16**: 777–802.

15 The right heart

The right heart tends to be a relatively neglected part of the standard transthoracic echo study, because:

- much of the right heart lies behind the sternum, making it difficult to image using ultrasound
- the anatomy and orientation of the right heart is relatively complex, compared with the left
- the right ventricle (RV) is trabeculated, which makes accurate measurements difficult.

Nonetheless, an assessment of right heart dimensions and function is an essential part of the standard echo study, not only to detect primary right heart disorders but also because right heart size and function can reveal a great deal about disorders affecting other parts of the heart (e.g. mitral valve disease, atrial septal defect (ASD)).

Right atrium

The right atrium (RA) receives venous blood returning from the upper body (via the superior vena cava, SVC), the lower body (via the inferior vena cava, IVC) and also from the myocardium (via the coronary sinus). It can best be seen in:

- parasternal RV inflow view (Fig. 6.3, p. 57)
- parasternal short axis view (aortic valve level) (Fig. 6.5, p. 60)
- apical 4-chamber view (Fig. 6.8, p. 63)
- subcostal view (Fig. 6.12, p. 67).

When studying the RA, assess and describe:

- RA size
- RA pressure
- normal variants (Eustachian valve/Chiari network)
- presence or absence of masses (tumour/thrombus)
- presence or absence of a pacing wire or venous catheter.

Right atrial size

Assessment of RA size can be challenging in view of the difficulty in imaging it clearly. In an apical 4-chamber view you can simply 'eyeball' the relative sizes of the left and right atria. The RA is normally no larger than the left – if it is larger, it is dilated.

To quantify RA size, in the apical 4-chamber view measure the RA minor axis from the lateral wall of the RA to the interatrial septum (perpendicular to the RA major axis, Fig. 15.1). Normal values are given in Table 15.1. Alternatively, perform planimetry of the RA in the apical 4-chamber view – a normal RA has an area $<20\ cm^2$.

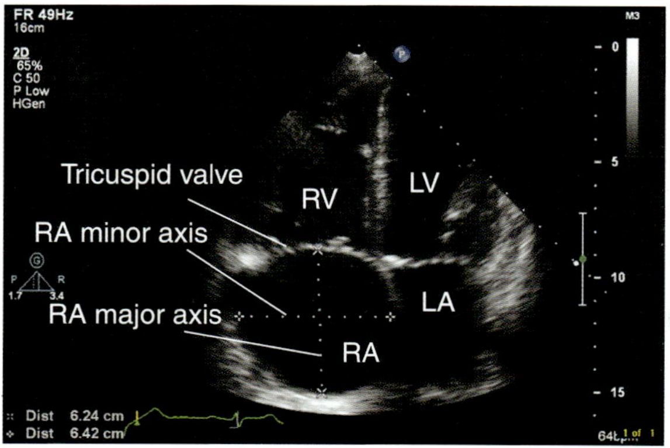

View	Apical 4-chamber
Modality	2-D

Fig. 15.1 Measurement of right atrial dimensions (LA = left atrium; LV = left ventricle; RA = right atrium; RV = right ventricle)

Table 15.1 Assessment of right atrial (RA) size

	Normal	Mildly dilated	Moderately dilated	Severely dilated
RA minor axis (cm)	2.9–4.5	4.6–4.9	5.0–5.4	⩾5.5
RA minor axis/BSA (cm/m^2)	1.7–2.5	2.6–2.8	2.9–3.1	⩾3.2

Reprinted from *Journal of the American Society of Echocardiography*, **18**, Lang RM, Bierig M, Devereux RB, *et al.*, Recommendations for chamber quantification, 1440–63, © 2005, with permission from Elsevier.

RA dilatation can result from RA pressure overload (e.g. pulmonary hypertension, restrictive cardiomyopathy, tricuspid stenosis), RA volume overload (e.g. tricuspid regurgitation, ASD) and chronic atrial fibrillation (AF).

Right atrial pressure

There are a number of ways of assessing RA pressure (RAP):

1. The RAP can be gauged by examining the patient's neck to assess their jugular venous pressure (JVP) – with the patient reclining supine at 45°, the height of the JVP above the sternal angle (in cm) is the same as RAP (in mmHg). However, the height of the JVP can be tricky to assess, particularly if the JVP is not clearly visible or if it is very high or low.
2. A 'constant' value of 10 mmHg can be 'assumed' as the RAP. However, RAP does vary, and so using a 'constant' value is rather a blunt instrument and can be potentially misleading.
3. The best approach is to estimate RAP using the IVC. In the subcostal window, look at the IVC and measure its diameter in both expiration and inspiration (Fig. 15.2). Normally the IVC measures 1.5–2.5 cm in diameter and decreases by >50 per cent in inspiration. The data in Table 15.2 will allow you to place an approximate value on RAP.

For example, if the IVC measures 2.8 cm in expiration and 1.8 cm in inspiration, a reduction of 36 per cent, the RAP would be estimated at 15–20 mmHg.

Another indicator of RAP is RA size, which is usually normal when RAP is ⩽10 mmHg, but becomes dilated at pressures above this (and, in general, the higher the RAP, the greater the dilatation). Similarly, the hepatic veins become increasingly dilated as RAP rises above 15 mmHg.

Eustachian valve and Chiari network

Where the IVC enters the RA there is often an embryological remnant, the **Eustachian valve**, which in fetal life directs oxygenated blood away from

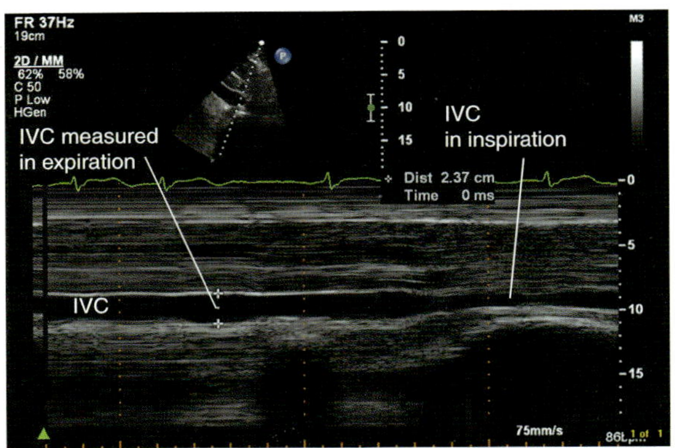

View	Subcostal (IVC view)
Modality	M-mode

Fig. 15.2 Measurement of inferior vena cava (IVC) diameter

Table 15.2 Assessment of right atrial pressure (RAP)

IVC size (cm)	IVC change with inspiration	Estimated RAP (mmHg)
Small (<1.5 cm)	Collapse	0–5
Normal (1.5–2.5 cm)	Decreased by >50%	5–10
Normal (1.5–2.5 cm)	Decreased by <50%	10–15
Dilated (>2.5 cm)	Decreased by <50%	15–20
Dilated (>2.5 cm)	No change	>20

IVC, inferior vena cava.

Reference ranges reproduced with permission of the British Society of Echocardiography and British Heart Foundation.

the tricuspid valve and towards the foramen ovale. The Eustachian valve can remain prominent in adult life and is a normal finding, but can be mistaken for a mass, thrombus or vegetation.

Similarly, a **Chiari network** is a fetal remnant and appears as a web-like structure extending into the RA with an attachment near the RA–IVC junction. It is present in around 2 per cent of the population as a normal variant but can be mistaken for a more sinister lesion.

Usually neither a prominent Eustachian valve nor a Chiari network is of any clinical significance, although there is some evidence that either remnant in combination with a patent foramen ovale may increase the risk of paradoxical (right-to-left) embolism.

Right atrial masses

Cardiac tumours and thrombi are described in Chapter 21. Renal cell carcinoma can extend from the kidney all the way up the IVC and into the RA.

Tricuspid valve

The tricuspid valve can best be seen in:

- parasternal RV inflow view (Fig. 6.3, p. 57)
- parasternal short axis view (aortic valve level) (Fig. 15.3)
- apical 4-chamber view (Fig. 6.8, p. 63)
- subcostal view (Fig. 6.12, p. 67).

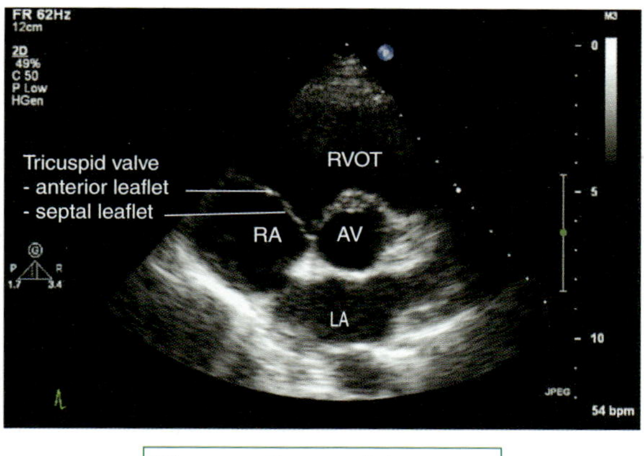

View	Parasternal short axis (aortic value level)
Modality	2-D

Fig. 15.3 Normal tricuspid valve (LA = left atrium; RA = right atrium; AV = aortic valve; RVOT = right ventricular outflow tract)

Tricuspid stenosis

Tricuspid stenosis is most commonly a consequence of previous rheumatic fever, and usually occurs together with mitral stenosis (indeed it is important not to 'miss' coexistent tricuspid stenosis in patients undergoing surgery for mitral stenosis). Rheumatic thickening of the tricuspid leaflets tends to be subtler than that of the mitral leaflets and so is harder to spot. Rarer causes of tricuspid stenosis include:

- carcinoid syndrome
- Ebstein's anomaly (see Chapter 22)
- 'functional' tricuspid stenosis as a result of obstruction of the valve by a large RA tumour, thrombus or vegetation.

Patients may present with fatigue, peripheral oedema or symptoms relating to an underlying cause (e.g. flushing in carcinoid syndrome) or coexistent condition (e.g. mitral stenosis). Physical signs include a prominent 'a' wave in the JVP, a tricuspid opening snap and a diastolic murmur at the left sternal edge.

Echo assessment of tricuspid stenosis

2-D and M-mode

Use 2-D and M-mode echo to assess the structure of the valve:

- Is the tricuspid valve normal, rheumatic or myxomatous?
- Is there evidence of Ebstein's anomaly (p. 307)?
- Are the valve leaflets (anterior, posterior, septal) normal? Is there thickening, and does this affects the tips or the body of the leaflet(s)?
- Is there leaflet calcification, and is this focal (anterior, posterior, septal) or diffuse?
- Is leaflet mobility normal or reduced? How much is it reduced?
- Is there any doming or prolapse of the leaflets?
- Is there any evidence of papillary muscle rupture?
- Are there any tricuspid valve vegetations or abscesses?
- Is the tricuspid annulus normal, dilated or calcified?

Colour Doppler

Use colour Doppler to look for any coexistent tricuspid regurgitation. The colour jet can also help in obtaining correct alignment of the probe for continuous wave (CW) and pulsed-wave (PW) Doppler recordings.

CW and PW Doppler

Use Doppler to record forward flow through the tricuspid valve from an apical 4-chamber view. Ignore traces obtained from ectopic beats (and the beat following an ectopic), and if the patient is in AF, you should average measurements taken from several beats. From the trace, measure the mean tricuspid valve gradient (trace the velocity time integral (VTI) of the tricuspid inflow).

Severity of tricuspid stenosis

Severity of tricuspid stenosis can be quantified by:

- mean tricuspid gradient
- tricuspid valve area.

The calculation of tricuspid valve area is somewhat controversial – estimation of valve area from pressure half-time (as for mitral stenosis) is not as well validated for tricuspid stenosis and many authors advise against using it for the tricuspid valve. If you do wish to use it, it can be calculated from:

$$\text{Tricuspid valve area (cm}^2\text{)} = \frac{190}{\text{Tricuspid presssure half-time (ms)}}$$

Table 15.3 summarizes the echo indicators of tricuspid stenosis severity.

Table 15.3 Indicators of tricuspid stenosis severity

	Normal	Severe
Tricuspid mean gradient (mmHg)	–	≥5
Tricuspid valve area (cm^2)	>7.0	<1.0

Reference ranges reproduced with permission of the British Society of Echocardiography and British Heart Foundation.

Tricuspid regurgitation

Tricuspid regurgitation is the flow of blood from the RV back through the tricuspid valve during systole. Tricuspid regurgitation can result from dysfunction of the tricuspid valve leaflets or their supporting structure. A trace amount of tricuspid regurgitation, in the absence of any structural heart disease, is a common finding in normal individuals. More significant tricuspid regurgitation can be the result of:

- rheumatic valve disease
- carcinoid syndrome
- infective endocarditis
- tricuspid valve prolapse
- Ebstein's anomaly (Chapter 22)
- tricuspid annular dilatation ('functional' tricuspid regurgitation, secondary to RV dilatation).

The presence of a pacing wire which passes through the tricuspid valve can also lead to a degree of regurgitation, by preventing full closure of the valve leaflets.

Significant tricuspid regurgitation can cause symptoms and signs of right-sided heart failure, with a prominent V wave in the jugular venous pressure, peripheral oedema, ascites and a distended pulsatile liver.

i CARCINOID SYNDROME AND THE HEART

Carcinoid tumours are rare and usually arise in the gastrointestinal system. If they metastasize they can produce the carcinoid syndrome, in which secretion of vasoactive substances such as 5-hydroxytryptamine causes flushing, diarrhoea and bronchospasm. These substances can also affect the heart, leading to the development of fibrous endocardial plaques, typically on the right-sided valves and chambers. The tricuspid and pulmonary valve leaflets characteristically become shortened and thickened, leading to stenosis and/or regurgitation and ultimately right heart failure.

Echo assessment of tricuspid regurgitation

2-D and M-mode

Use 2-D and M-mode echo to assess the structure of the valve as described for tricuspid stenosis (above). Remember to look at the whole valve apparatus (tricuspid annulus, papillary muscles and chordae), not just the leaflets.

Colour Doppler

Use colour Doppler to examine the jet of tricuspid regurgitation in the parasternal and apical (Fig. 15.4) views. Describe:

- the extent of the regurgitant jet within the RA (trace the area of the jet in the apical 4-chamber view)
- the position of the jet in relation to the tricuspid leaflets (e.g. central jet, or evidence of regurgitation through a leaflet perforation)
- the direction of travel of the regurgitant jet within the atrium (central or directed towards the interatrial septum or the RA free wall).

Measure the width of the vena contracta (VC) – the narrowest region of colour flow at the level of the tricuspid valve – in the apical 4-chamber view and with the Nyquist limit set at 50–60 cm/s.

CW and PW Doppler

Record the CW Doppler trace with the probe carefully aligned with the direction of the regurgitant jet (Fig. 15.5). The CW Doppler trace is soft in

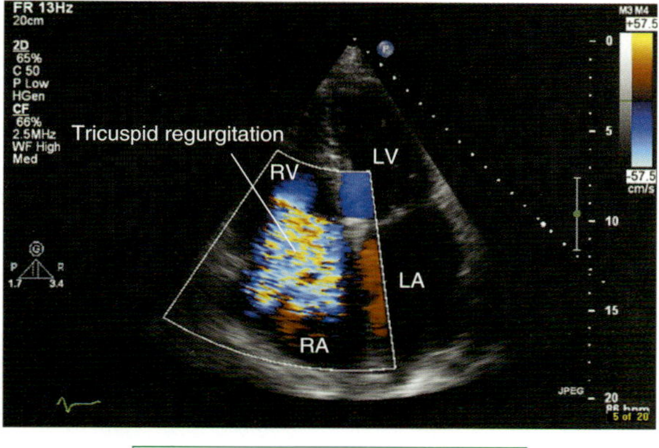

View	Apical 4-chamber
Modality	Colour Doppler

Fig. 15.4 Severe tricuspid regurgitation (LA = left atrium; RA = right atrium; LV = left ventricle; RV = right ventricle)

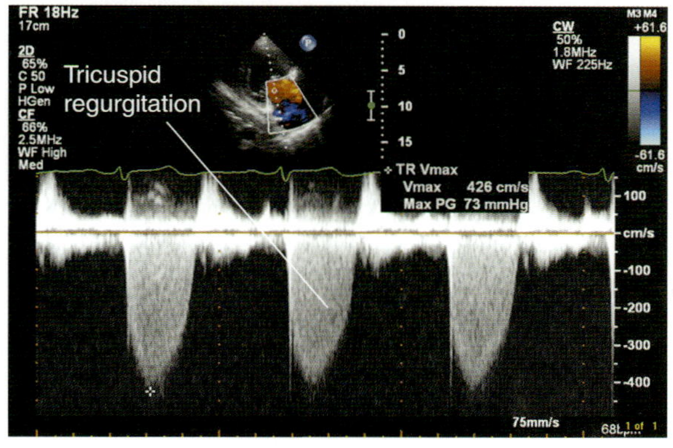

View	Parasternal right ventricular inflow
Modality	CW Doppler

Fig. 15.5 Moderate tricuspid regurgitation (TR), showing measurement of peak velocity (TR V_{max}) (PG = pressure gradient)

mild tricuspid regurgitation and denser in moderate or severe regurgitation. Look at the contour of the regurgitant jet – in mild tricuspid regurgitation the shape of the waveform is parabolic, but in severe regurgitation the shape becomes more triangular with an early peak.

The peak velocity of the tricuspid regurgitant jet reflects RV systolic pressure and can be used to calculate pulmonary artery systolic pressure (see below).

Use PW Doppler to assess hepatic vein flow, ideally in the central hepatic vein, in the subcostal window (Fig. 15.6). Hepatic vein flow is normally directed towards the RA throughout the cardiac cycle, with the systolic component being predominant. Systolic hepatic vein flow becomes blunted in moderate tricuspid regurgitation and reversed in severe regurgitation.

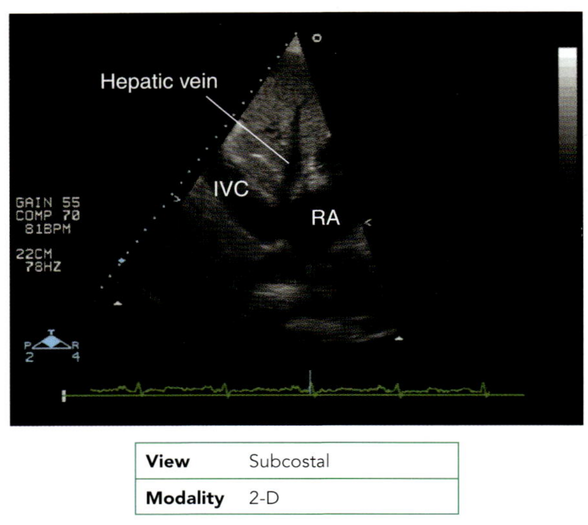

View	Subcostal
Modality	2-D

Fig. 15.6 Hepatic veins (IVC = inferior vena cava; RA = right atrium)

PISA assessment

The proximal isovelocity surface area (PISA) principle can be used for tricuspid regurgitation as for mitral regurgitation (Chapter 14):

1. Using colour Doppler in the apical 4-chamber view, narrow down the sector width and minimize the depth before zooming in on the location of the regurgitant jet through the tricuspid valve. Adjust the aliasing velocity by adjusting the zero point on the colour flow scale until you see a clear hemisphere of converging blood flow on the ventricular side of the valve, usually at a setting of 20–40 cm/s. There should be a clear interface between red- and blue-coloured flow, and the velocity of blood flow at this point equals the aliasing velocity (in cm/s).

2. Measure the radius (r) of this hemisphere by taking a measurement from the edge of the hemisphere (i.e. the red–blue interface) to the centre of the valve orifice. Use this to calculate PISA, the surface area of this hemisphere, in cm^2:

$$PISA = 2\pi r^2$$

3. The regurgitant flow rate, in mL/s, can be calculated from:

$$\text{Regurgitant flow rate} = \text{PISA} \times \text{aliasing velocity}$$

For the purposes of estimating severity, it is sufficient just to measure the PISA radius. A radius >0.9 cm indicates severe regurgitation. The PISA technique should not be used if a clear symmetrical hemisphere cannot be obtained or if the jet of tricuspid regurgitation is eccentric.

Associated features

If tricuspid regurgitation is present you should:

- assess any coexistent tricuspid stenosis
- assess any coexistent disease affecting the other valves (as patients undergoing tricuspid valve surgery may also require any other valvular abnormalities to be corrected at the same time)
- assess the size of the RA, RV and IVC – these chambers are usually dilated if tricuspid regurgitation is severe
- Assess RV dimensions and function
- Calculate pulmonary artery systolic pressure (see below) to assess if there is pulmonary hypertension.

Severity of tricuspid regurgitation

Severity of tricuspid regurgitation can be assessed by:

- jet area
- VC width
- PISA radius
- CW Doppler jet density/contour
- RA/RV/IVC size
- hepatic vein flow.

Table 15.4 summarizes the echo indicators of tricuspid regurgitation severity.

Table 15.4 Indicators of tricuspid regurgitation severity

	Mild	Moderate	Severe
2-D			
RA/RV/IVC size	Normal	Normal/dilated	Usually dilated
Colour Doppler			
Jet area (cm^2)	<5	5–10	>10
Vena contracta width (cm)	Not defined	<0.7	≥0.7
PISA radius (cm)	≤0.5	0.6–0.9	>0.9
CW Doppler			
CW jet density	Soft	Dense	Dense
CW jet contour	Parabolic	Variable	Triangular early peaking
PW Doppler			
Hepatic vein flow	Systolic dominance	Systolic blunting	Systolic reversal

CW, continuous wave; IVC, inferior vena cava; PISA, proximal isovelocity surface area; RA, right atrium; RV, right ventricle.

Reference ranges reproduced with permission of the British Society of Echocardiography and British Heart Foundation.

SAMPLE REPORT

The tricuspid valve is rheumatic in appearance with a central jet of regurgitation. There is a dense CW Doppler trace with a triangular early-peaking contour. On colour flow the regurgitant jet area is 13 cm^2, with a vena contracta width of 0.9 cm and a PISA radius of 1.2 cm. The RA, RV and IVC are moderately dilated and there is systolic flow reversal in the hepatic vein. The pulmonary artery systolic pressure is normal at 24 mmHg. The appearances are in keeping with severe tricuspid regurgitation secondary to rheumatic valve disease.

Management of tricuspid regurgitation

Treatment with diuretics will provide symptomatic relief for patients with symptoms of fluid overload secondary to tricuspid regurgitation. Surgical repair/replacement may be necessary for severe tricuspid regurgitation (particularly in combination with surgery for coexistent mitral valve disease), or if the valve is abnormal because of infective endocarditis or Ebstein's anomaly.

Right ventricle

The RV can be challenging to assess by echo because of its shape and extensive trabeculation. The RV can best be seen in:

- parasternal long axis view (Fig. 6.2, p. 56)
- parasternal RV inflow view (Fig. 6.3, p. 57)
- parasternal RV outflow view (Fig. 6.4, p. 58)
- parasternal short axis view (aortic valve level) (Fig. 6.5, p. 60)
- parasternal short axis view (mitral valve level) (Fig. 6.6, p. 61)
- parasternal short axis view (papillary muscle level) (Fig. 6.7, p. 61)
- apical 4-chamber view (Fig. 6.8, p. 63)
- subcostal long axis view (Fig. 6.12, p. 67).

An RV assessment should include:

- RV dimensions
  - cavity size
  - wall thickness
- global systolic function
- regional systolic function
- RV masses or thrombus (see Chapter 21).

Right ventricular dimensions

Assessment of RV dimensions is commonly made qualitatively by 'eyeball', particularly in the apical 4-chamber view. In this view, the RV is normally around two-thirds the size of the left ventricle (LV); if the two ventricles appear to be the same size, the RV is dilated.

RV size can also be assessed quantitatively, and because of its complex morphology it is possible to obtain RV diameters from several different points. Use 2-D imaging to take measurements at **end-diastole** as follows:

- apical 4-chamber view (Fig. 15.7)
  - basal RV diameter (RVD1)
  - mid RV diameter (RVD2)
  - RV base-to-apex (long axis) length (RVD3)
- parasternal short axis view – aortic valve level (Fig. 15.8)
  - RV outflow tract (RVOT) diameter at aortic valve (AV) level (RVOT1)
  - RVOT diameter at pulmonary valve (PV) annulus level (RVOT2)
  - main pulmonary artery diameter (PA1).

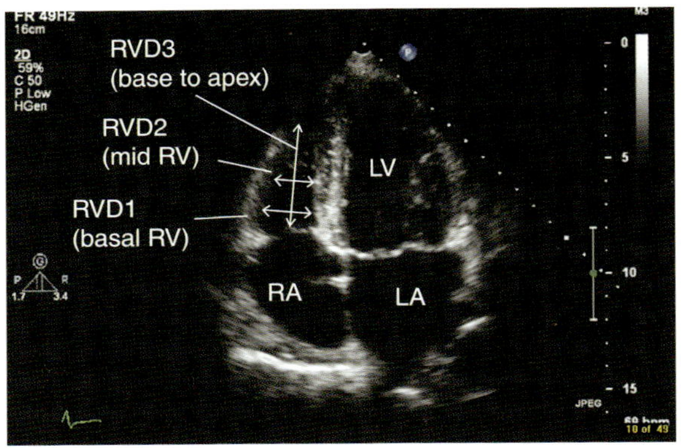

View	Apical 4-chamber
Modality	2-D

Fig. 15.7 Measurement of right ventricular dimensions (RVD) in apical 4-chamber view (LA = left atrium; RA = right atrium; LV = left ventricle)

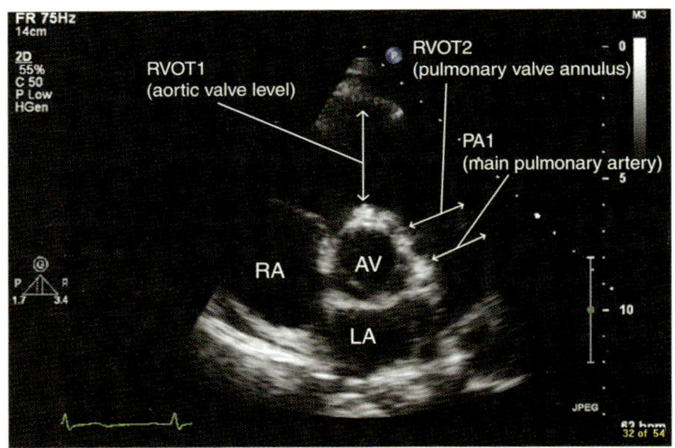

View	Parasternal short axis (aortic valve level)
Modality	2-D

Fig. 15.8 Measurement of right ventricular dimensions in parasternal short axis view (AV = aortic valve; LA = left atrium; PA1 = main pulmonary artery diameter; RA = right atrium; RVOT = right ventricular outflow tract)

The reference ranges for RV, RVOT and PA dimensions are listed in Table 15.5.

Table 15.5 RV, RVOT and PA dimensions – reference ranges

	Normal	Mild	Moderate	Severe
Apical 4-chamber view				
Basal RV diameter (RVD1) (cm)	2.0–2.8	2.9–3.3	3.4–3.8	⩾3.9
Mid RV diameter (RVD2) (cm)	2.7–3.3	3.4–3.7	3.8–4.1	⩾4.2
Base-to-apex length (RVD3) (cm)	7.1–7.9	8.0–8.5	8.6–9.1	⩾9.2
Parasternal short axis view				
RVOT at AV level (RVOT1) (cm)	2.5–2.9	3.0–3.2	3.3–3.5	⩾3.6
RVOT at PV annulus (RVOT2) (cm)	1.7–2.3	2.4–2.7	2.8–3.1	⩾3.2
Main PA (PA1) (cm)	1.5–2.1	2.2–2.5	2.6–2.9	⩾3.0

PA, pulmonary artery; PV, pulmonary valve; RV, right ventricle; RVOT, right ventricular outflow tract.

Reference ranges reproduced with permission of the British Society of Echocardiography and British Heart Foundation.

The thickness of the RV wall is ideally measured, at end-diastole, from the anterior wall of the RVOT in the parasternal long axis view (Fig. 15.9), or alternatively using the RV wall in the subcostal view. The normal RV wall thickness is <5 mm.

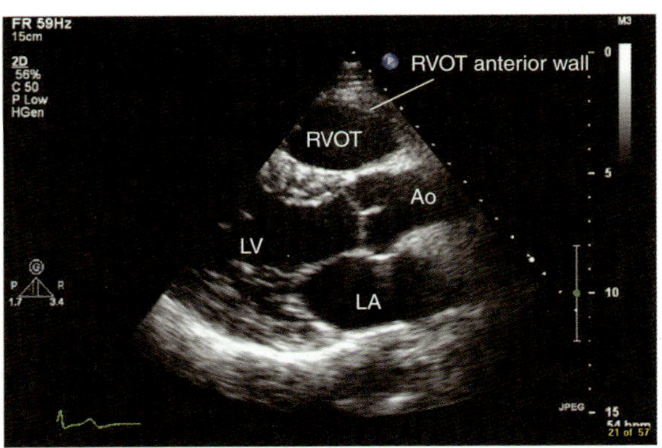

View	Parasternal long axis
Modality	2-D

Fig. 15.9 Assessment of the right ventricular outflow tract (RVOT) anterior wall (Ao = aorta; LA = left atrium; LV = left ventricle)

RV area can be measured in the apical 4-chamber view, tracing around the endocardial border to obtain an outline of the cavity area. Area should be measured at end-diastole and end-systole to allow quantitative assessment of RV function (see below). The reference ranges for RV area are listed in Table 15.6.

Table 15.6 Right ventricle (RV) area – reference ranges

	Normal	Mild	Moderate	Severe
RV end-diastolic area (cm^2)	11–28	29–32	33–37	⩾38
RV end-systolic area (cm^2)	7.5–16	17–19	20–22	⩾23

Reference ranges reproduced with permission of the British Society of Echocardiography and British Heart Foundation.

Although RV volume can be estimated using area–length or Simpson's rule methods, as for the LV, the more complex geometry of the RV means that simplifying assumptions have to be made about RV morphology. Volume calculations are therefore used infrequently.

Right ventricular function

Assessment of RV function is often made qualitatively, using 'eyeball' assessment of RV contractility from several different views. Inspect the RV carefully for evidence of regional wall motion abnormality (normokinesia, hypokinesia, akinesia, dyskinesia) and describe the region(s) affected (RV free wall, RV apex, interventricular septum (IVS), RVOT anterior wall). A more quantitative approach to RV function can also be taken, using one or more of the following parameters:

- fractional area change
- tricuspid annular plane systolic excursion
- Tei index.

Fractional area change

To calculate RV fractional area change:

1. In the apical 4-chamber view, trace the RV endocardium to obtain an area measurement (in cm^2) at end-diastole and end-systole.
2. RV fractional area change can then be calculated (as a percentage) from:

$$\text{RV fractional area change} = \frac{\text{End-diastolic area} - \text{End-systolic area}}{\text{End-diastolic area}} \quad (\times\ 100 \text{ to express as a percentage})$$

Reference ranges are given in Table 15.7.

Tricuspid annular plane systolic excursion

Tricuspid annular plane excursion (TAPSE) is a simple and well-validated method of assessing RV function. The underlying principle is based on measuring how much the lateral tricuspid annulus moves vertically during systole – the more impaired the RV, the less annular displacement is seen. To measure TAPSE:

1. Obtain an apical 4-chamber view of the RV.
2. Using M-mode, place the cursor so that it passes through the lateral tricuspid annulus. Obtain an M-mode trace.
3. Measure the vertical displacement of the lateral tricuspid annulus from the M-mode trace (Fig. 15.10).

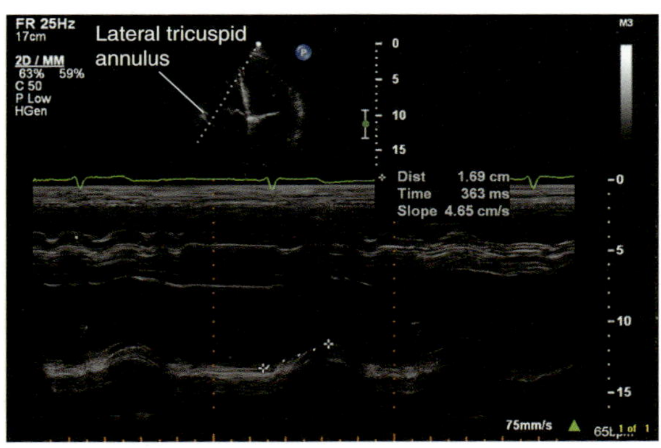

View	Apical 4-chamber
Modality	M-mode

Fig. 15.10 Measurement of tricuspid annular plane systolic excursion

Reference ranges are given in Table 15.7.

Table 15.7 Right ventricle (RV) function – reference ranges

	Normal	Mild disease	Moderate disease	Severe disease
RV fractional area change (%)	32–60	25–31	18–24	≤17
TAPSE (mm)	16–20	11–15	6–10	≤5

TAPSE, tricuspid annular plane systolic excursion.

Reference ranges reproduced with permission of the British Society of Echocardiography and British Heart Foundation.

Tei index

The Tei index (myocardial performance index) is a measure of myocardial function that takes into account both systolic and diastolic function and is independent of heart rate (but cannot be used in an irregular rhythm such as AF). It is based upon the ratio between the sum of RV isovolumic contraction time (ICT) and isovolumic relaxation time (IRT), divided by ejection time (ET). To calculate the Tei index (Fig. 15.11):

1. Use PW Doppler to obtain a trace of forward flow through the tricuspid valve, and measure the duration (in s) of RV systole. This is measured from the end of the forward flow trace in one cardiac cycle to the start of the forward flow trace in the next cycle. This is 'a' and represents ICT, ET and IRT.
2. Use PW Doppler to obtain a trace of forward flow through the pulmonary valve, and measure the duration (in s) of ejection. This is measured from the start to the end of a single forward flow trace in one cardiac cycle. This is 'b' and represents ET alone.

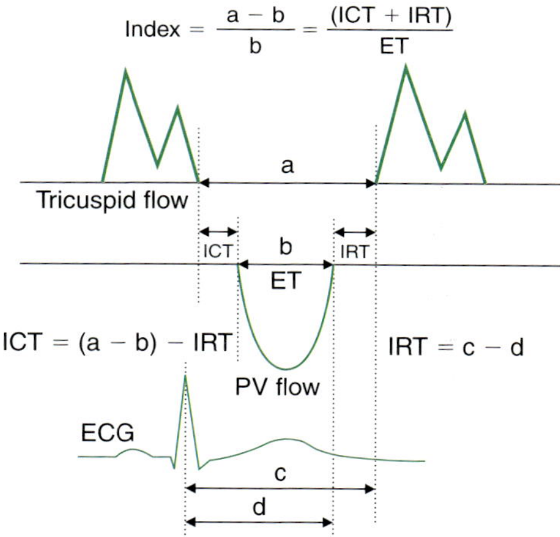

Fig. 15.11 Measurement and calculation of the Tei index (ICT = isovolumic contraction time; IRT = isovolumic relaxation time; ET = ejection time PV = pulmonary valve) (Adapted from *Journal of the American College of Cardiology*, **28**, Tei C, *et al.*, Doppler index combining systolic and diastolic myocardial performance: clinical value in cardiac amyloidosis, 658–64, © 1996, with permission from Elsevier)

3. Calculate the Tei index from:

$$\text{Tei index} = \frac{a-b}{b}$$

A normal Tei index is <0.40, with higher values indicating worsening RV function. The Tei index principle can also be used to assess LV function as well as RV function.

VOLUME AND PRESSURE OVERLOAD

Assessing the IVS in the parasternal short axis view can provide useful information about RV haemodynamics. Normally septal motion is dominated by the LV, and the septum bulges towards the RV in the short axis views. If the RV is overloaded this septal bulge starts to flatten, and in the short axis views this gives the LV a 'D' shape rather than its usual circular appearance. In the presence of chronic RV **volume** overload (e.g. severe tricuspid regurgitation), the RV is dilated and the septum is pushed towards the LV in diastole. In RV **pressure** overload (e.g. severe pulmonary hypertension), the RV is hypertrophied and the septum is pushed towards the LV in systole. Coexistent volume and pressure overload will flatten the septum in both systole *and* diastole.

Pulmonary valve

The pulmonary valve can best be seen in:

- parasternal RV outflow view (Fig. 6.4, p. 58)
- parasternal short axis view (aortic valve level) (Fig. 6.5, p. 60)
- subcostal short axis view.

Beyond the pulmonary valve it is possible to visualize the main pulmonary artery ('pulmonary trunk'), sometimes to the point of its bifurcation into left and right pulmonary arteries (often best seen in the parasternal RV outflow view).

Pulmonary stenosis

Pulmonary stenosis is most commonly a congenital defect, often presenting in infancy or childhood, although it can also result from previous rheumatic fever or from carcinoid syndrome (see above).

Patients are often asymptomatic and are diagnosed when an incidental heart murmur is found during examination. Symptomatic patients may have fatigue, breathlessness, presyncope/syncope, symptoms of RV dysfunction or symptoms relating to an underlying cause (e.g. flushing in carcinoid syndrome), or cyanosis (when there is a coexistent right-to-left shunt). Physical signs include a widely split second heart sound and an ejection systolic murmur in the pulmonary area, and in severe stenosis there may be evidence of RV hypertrophy.

Echo assessment of pulmonary stenosis

2-D and M-mode

Use 2-D echo to assess the pulmonary valve and surrounding structures:

- Is it a tricuspid pulmonary valve, or is it bicuspid or dysplastic?
- Is there any thickening or calcification of the cusps? Is this diffuse or focal? If focal, which area of each cusp is affected?
- Is cusp mobility normal or reduced? How much is it reduced?
- Is there any doming of the cusps?
- Is there any evidence of infundibular or supravalvular stenosis? Is there any stenosis in the branch pulmonary arteries?
- Are there any vegetations or masses attached to the valve?
- Is there any thrombus (pulmonary embolism) visible in the main pulmonary artery or its branches?

Although it is possible to obtain an M-mode recording of the motion of the individual pulmonary valve cusps in the parasternal short axis view, this is seldom necessary in everyday practice.

Colour Doppler

Use colour Doppler to map any regurgitant blood flow proximal to the pulmonary valve:

- Is there any pulmonary regurgitation?
- Which part of the valve does it arise from?
- How extensive is it?

CW and PW Doppler

Use CW Doppler to obtain a trace of forward flow through the pulmonary valve (Fig. 15.12). You should obtain traces from the parasternal right ventricular outflow view and the parasternal short axis view (aortic valve level).

The CW Doppler trace will give peak transpulmonary velocity (V_{max}), which relates to peak transpulmonary pressure gradient (ΔP_{max}) via the simplified Bernoulli equation:

$$\Delta P_{max} = 4 \times V^2{}_{max}$$

If peak velocity in the RVOT is >1.0 m/s, the full Bernoulli equation should be used for greater accuracy:

$$\Delta P_{max} = 4 \times (V_2{}^2 - V_1{}^2)$$

where V_2 is the peak transpulmonary velocity, assessed by CW Doppler, and V_1 is the peak RVOT velocity, assessed by PW Doppler.

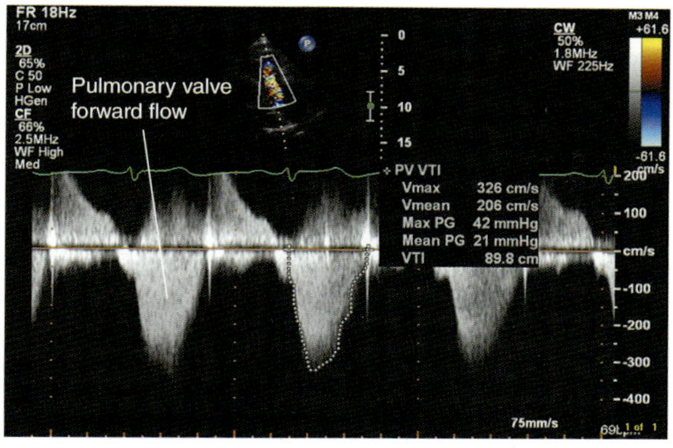

View	Parasternal short axis (aortic valve level)
Modality	CW Doppler

Fig. 15.12 Moderate pulmonary stenosis (PG = pressure gradient; PV = pulmonary valve; V_{max} = peak velocity; V_{mean} = mean velocity; VTI = velocity time integral)

The mean transpulmonary pressure gradient (ΔP_{mean}) can be obtained by tracing the Doppler envelope, from which the echo machine can calculate a mean value by averaging the instantaneous gradients throughout the trace. Calculation of the pulmonary valve effective orifice area is not usually necessary, but if it is required then the continuity equation can be used (as for aortic stenosis, see Chapter 13).

If you suspect infundibular or supravalvular stenosis, use PW Doppler to assess blood flow at different levels above and below the valve to detect where the main flow acceleration occurs. If colour Doppler reveals pulmonary regurgitation, record a trace using CW Doppler to assess the density of the regurgitant signal (more dense = more severe) and also the angle of the downward (deceleration) slope (steeper slope = more severe).

Associated features

Pulmonary stenosis is often associated with other congenital heart disorders, and so you should look carefully for any other structural heart defects (e.g. tetralogy of Fallot). In addition:

- assess any coexistent pulmonary regurgitation
- assess any coexistent tricuspid valve disease (carcinoid syndrome can affect both tricuspid and pulmonary valves)

- assess RV dimensions and function. Obstruction to RV outflow by the pulmonary valve raises RV pressure, leading to RV hypertrophy and subsequently dilatation and impaired function
- assess pulmonary artery dimensions (pulmonary artery dilatation is a common finding in pulmonary stenosis).

Severity of pulmonary stenosis

Severity of pulmonary stenosis can be quantified by P_{max} (Table 15.8).

Table 15.8 Indicators of pulmonary stenosis severity

	Mild	Moderate	Severe
Pulmonary P_{max} (mmHg)	<40	40–75	>75

Reference ranges reproduced with permission of the British Society of Echocardiography and British Heart Foundation.

SAMPLE REPORT

The pulmonary valve cusps are thin but the commissures are partially fused with 'doming' of the valve during systole. The transpulmonary peak velocity is 4.8 m/s (peak gradient 92 mmHg, mean gradient 56 mmHg). There is mild pulmonary regurgitation. The tricuspid, mitral and aortic valves are normal. There is moderate RV hypertrophy with good systolic function. The main pulmonary artery is mildly dilated. The findings are consistent with severe pulmonary stenosis.

Pulmonary regurgitation

Pulmonary regurgitation is the flow of blood from the pulmonary artery back through the pulmonary valve during diastole. A trace amount of pulmonary regurgitation, in the absence of any structural heart disease, is a common finding in normal individuals. More significant pulmonary regurgitation can be the result of:

- rheumatic valve disease
- infective endocarditis
- idiopathic dilatation of the pulmonary annulus
- pulmonary artery dilatation (e.g. in pulmonary hypertension)
- carcinoid syndrome
- congenital absence of one or more cusps
- pulmonary valvuloplasty.

Significant pulmonary regurgitation leads to RV volume overload and can cause symptoms and signs of right-sided heart failure.

Echo assessment of pulmonary regurgitation

2-D and M-mode

Use 2-D and M-mode echo to assess the structure of the valve as described for pulmonary stenosis (above).

Colour Doppler

Use colour Doppler to examine the jet of pulmonary regurgitation and describe the jet size. In mild pulmonary regurgitation the jet is narrow (<1.0 cm), whereas in moderate or severe regurgitation the jet is wider.

CW and PW Doppler

Record a CW Doppler trace with the probe carefully aligned with the direction of the regurgitant jet (Fig. 15.13). The CW Doppler trace is soft in mild pulmonary regurgitation, and denser in moderate or severe regurgitation. Look at the contour of the regurgitant jet – in mild pulmonary regurgitation the deceleration rate of the jet is slow, becoming steeper with more severe degrees of regurgitation.

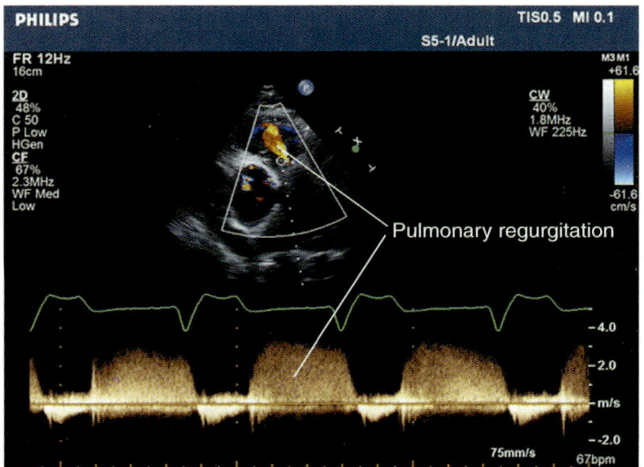

View	Parasternal short axis (aortic valve level)
Modality	Colour and CW Doppler

Fig. 15.13 Pulmonary regurgitation (Figure reproduced with permission of Philips)

Use PW Doppler to assess the VTI of forward flow in the RVOT (in the parasternal view) and also in the LVOT (in the apical 5-chamber view). The ratio of $RVOT_{VTI}/LVOT_{VTI}$ increases with increasing severity of pulmonary regurgitation. Measurement of the peak velocity of the jet of pulmonary regurgitation allows calculation of pulmonary artery diastolic pressure (p. 219).

Regurgitant volume and fraction

The volume of blood entering the RV via the tricuspid valve during diastole should normally equal the volume of blood leaving it via the RVOT (stroke volume) during systole. In the presence of pulmonary regurgitation, RVOT outflow will be greater than tricuspid valve inflow as the systolic RVOT outflow will consist of the blood that has entered via the tricuspid valve plus the blood that entered the ventricle via pulmonary regurgitation during diastole. The difference between RVOT outflow and tricuspid valve inflow gives the regurgitant volume:

1. In the apical 4-chamber view, measure the diameter of the tricuspid annulus in cm, and then use this to calculate the CSA of the tricuspid valve in cm^2. This calculation makes the assumption that the tricuspid orifice is circular:

$$CSA_{TV} = 0.785 \times (\text{tricuspid annulus diameter})^2$$

2. In the apical 4-chamber view, measure the VTI of tricuspid valve inflow (using PW Doppler) to give VTI_{TV}, in cm. It is generally easiest to place the sample volume at the valve tips (some place it at the level of the tricuspid valve annulus).
3. The stroke volume of the tricuspid valve (SV_{TV}), in mL/beat, can then be calculated from:

$$SV_{TV} = CSA_{TV} \times VTI_{TV}$$

4. In the parasternal short axis view (aortic valve level), measure the diameter of the RVOT at the level of the pulmonary valve annulus (RVOT2) in cm, and then use this to calculate the cross-sectional area (CSA) of the RVOT in cm^2:

$$CSA_{RVOT} = 0.785 \times (\text{RVOT diameter})^2$$

5. At the same point in the parasternal short axis view, measure the VTI of RVOT outflow (using PW Doppler) to give VTI_{RVOT}, in cm.

6. The stroke volume of the RVOT (SV_{RVOT}), in mL/beat, can then be calculated from:

$$SV_{RVOT} = CSA_{RVOT} \times VTI_{RVOT}$$

7. Pulmonary regurgitant volume (RV) can be calculated from:

$$RV = SV_{RVOT} - SV_{TV}$$

8. Pulmonary regurgitant fraction (RF) can be calculated from:

$$RF = \frac{RV}{SV_{TV}} \text{ (× 100 to express as a percentage)}$$

This measurement is not valid if there is significant tricuspid regurgitation, and any error in measurement of tricuspid valve orifice area or RVOT diameter can have a large impact on the result.

Associated features

If pulmonary regurgitation is present you should:

- assess any coexistent pulmonary stenosis
- assess any coexistent disease affecting the other valves
- assess RV dimensions and function – the RV may become dilated due to volume overload if pulmonary regurgitation is severe
- assess flow in the pulmonary artery (diastolic flow reversal indicates severe pulmonary regurgitation)
- calculate pulmonary artery systolic and diastolic pressure (see below) to assess if there is pulmonary hypertension.

Severity of pulmonary regurgitation

Severity of pulmonary regurgitation can be assessed by:

- jet size
- RF
- CW Doppler jet density
- CW Doppler jet deceleration rate
- $RVOT_{VTI}/LVOT_{VTI}$ ratio.

Table 15.9 summarizes the echo indicators of pulmonary regurgitation severity.

Table 15.9 Indicators of pulmonary regurgitation severity

	Mild	Moderate	Severe
Jet size	Narrow, <1.0 cm	Intermediate	Wide, large
Regurgitant fraction (%)	<40	40–60	>60
CW jet density	Soft	Dense	Dense
CW jet deceleration rate	Slow	Variable	Steep
$RVOT_{VTI}/LVOT_{VTI}$	↑	↑ ↑	↑ ↑ ↑

CW, continuous wave; LVOT, left ventricular outflow tract; RVOT, right ventricular outflow tract; VTI, velocity time integral.

Reference ranges reproduced with permission of the British Society of Echocardiography and British Heart Foundation.

SAMPLE REPORT

The pulmonary valve cusps are thin and mobile. The main pulmonary artery is moderately dilated at 2.8 cm. There is a wide jet of pulmonary regurgitation on colour Doppler. On CW Doppler the regurgitant jet is dense with a steep deceleration rate and on PW Doppler there is a high ratio in velocity time integral between the right and left ventricular outflow tracts. There is diastolic flow reversal in the pulmonary artery. The pulmonary regurgitant fraction is 68 per cent. The RV is moderately dilated with impaired function. There is pulmonary hypertension (pulmonary artery pressure 72/28 mmHg). The findings indicate severe pulmonary regurgitation secondary to moderate pulmonary artery dilatation and pulmonary hypertension.

Pulmonary hypertension

Pulmonary hypertension refers to an increase in blood pressure within the pulmonary vasculature. It is defined haemodynamically as a:

- mean pulmonary artery pressure >25 mmHg at rest (with a normal or near-normal pulmonary capillary wedge pressure ≤15 mmHg), or
- mean pulmonary artery pressure >30 mmHg during exercise.

It should be remembered that these definitions refer to *mean* pulmonary artery pressure, not the systolic pressure, and are based on cardiac catheter studies. On echo, mild pulmonary hypertension is regarded as a pulmonary artery systolic pressure of 36–50 mmHg.

Causes of pulmonary hypertension

Pulmonary hypertension results from an increased resistance to blood flow through the pulmonary vasculature. The World Health Organization categorizes the causes of pulmonary hypertension into five groups:

- **pulmonary arterial hypertension** (e.g. idiopathic, familial, collagen vascular disease, congenital systemic-to-pulmonary shunts)
- **pulmonary venous hypertension**, as a consequence of left heart disease (e.g. mitral valve disease, aortic valve disease, LV failure)
- **lung diseases and/or hypoxaemia** (e.g. chronic obstructive pulmonary disease, interstitial lung disease, sleep-disordered breathing)
- **chronic thrombotic and/or embolic disease** (e.g. pulmonary embolism)
- **miscellaneous causes** (e.g. sarcoidosis, lymphangiomatosis).

It is important to be aware of the potential causes of pulmonary hypertension, so that a search can be made for any clues to the underlying cause whenever pulmonary hypertension is detected on echo.

Clinical features of pulmonary hypertension

The clinical features of pulmonary hypertension are summarized in Table 15.10. As well as symptoms and signs relating to the pulmonary hypertension itself, the patient may also have clinical features specific to the underlying cause and therefore a detailed history and clinical examination are necessary in every case.

Table 15.10 Clinical features of pulmonary hypertension

Symptoms	Signs
Symptoms are often of very gradual onset	Elevated jugular venous pressure
Breathlessness	Parasternal heave
Fatigue	Loud pulmonary component to second heart sound (P_2)
Cough	Tricuspid regurgitation
Dizziness and syncope	Peripheral oedema
Peripheral oedema	Ascites

Echo assessment of pulmonary hypertension

Echo provides a valuable non-invasive method for estimating pulmonary artery pressure.

Pulmonary artery systolic pressure

The technique for measuring pulmonary artery systolic pressure (PASP) relies upon the presence of tricuspid regurgitation. Fortunately, at least two-thirds of normal individuals have a detectable degree of tricuspid regurgitation (and it is even commoner in those with pulmonary hypertension). You can assess tricuspid regurgitation using CW Doppler in:

- parasternal RV inflow view (Fig. 6.3, p. 57)
- parasternal short axis view (aortic valve level) (Fig. 6.5, p. 60)
- apical 4-chamber view (Fig. 6.8, p. 63).

It is a good idea to assess the tricuspid regurgitation in as many of these views as possible. Using CW Doppler, measure the peak velocity of *regurgitant* flow through the tricuspid valve (TR V_{max}) in m/s. Figure 15.5 (p. 199) shows a CW Doppler trace of a tricuspid regurgitation jet with a V_{max} of 4.26 m/s. The tricuspid regurgitation is driven by, and therefore reflects, the pressure gradient between right ventricular systolic pressure (RVSP) and RAP, and this pressure gradient can be calculated using the simplified Bernoulli equation:

$$\text{RVSP} - \text{RAP} = 4 \times (\text{TR } V_{max})^2$$

For example, if the peak velocity of the TR jet is 4.26 m/s then:

$$\text{RVSP} - \text{RAP} = 4 \times (4.26)^2$$

$$\text{RVSP} - \text{RAP} = 4 \times 18.15$$

$$\text{RVSP} - \text{RAP} = 73\,\text{mmHg}$$

Now you know the pressure *difference* between the RV and the RA. The next step is to estimate the *actual* systolic pressure in the RV, and to do that you need to know what the RAP is. The estimation of RAP from IVC diameter has been described earlier in this chapter (p. 193). If assessment of the IVC gives an estimated RAP of 15–20 mmHg then, continuing with our example from above:

$$\text{RVSP} - \text{RAP} = 73\,\text{mmHg}$$

$$\text{RVSP} = 73\,\text{mmHg} + \text{RAP}$$

$$\text{RVSP} = 73 + 15\text{–}20\,\text{mmHg}$$

$$\text{RVSP} = 88\text{–}93\,\text{mmHg}$$

The patient therefore has an estimated RVSP of approximately 90 mmHg. Assuming there is no significant pulmonary stenosis, the

RVSP is approximately equal to the pulmonary artery systolic pressure (PASP):

$$PASP = RVSP$$

$$PASP = 88\text{–}93\ \text{mmHg}$$

(If there *is* coexistent pulmonary stenosis, then the RVSP will be higher than PASP, and the difference will be equal to the peak pressure gradient across the stenosis.)

Pulmonary artery diastolic pressure

Estimation of pulmonary artery diastolic pressure (PADP) relies on the presence of pulmonary regurgitation. You can assess pulmonary regurgitation using CW Doppler in:

- parasternal RV outflow view (Fig. 6.4, p. 58)
- parasternal short axis view (aortic valve level) (Fig. 6.5, p. 60).

Using CW Doppler, measure the peak velocity of *regurgitant* flow through the pulmonary valve (PR velocity) in m/s. The pulmonary regurgitation is driven by, and therefore reflects, the diastolic pressure gradient between the pulmonary artery (PADP) and the right ventricle (RVDP), and this pressure gradient can be calculated using the simplified Bernoulli equation:

$$PADP - RVDP = 4 \times (\text{PR velocity})^2$$

For example, if the peak velocity of the pulmonary regurgitation jet is 1.1 m/s then:

$$PADP - RVDP = 4 \times (1.1)^2$$

$$PADP - RVDP = 4 \times 1.2$$

$$PADP - RVDP = 4.8\ \text{mmHg}$$

Now you know the diastolic pressure *difference* between the pulmonary artery and the RV. The next step is to estimate the *actual* diastolic pressure in the RV, and this is taken to be the same as RA pressure (estimated using the IVC technique, as outlined above). For example, if the IVC is normal then the RAP would be estimated at 5–10 mmHg, and so the RVDP would be 5–10 mmHg too. Continuing with our example:

$$PADP - RVDP = 4.8\ \text{mmHg}$$

$$PADP = 4.8\ \text{mmHg} + RVDP$$

$$PADP = 4.8 + 5\text{–}10\,\text{mmHg}$$

$$PADP = 9.8\text{–}14.8\,\text{mmHg}$$

The patient therefore has a PADP of approximately 10–15 mmHg.

Mean pulmonary artery pressure

Once you have estimated PASP and PADP, you can calculate mean pulmonary artery pressure as follows:

$$\text{Mean pulmonary artery pressure} = \frac{(\text{PASP} + \text{PADP})}{3}$$

Associated features

If pulmonary hypertension is present your echo study should include a careful search for potential causes, for example:

- mitral and/or aortic valve disease
- left-to-right shunts (e.g. ASD, VSD)
- LV dysfunction
- pulmonary emboli.

You must also look for, and report upon, any consequences of pulmonary hypertension:

- pulmonary artery dilatation
- pulmonary and/or tricuspid regurgitation
- RV dilatation and impairment
- RA dilatation.

SAMPLE REPORT

The RV is severely dilated and impaired, and there is severe functional tricuspid regurgitation into a dilated right atrium. The tricuspid regurgitation gradient is 68 mmHg. There is moderate pulmonary regurgitation with a regurgitation gradient of 10 mmHg. The IVC is dilated at 2.8 cm and decreases to 1.8 cm on inspiration, giving an estimated right atrial pressure of 15–20 mmHg. The estimated pulmonary artery pressure is therefore 83–88 mmHg/25–30 mmHg, indicating severe pulmonary hypertension. The patient also has severe mitral stenosis.

Management of pulmonary hypertension

Treatment options for pulmonary hypertension include identification and treatment of any underlying causes (e.g. valvular heart disease, pulmonary emboli). Oral anticoagulants, diuretics, oxygen therapy, digoxin and calcium-channel blockers may all have a role to play. Endothelin receptor antagonists can also be useful. Surgical options include balloon atrial septostomy or lung/heart–lung transplantation.

FURTHER READING

Fox DJ, Khattar RS. Carcinoid heart disease: presentation, diagnosis, and management. *Heart* 2004; **90**: 1224–8.

Ionescu A. *British Society of Echocardiography Distance Learning Module 10: The Echocardiographic Assessment of the Right Heart in the Adult*. Accessible from the BSE website (www.bsecho.org).

Lang RM, Bierig M, Devereux RB, *et al*. Recommendations for chamber quantification: a report from the American Society of Echocardiography's Guidelines and Standards Committee and the Chamber Quantification Writing Group, developed in conjunction with the European Association of Echocardiography, a branch of the European Society of Cardiology. *J Am Soc Echocardiogr* 2005; **18**: 1440–63.

National Pulmonary Hypertension Centres of the UK and Ireland. Consensus statement on the management of pulmonary hypertension in clinical practice in the UK and Ireland. *Heart* 2008; **94**(suppl 1): i1–4.

Simonneau G, Galie N, Rubin LJ, *et al*. Clinical classification of pulmonary hypertension. *J Am Coll Cardiol* 2004; **43**: 5–12.

Tei C, Dujardin KS, Hodge DO, *et al*. Doppler index combining systolic and diastolic myocardial performance: clinical value in cardiac amyloidosis. *J Am Coll Cardiol* 1996; **28**: 658–64.

16 Heart valve repair and replacement

Valvular heart disease can be treated in a variety of ways:

- valve replacement, in which an artificial (prosthetic) heart valve is implanted surgically to replace an abnormal (regurgitant or stenotic) valve
- valve repair, in which a regurgitant valve is corrected surgically, preserving the original valve rather than replacing it
- percutaneous techniques, which include percutaneous balloon valvuloplasty (in which a stenotic valve is 'stretched' with a balloon) and, more recently, transcatheter aortic valve implantation (in which an abnormal aortic valve is replaced with a new valve deployed percutaneously rather than with cardiothoracic surgery).

It is important to be aware of the different valvular procedures that patients undergo, as patients will require follow-up echo studies to confirm the success of the procedure and to monitor their repaired/replaced valve for any subsequent dysfunction. It's particularly useful to undertake a detailed 'baseline' echo study around 6–8 weeks after valve surgery to act as a comparator for subsequent studies.

Prosthetic valves

Each year approximately 6000 people in the UK (and 60 000 in the USA) undergo surgery to implant a prosthetic heart valve. Prosthetic valves fall into one of two categories:

- Mechanical valves – in which the valve is constructed using artificial materials.
- Biological valves – in which the valve contains biological material, derived either from a natural valve or fashioned from pericardium. Biological valves are also sometimes called 'tissue valves' or 'bioprosthetic valves'.

Before undertaking an echo assessment of a prosthetic valve, it is essential to know the type of valve implanted. The request form should therefore state:

- the type of prosthetic valve (e.g. biological, mechanical) and its specific name (e.g. Bjork-Shiley)
- the size of prosthetic valve (which is its internal diameter, stated in mm)
- the date of implantation
- current clinical details (e.g. new diastolic murmur)
- a specific question to be addressed (e.g. valve dehiscence?).

Details of the type of valve can usually be obtained from the original operation note.

Echo assessment of mechanical valves

A mechanical valve consists of three parts: the **sewing ring** (which is like the 'annulus' of the valve, used by the surgeon to sew the valve into position), the **occluder** (the moving part of the valve which opens and closes during the cardiac cycle) and the **retaining mechanism** (which is attached to the sewing ring and holds the occluder in position).

There are three types of mechanical valve (Fig. 16.1):

- Ball and cage valves, consisting of a silastic ball occluder which can move up and down within the cage-like retaining mechanism – this was the earliest type of mechanical valve, introduced during the 1960s
- Tilting disc valves, in which a single disc occluder tilts within its occluder
- Bileaflet valves, in which two semicircular disc occluders open and close on hinges – these are now the most commonly used prosthetic valves.

The advantage of mechanical valves is their long-term durability (although some earlier valves were prone to catastrophic failure). The main disadvantage

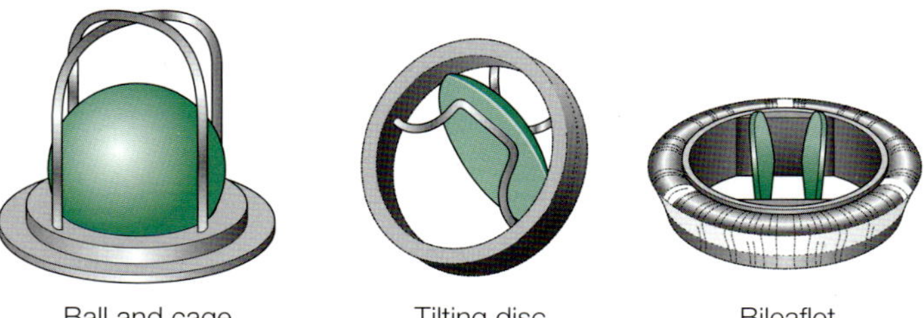

Fig. 16.1 Types of mechanical heart valve

of mechanical valves is that, because they are constructed from artificial materials, they can be a source of thrombus formation. Patients with mechanical valves therefore require lifelong anticoagulation with drugs such as warfarin, which can be a major drawback, particularly in patients at risk of bleeding or women of child-bearing age who wish to become pregnant.

Mechanical valve structure

Mechanical valves can be challenging to assess on echo because of the reverberation caused by the materials in the valve (Fig. 16.2). Mitral prostheses are usually best assessed from the apical window, aortic prostheses from the apical and parasternal windows. Transoesophageal echo (TOE) can help, particularly for prosthetic valves in the mitral position (see box).

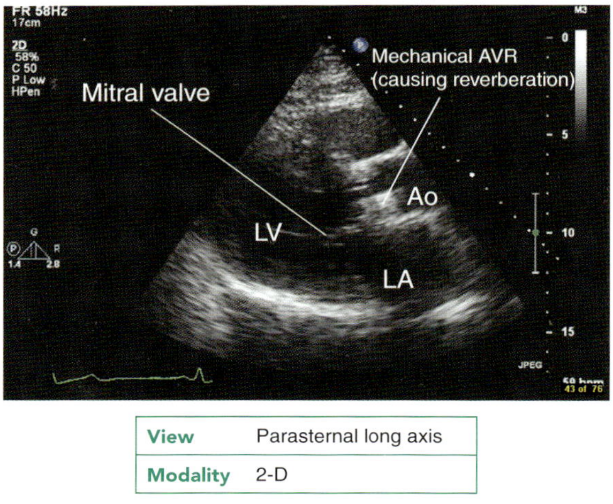

View	Parasternal long axis
Modality	2-D

Fig. 16.2 Normal mechanical aortic valve replacement (AVR) (Ao = aorta; LA = left atrium; LV = left ventricle)

As far as possible, examine the structure of the mechanical valve, asking the following questions:

- Is the valve well seated, or does it appear to be 'rocking'? A rocking valve prosthesis indicates a degree of separation ('dehiscence') of the valve's sewing ring from the rest of the heart – look carefully for associated paravalvular regurgitation.
- Is there a normal range of movement of the valve occluder(s)? Occluder motion can be obstructed by thrombus or pannus (excessive fibrous or

'scar' tissue around the valve). Obstruction to occluder opening causes stenosis, while obstruction to occluder closure causes regurgitation.

- Are there any masses associated with the valve, and are the masses mobile or immobile? Pannus is an immobile mass, whereas thrombus or vegetations are usually (but not always) mobile. Prosthetic valve masses usually require a TOE study for full characterization.

Sometimes very small bubbles are seen near a mechanical valve just as its occluder closes (Fig. 16.3). These microbubbles are caused by cavitation of blood by the occluder, and are regarded as a harmless finding.

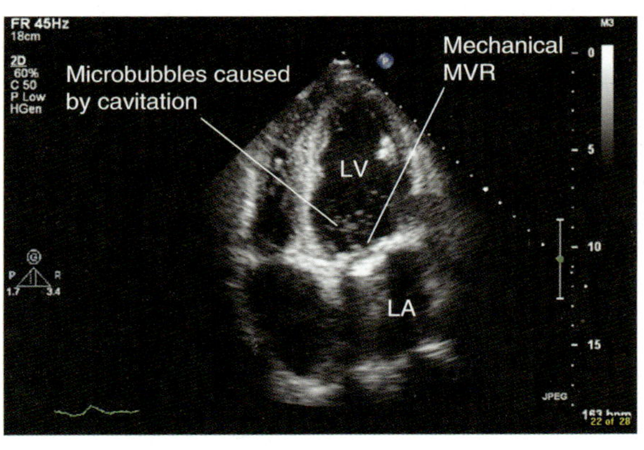

View	Apical 4-chamber
Modality	2-D

Fig. 16.3 Normal mechanical mitral valve replacement (MVR) showing cavitation (LA = left atrium; LV = left ventricle)

If the valve prosthesis cannot be imaged adequately, state this in your report so that appropriate alternative imaging can be arranged.

TOE AND MECHANICAL VALVE ASSESSMENT

TOE can play a valuable role in the assessment of mechanical valves, particular in the mitral position. TOE provides good resolution of the left atrium and the mitral valve, and so can provide useful information on the function of a mechanical mitral valve prosthesis. TOE is less useful for imaging mechanical aortic valves, particularly when a mechanical mitral valve is also present.

Mechanical valve function

Forward flow

All prosthetic valves exhibit a degree of 'patient–prosthesis mismatch', in that the prosthetic valve tends to have a smaller effective orifice area than the native valve it replaces, and so some degree of obstruction to blood flow is to be expected. As for native valves, assess forward flow by measuring:

- gradient (peak and mean) – but beware the problem of pressure recovery (see box)
- pressure half-time (for mitral prostheses)
- effective orifice area (based on pressure half-time for mitral prostheses and the continuity equation for aortic prostheses).

PRESSURE RECOVERY

The phenomenon of pressure recovery is complex, but in essence it describes how pressure increases downstream of a stenosis because of the conversion ('recovery') of kinetic energy into potential energy. The practical upshot of pressure recovery is that measured pressure gradients across prosthetic valves can appear misleadingly high, particularly for aortic valves. The phenomenon has been found in both mechanical and biological valves. Calculation of effective orifice area for a prosthetic valve is often more useful than valve gradient alone, and serial measurements are particularly helpful for identifying 'true' prosthetic valve stenosis.

The normal ranges of prosthetic valve forward flow parameters vary according to the type and size of the valve concerned, and tables of normal values can be obtained either from the prosthetic valve's manufacturer or by referring to published tables in the literature (the paper by Rosenhek *et al.* is particularly useful – see Further Reading below).

Obstruction to forward flow occurs if motion of the valve occluder is obstructed (by thrombus, pannus, vegetations or mechanical failure), so that the occluder cannot open properly, or if there is subvalvular or supravalvular obstruction from pannus formation. Inspect the valve carefully to assess occluder motion where possible. If obstruction occurs intermittently, a prolonged period of Doppler interrogation may be required.

Regurgitant flow

A small amount of regurgitation is normal for mechanical valve prostheses. There is an initial regurgitant flow as the occluder closes and blood is pushed backwards by it. Then, once the occluder is closed, there is a further regurgitant flow which is intended to 'wash' over the prosthesis and reduce the risk of thrombus formation. These normal regurgitant jets are usually small – the precise extent and location of the regurgitant jet(s) depends on the type of valve.

Abnormal regurgitation through the orifice of the prosthetic valve may occur if the occluder fails to close properly, either because closure is obstructed (e.g. by thrombus, vegetations or pannus) or because of mechanical failure of the occluder itself. Regurgitation through a prosthetic valve orifice is called **transvalvular regurgitation**. Regurgitation may also occur around the valve, due to dehiscence of part of the sewing ring – this is **paravalvular regurgitation**. Use colour Doppler to examine the location and extent of any abnormal regurgitation, and describe it as fully as possible. Regurgitation from mitral prostheses can be difficult to see with transthoracic echo and a TOE study may be required.

Echo assessment of biological valves

As with a mechanical valve, biological valves contain a sewing ring which the surgeon uses to sew the valve into position. From the sewing ring projects a framework consisting of a number of struts, commonly called stents, to which the valve leaflets are attached. These stents take up space and thus can cause a degree of obstruction to blood flow through the valve. Valves which lack this supporting framework, called 'stentless valves' are available and offer a greater orifice area (for the same overall size of valve), reducing the gradient across the prosthetic valve.

There are three types of biological valve:

- Xenograft valves, in which the valve is fashioned from a porcine valve or from bovine pericardium
- Homograft valves, which are human valves obtained from cadavers
- Autograft valves, in which a patient's own pulmonary valve is used to replace their aortic valve (and the pulmonary valve is itself replaced with a xenograft or homograft valve) – this is known as the Ross procedure.

Unlike mechanical valves, biological valves do not require long-term anticoagulation. However, they do not have the durability of mechanical valves and there is a significant failure rate from 8–10 years onwards after implantation. Failure can occur as a result of gradual calcification of the valve, causing stenosis, or from regurgitation.

Biological valve structure

Stentless bioprosthetic valves can look very similar to native valves on echo. For stented valves the stents can be very obvious (Figs 16.4, 16.5) and can cause shadowing of the ultrasound beam.

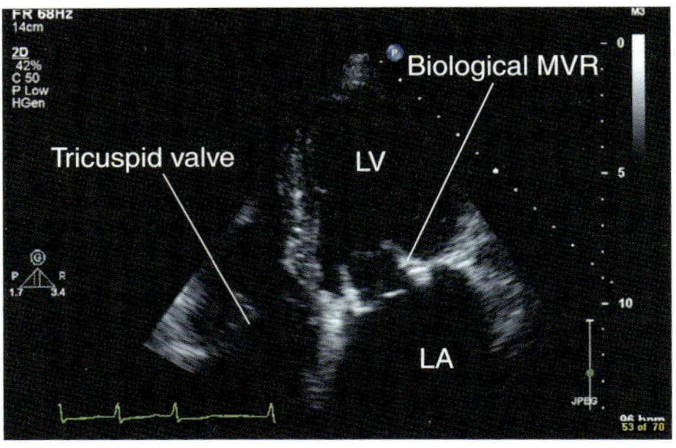

View	Apical 4-chamber
Modality	2-D

Fig. 16.4 Normal biological mitral valve replacement (MVR) (LA = left atrium; LV = left ventricle)

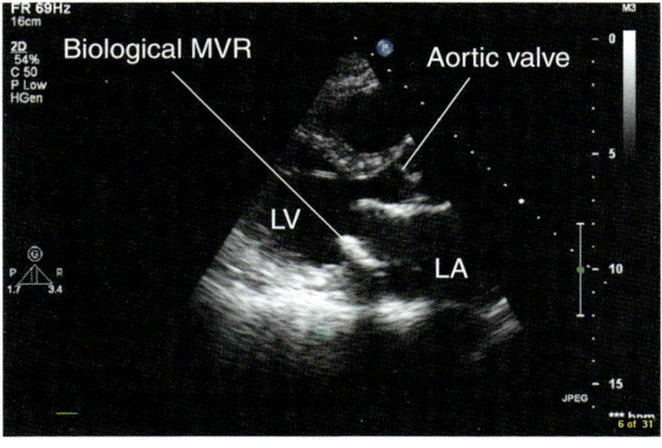

View	Parasternal long axis
Modality	2-D

Fig. 16.5 Normal biological mitral valve replacement (MVR) (LA = left atrium; LV = left ventricle)

Examine the structure of the biological valve, asking the following questions:

- Is the valve well seated, or does it appear to be 'rocking'? As for mechanical valves, a rocking biological valve indicates dehiscence of the sewing ring, so check for associated paravalvular regurgitation.
- Do the valve leaflets appear thin and mobile? Biological valve leaflets become fibrotic and calcified with time, developing a thickened appearance on echo with reduced mobility.
- Are there any masses associated with the valve (pannus, thrombus, vegetations)?

If the valve prosthesis cannot be imaged adequately, state this in your report so that appropriate alternative imaging can be arranged.

Biological valve function

Forward flow

As with mechanical valves, biological valves have a smaller effective orifice area than the native valves they replace (although less so with stentless valves). As time passes, biological valve leaflets tend to become deformed as a result of fibrosis, and this can result in stenosis, with an increase in the gradient across the valve (and a decrease in the effective orifice area). As for native valves, assess forward flow by measuring:

- gradient (peak and mean)
- pressure half-time (for mitral prostheses)
- effective orifice area (based on pressure half-time for mitral prostheses and the continuity equation for aortic prostheses).

The normal ranges of prosthetic valve forward flow parameters vary according to the type and size of the valve concerned, and tables of normal values can be obtained either from the prosthetic valve's manufacturer or by referring to published tables in the literature (the paper by Rosenhek *et al.* is particularly useful – see Further Reading below).

Regurgitant flow

Up to half of normal biological valve prostheses have a mild degree of transvalvular regurgitation. Abnormal transvalvular regurgitation may occur if the valve has developed fibrocalcific degeneration, or if there has been acute leaflet rupture. Paravalvular regurgitation may occur around the valve due to dehiscence of part of the sewing ring (Fig. 16.6), as for mechanical valves. Use Doppler interrogation to examine the location and extent of any abnormal regurgitation, and describe it as fully as possible.

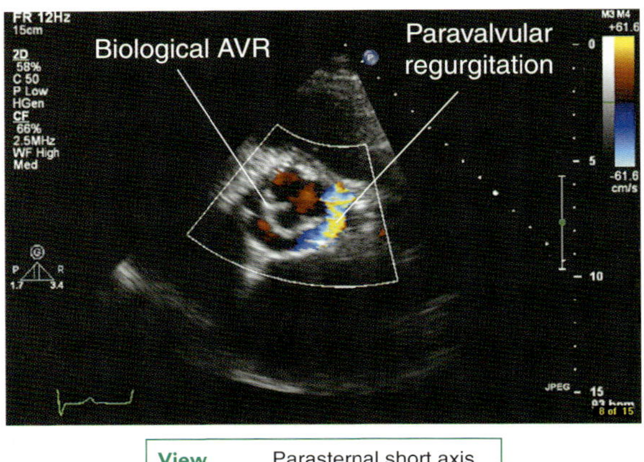

View	Parasternal short axis
Modality	Colour Doppler

Fig. 16.6 Biological aortic valve replacement (AVR) with paravalvular regurgitation

SAMPLE REPORT

There is a biological stented aortic valve replacement *in situ* (stated to be a 23 mm Carpentier-Edwards prosthesis, implanted 3 years ago, on the request form). The valve is well seated. There are no associated masses. The valve cusps are thin and mobile, with a peak gradient of 25 mmHg (mean 13 mmHg) and an effective orifice area of 1.9 cm^2 (calculated from the continuity equation). There is no transvalvular or paravalvular regurgitation. The findings indicate a normally functioning biological aortic valve replacement.

Valve repair

Mitral valve repair is, where feasible, the preferred surgical option for mitral regurgitation with better long-term outcomes than valve replacement. The operation usually involves resection of a wedge of redundant mitral tissue and, where necessary, inserting an annuloplasty ring to reinforce the mitral annulus and repairing/replacing damaged chordae tendineae. An alternative technique is the so-called Alfieri or 'edge-to-edge' repair, in which the central points of the two mitral leaflets are sutured together to create a double-orifice mitral valve.

Echo assessment of valve repair

When performing an echo following mitral valve repair (Fig. 16.7), assess:

- mitral valve morphology, looking in particular at leaflet mobility and for the presence of an annuloplasty ring and/or repaired/replaced chordae
- mitral valve flow, looking for evidence of stenosis or regurgitation as for a native valve.

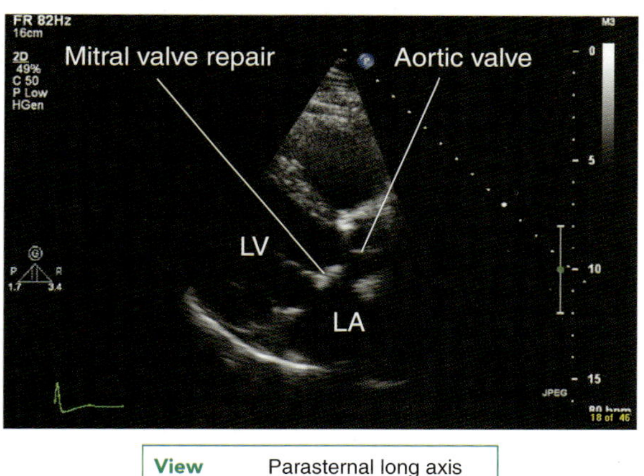

View	Parasternal long axis
Modality	2-D

Fig. 16.7 Normal mitral valve repair (LA = left atrium; LV = left ventricle)

Percutaneous techniques

Percutaneous techniques for valvular intervention include percutaneous balloon mitral valvuloplasty (PBMV) and transcatheter aortic valve implantation (TAVI).

Percutaneous balloon mitral valvuloplasty

PBMV is a technique in which a balloon is passed to the heart via a femoral vein and a deliberate puncture is made in the interatrial septum to allow access to the left atrium. The balloon is then passed across the stenosed mitral valve and inflated to relieve the stenosis. The technique works primarily through commissural splitting, and it is important to assess the mitral valve (and particularly the commissures) to select patients most likely to benefit from this procedure.

Echo assessment for PBMV is formalised in the Wilkins score, which grades the valve's suitability according to four criteria: leaflet mobility, valvular thickening, subvalvular thickening and valvular calcification. Each criterion is scored from 1 to 4, and a total score >8 indicates a low probability of successful PBMV. Full assessment will entail a TOE. Patients not suitable for PBMV include those with:

- significant mitral regurgitation
- bilateral commissural calcification
- thrombus on the interatrial septum, protruding into the atrial cavity or obstructing the mitral orifice.

The presence of unilateral commissural calcification or thrombus in the left atrial appendage is a relative contraindication to PBMV.

Following PBMV the valve should be assessed carefully for any residual stenosis or for the development of mitral regurgitation, and for any residual atrial septal defect. Note that mitral valve pressure half-time is *not* a reliable way to assess mitral stenosis in the 72 h following PBMV. During this period the improvement in transmitral flow following the procedure causes an increase in left atrial (and a decrease in left ventricular) compliance, which affects pressure half-time measurements. Once chamber compliance has stabilised after 72 h, pressure half-time can be used once again.

Transcatheter aortic valve implantation (TAVI)

For many years balloon valvuloplasty has been available to treat aortic stenosis in patients for whom conventional surgery is contraindicated. More recently, there has been growing interest in new techniques not just to dilate a stenosed aortic valve but also to replace the aortic valve via a transcatheter approach, particularly in elderly patients with aortic stenosis who have multiple comorbidities and for whom conventional aortic valve surgery would present a high risk. TAVI can be performed either via the femoral artery (transluminal approach) or via a direct puncture at the left ventricular apex (transapical approach). A balloon is placed across the stenosed aortic valve and inflated to dilate it. A replacement valve, which is mounted within a stent, is then deployed using either a balloon or a self-expanding system.

Following TAVI, echo is important is assessing the function of the prosthetic aortic valve and checking for any complications of the procedure (such as pericardial effusion/cardiac tamponade).

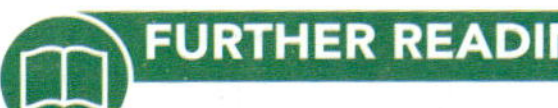

FURTHER READING

Bloomfield P. Choice of heart valve prosthesis. *Heart* 2002; **87**: 583–9.

British Society of Echocardiography Distance Learning Module 8: The Echocardiographic Assessment of Prosthetic Heart Valves. Accessible from the BSE website (www.bsecho.org).

Prendergast BD, Shaw TRD, Iung B, *et al.* Contemporary criteria for the selection of patients for percutaneous balloon mitral valvuloplasty. *Heart* 2002; **87**: 401–4.

Rosenhek R, Binder T, Maurer G, *et al.* Normal values for Doppler echocardiographic assessment of heart valve prostheses. *J Am Soc Echocardiogr* 2003; **16**: 1116–27.

17 Endocarditis

Endocarditis refers to inflammation of the endocardium, the inner layer of the heart (including the heart valves). Endocarditis can be:

- infective (e.g. bacterial, fungal)
- non-infective (e.g. Libman–Sacks endocarditis in systemic lupus erythematosus).

The characteristic lesion in endocarditis is the vegetation, a mass of inflammatory material which can include fibrin, platelets, red and white blood cells and (where present) micro-organisms.

Infective endocarditis

In the past, infective endocarditis has been classified as acute or subacute ('SBE', subacute bacterial endocarditis) but this terminology is outdated and should no longer be used. Although infective endocarditis is rare (fewer than 10 cases per 100 000 population every year) it is nevertheless a serious and dangerous condition, with a mortality of around 20 per cent.

Infective endocarditis starts with organisms reaching the endocardium either via a bacteraemia or directly via surgery or device placement. The organisms adhere to the endocardium and as they invade the local tissues a vegetation begins to form. Left untreated, they cause local tissue destruction (e.g. valvular regurgitation) and can also lead to abscess and/or fistula formation.

The single most common causative organism is *Staphylococcus aureus*; other commonly encountered organisms are listed in Table 17.1.

Table 17.1 Common causes of infective endocarditis

Bacterial	*Staphylococcus aureus* *Streptococcus viridans* *Streptococcus intermedius* *Pseudomonas aeruginosa* HACEK organisms *Bartonella* *Coxiella burnetii*
Fungal	*Candida* *Aspergillus* *Histoplasma*

Clinical features of infective endocarditis

The clinical features of infective endocarditis (Table 17.2) can be subtle and sometimes will have been present for several weeks, so a high index of suspicion is needed to avoid missing the diagnosis. Be particularly alert to the possibility of infective endocarditis in those at risk (see above), and/or those with a history of invasive procedures or intravenous drug use.

Table 17.2 Clinical features of infective endocarditis

Symptoms	Signs
Fever Fatigue Anorexia Weight loss Flu-like symptoms	Fever Heart murmur Splinter haemorrhages Janeway lesions Osler's nodes Roth spots Peripheral emboli

The Duke (or modified Duke) criteria can be helpful in cases of diagnostic uncertainty (Durack *et al.* 1994). Blood cultures are the mainstay of diagnosis, and at least three sets should be taken from different sites at different times. Blood cultures may be negative because of prior antibiotic treatment or the presence of fastidious (difficult to culture) organisms.

Echocardiography plays a valuable role in identifying:

- presence of vegetations
- valvular destruction
- associated abscess, fistula or perforation.

'Major' echo criteria supporting a diagnosis of infective endocarditis are the presence of oscillating structures (vegetations), the presence of an abscess, new valvular regurgitation and dehiscence of a prosthetic valve.

Transthoracic echo (TTE) can, at best, detect vegetations down to a minimum size of 2 mm (and is known to miss the majority of vegetations <5 mm). The superior image quality of transoesophageal echo (TOE) makes it more sensitive and specific than TTE, particularly in cases of prosthetic valve endocarditis and in the detection of abscesses. TTE has an overall sensitivity in detecting vegetations of ≈50 per cent, whereas the sensitivity of TOE is ⩾90 per cent. TOE should be considered in cases where the TTE is negative or inconclusive (particularly if the clinical suspicion of infective endocarditis is high), or where there is a suspicion of prosthetic valve endocarditis, right heart endocarditis or a cardiac abscess. It is important to note that a negative echocardiogram (even TOE) does *not* rule out a diagnosis of infective endocarditis and it is prudent to include this, when appropriate, in your echo report.

VEGETATIONS AND JET LESIONS

Vegetations occur most commonly on heart valves. However, they can also occur anywhere where a high velocity jet of blood flow ('jet lesion') occurs between a high-pressure and low-pressure chamber, impinging on the endocardium and potentially resulting in endothelial injury and establishing a focus for infection. Examples include the high velocity jets found in ventricular septal defect (VSD) or persistent ductus arteriosus (PDA).

Echo assessment of infective endocarditis

A full echo study should be performed and any structural abnormalities that predispose to infective endocarditis noted. According to the National Institute for Health and Clinical Excellence (2008), patients at risk of developing infective endocarditis include those with:

- acquired valvular disease including stenosis or regurgitation
- valve replacement
- structural congenital heart disease, including surgically corrected or palliated conditions (except isolated atrial septal defect and fully repaired VSD or PDA, and endothelialized closure devices)

- hypertrophic cardiomyopathy
- previous infective endocarditis.

Look carefully for any features of infective endocarditis:

- vegetations
- valvular destruction
- abscess
- fistula.

Vegetations

The characteristic echo appearance of a vegetation is of an echogenic mass, irregular in shape, attached to the 'upstream' side of a valve leaflet (i.e. the atrial side in the case of the mitral and tricuspid valves, the ventricular side for the aortic and pulmonary valves). Vegetations can be attached to any part of the valve, but most commonly at the coaptation line. Vegetations move with the leaflet but in a more chaotic ('oscillating') manner. It is common for a vegetation to prolapse through the valve as it opens.

Vegetations vary in size, often being just a few mm in diameter but sometimes reaching 2–3 cm. Vegetations resulting from fungal infections (e.g. *Candida*, *Aspergillus*) are usually much bigger than bacterial vegetations, and can be so big that they are mistaken for a cardiac tumour. Fungal endocarditis is rare and is more likely to occur in patients who are immunosuppressed.

In order of decreasing frequency, the valves affected by infective endocarditis are the mitral (Fig. 17.1), aortic, tricuspid and pulmonary. More than one valve can be affected. Right heart endocarditis is much commoner in patients who are intravenous drug users, and can also occur in association with right-sided devices such as pacemaker leads.

If vegetations are present, describe their:

- location (which valve(s), and which parts of the valve, are affected)
- mobility (e.g. immobile, oscillating)
- size.

Because infective endocarditis usually occurs on a valve that is already abnormal, you must also describe any underlying valvular disease as well as looking for any evidence that the infection is causing valvular destruction (see below).

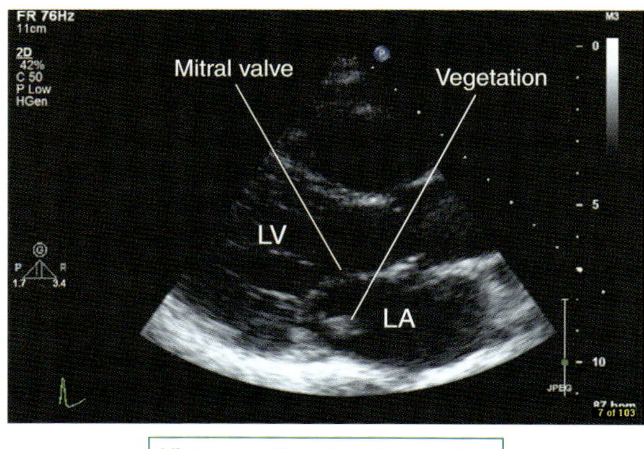

View	Parasternal long axis
Modality	2-D

Fig. 17.1 Vegetation on mitral valve (LA = left atrium; LV = left ventricle)

! PITFALLS IN THE ECHO ASSESSMENT OF VEGETATIONS

Infective endocarditis commonly occurs on a heart valve that is already abnormal, and a pre-existing abnormality (e.g. myxomatous mitral valve disease, nodular aortic cusp thickening) can be mistaken for vegetations, or can make the recognition of existing vegetations more difficult. Patients who are left with sterile vegetations following a previously treated episode of endocarditis can pose a difficult diagnostic challenge.

Cardiac tumours and thrombi can also be mistaken for vegetations (and vice versa). Benign structures that can be mistaken for vegetations include Lambl's excrescences and the Eustachian valve (see Chapter 21). Remember too that not all vegetations are infective in nature (p. 241).

Valvular destruction

Infective endocarditis can cause valvular destruction, leading to regurgitation either through distorting normal valve closure or through perforation of a valve leaflet (Fig. 17.2). Valvular regurgitation should be assessed and described as for native valvular regurgitation, as outlined in Chapters 13–15. Valvular stenosis as a result of infective endocarditis is much rarer, and usually results from obstruction of the valve orifice by a large vegetation.

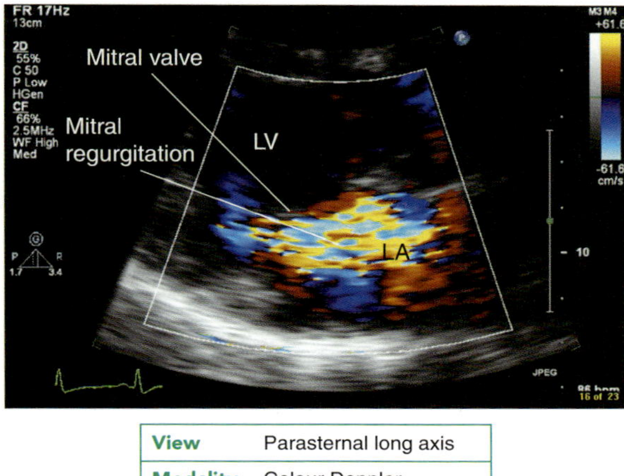

View	Parasternal long axis
Modality	Colour Doppler

Fig. 17.2 Mitral regurgitation as a result of infective endocarditis (LA = left atrium; LV = left ventricle)

PROSTHETIC VALVE ENDOCARDITIS

Prosthetic valve endocarditis can be challenging to diagnose, particularly using TTE. Imaging of the valve itself is often suboptimal because of shadowing and reverberation of the echo signal by the prosthesis. Furthermore, prosthetic valve infections typically occur at the sewing ring rather than on the leaflets, making it harder to identify any vegetations. Look carefully for any signs of dehiscence ('splitting open') of the sewing ring around the valve, allowing regurgitant blood flow *around* the valve prosthesis (paravalvular regurgitation).

A TOE study is therefore usually appropriate in order to obtain better resolution of the prosthesis and any associated abnormalities. Prosthetic valve endocarditis is difficult to treat with antibiotics alone and early re-do surgery is usually required, particularly in the first 12 months after the valve was first implanted.

Abscess

A valvular infection can spread to involve surrounding tissues, particularly in prosthetic valve endocarditis. On echo, an abscess appears as an echolucent or echodense area in the valve annulus or surrounding tissues. TOE has a much greater sensitivity for detecting perivalvular abscesses than TTE.

Abscesses occur more commonly around the aortic valve than the mitral valve, although an aortic root abscess can sometimes spread to affect the anterior mitral valve leaflet. A mitral valve abscess typically affects the posterior annulus, appearing on echo as a thickened and echodense region.

If an abscess is present, describe its:

- location (which valve is affected, and where the abscess lies in relation to the valve)
- size.

Fistula

An aortic root abscess (or pseudoaneurysm) may rupture into a neighbouring chamber (usually the right ventricle, but sometimes one of the atria) to form an abnormal communication or fistula. Fistulas can be multiple.

A fistula can be demonstrated using colour Doppler and continuous wave (CW) Doppler to show abnormal flow arising in the aortic root and flowing through the fistula. Describe where the fistula arises and which chambers it connects. Describe too its haemodynamic effects, such as consequent chamber dilatation and/or dysfunction.

SAMPLE REPORT

The aortic valve cusps are thickened with mildly reduced mobility and there is mild aortic stenosis (peak gradient 24 mmHg). There is a mobile 'oscillating' echogenic nodule, measuring 7 mm in diameter, attached to the ventricular surface of the right coronary cusp. There is moderate aortic regurgitation into a non-dilated left ventricle, with good systolic function. No evidence of abscess or fistula formation is seen. The appearances are in keeping with a vegetation on the aortic valve.

Management of infective endocarditis

The treatment of infective endocarditis usually requires a prolonged (4–6 week) course of antibiotics, chosen where possible according to the antibiotic sensitivities of the causative organism. Cardiac surgery is necessary in about half of patients with infective endocarditis. Ideally, in stable patients, surgery should be performed only once the infection has been successfully treated with antibiotics to minimize the risk of recurrent infection. However, it is not always possible to delay surgery if patients are unstable or at high risk of complications (e.g. embolization). Early surgery should be considered for:

- haemodynamic instability/heart failure as a result of acute aortic or mitral regurgitation
- persistent infection (fever and bacteraemia despite treatment with appropriate antibiotics for 7–10 days)
- development of a perivalvular abscess or fistula
- infective endocarditis on a prosthetic valve
- fungal infections
- difficult to treat organisms (e.g. *Brucella*)
- high embolic risk:
  - recurrent emboli despite appropriate antibiotics
  - large vegetation (>10 mm) and a single embolic event
  - very large mobile vegetation (>15 mm).

Follow-up echo

Patients being treated for infective endocarditis require regular follow-up echo studies to monitor progress and to watch for complications. With effective treatment the vegetations may gradually shrink and become less mobile. The sudden disappearance of a vegetation between studies should raise a suspicion that the vegetation has broken free and embolized elsewhere.

Even when an episode of infective endocarditis has been fully treated, (sterile) vegetations may remain visible on echo. This can make the diagnosis of recurrent infection challenging in patients who have suffered an episode of endocarditis previously – clinical evidence of active infection, particularly on blood cultures, is the key to diagnosis in such cases.

Prevention of infective endocarditis

Patients at risk of infective endocarditis (see above) should receive guidance on good oral hygiene and how to recognize the symptoms of infective endocarditis, and also information on the risks of invasive procedures, but antibiotic prophylaxis is no longer routinely recommended.

Non-infective endocarditis

Not all vegetations occur as a result of infection, a fact that emphasises the importance of taking the patient's clinical history (and in particular the results of blood cultures) into account when making a diagnosis of infective (versus non-infective) endocarditis.

Non-infective endocarditis has also been termed non-bacterial thrombotic endocarditis (NBTE) or, historically, marantic endocarditis. The vegetations that occur are sterile, and are composed mainly of fibrin and platelets. Non-infective endocarditis can result from:

- trauma to the valve leaflets (e.g. from an intracardiac catheter)
- circulating immune complexes
- vasculitis
- hypercoagulability
- mucin-producing adenocarcinomas.

Non-infective endocarditis occurring in systemic lupus erythematosus is called Libman–Sacks endocarditis (also known as 'verrucous' endocarditis), and in this condition, the vegetations mainly consist of immune complexes and mononuclear cells. The mitral and aortic valves are most commonly affected, although just about any part of the endocardium can be involved. The vegetations are usually small, irregular and immobile (compared with the vegetations in infective endocarditis). Libman–Sacks endocarditis is usually asymptomatic, but can present with valvular regurgitation or, less commonly, stenosis. There is also a risk of embolization, although this is uncommon.

FURTHER READING

Beynon RP, Bahl VK, Prendergast BD. Infective endocarditis. *BMJ* 2006; **333**: 334–9.

Durack DT, Lukes AS, Bright DK. New criteria for diagnosis of infective endocarditis: utilization of specific echocardiographic findings. Duke Endocarditis Service. *Am J Med* 1994; **96**: 200–9.

Evangelista A, González-Alujas MT. Echocardiography in infective endocarditis. *Heart* 2004; **90**: 614–17.

Habib G. Management of infective endocarditis. *Heart* 2006; **92**: 124–30.

National Institute for Health and Clinical Excellence. *Prophylaxis Against Infective Endocarditis.* NICE clinical guideline No. 64, 2008. Available at: www.nice.org.uk/CG064 (accessed 8 December 2008).

The Task Force on Infective Endocarditis of the European Society of Cardiology. Guidelines on the prevention, diagnosis and treatment of infective endocarditis: executive summary. *Eur Heart J* 2004; **25**: 267–76.

18 The cardiomyopathies

Classification of the cardiomyopathies

In 1995, a classification scheme for the cardiomyopathies was proposed by the World Health Organization (WHO). This scheme defined cardiomyopathies as 'diseases of the myocardium associated with cardiac dysfunction' and categorized them as follows:

- dilated cardiomyopathy (DCM)
- hypertrophic cardiomyopathy (HCM)
- restrictive cardiomyopathy
- arrhythmogenic right ventricular (RV) cardiomyopathy
- unclassified cardiomyopathies (e.g. isolated ventricular non-compaction).

The WHO classification also recognized an overlapping group of 'specific' cardiomyopathies, in which a particular case of cardiomyopathy could be attributed to a specific underlying aetiology. Examples include:

- ischemic cardiomyopathy
- valvular cardiomyopathy
- hypertensive cardiomyopathy
- metabolic cardiomyopathy
- peripartum cardiomyopathy.

The advent of molecular genetics has provided new insights into the pathophysiology of the cardiomyopathies, and in some respects the WHO classification is now somewhat outdated. In 2006, the American Heart Association (AHA) proposed a new scheme in which cardiomyopathies are defined as: 'a heterogeneous group of diseases of the myocardium associated with mechanical and/or electrical dysfunction that usually (but not invariably) exhibit inappropriate ventricular hypertrophy or dilatation and are due to a variety of causes that frequently are genetic. Cardiomyopathies either are confined to the heart or are part of generalized systemic disorders, often leading to cardiovascular death or progressive heart failure-related disability.'

According to the AHA classification, cardiomyopathies can be classified as primary (mainly or only affecting the heart) or secondary (where the cardiomyopathy is part of a wider multisystem disorder):

- primary cardiomyopathies
  - genetic (e.g. HCM, arrhythmogenic RV cardiomyopathy, isolated ventricular non-compaction)
  - acquired (e.g. post-myocarditis, stress-related, peripartum, tachycardia-induced)
  - mixed (e.g. DCM, restrictive cardiomyopathy)
- secondary cardiomyopathies
  - infiltrative (e.g. amyloidosis)
  - storage (e.g. haemochromatosis, Fabry's disease)
  - toxicity (e.g. drugs)
  - endomyocardial (e.g. endomyocardial fibrosis)
  - inflammatory (e.g. sarcoidosis)
  - endocrine (e.g. diabetes mellitus, acromegaly)
  - cardiofacial (e.g. Noonan syndrome)
  - neuromuscular/neurological (e.g. Friedreich's ataxia)
  - nutritional deficiencies (e.g. beriberi, scurvy)
  - autoimmune/collagen (e.g. systemic lupus erythematosus)
  - electrolyte imbalance
  - consequence of cancer therapy (e.g. anthracyclines).

The echo assessment of any cardiomyopathy requires a detailed study with a particular emphasis on chamber morphology, dimensions and function (including ventricular systolic and diastolic function), as outlined in Chapters 11, 12 and 15, together with a full assessment of valvular function. In addition, you will need to look for the specific features relating to the cardiomyopathy in question. This chapter describes the key features of the cardiomyopathies most likely to be encountered in everyday practice.

Dilated cardiomyopathy

DCM is characterized by dilatation and systolic impairment of the left ventricle (LV), usually accompanied by dilatation of the RV and the atria. DCM can result from a number of conditions, including:

- myocarditis
- alcohol

- prolonged tachycardia (tachycardia-induced cardiomyopathy)
- pregnancy (peripartum cardiomyopathy).

Familial DCM is also recognized, defined by the presence of DCM in two or more individuals in the same family. DCM is also seen in X-linked diseases such as Becker and Duchenne muscular dystrophies. DCM without an identifiable cause is called idiopathic DCM. LV dilatation and impairment secondary to ischaemic, valvular or hypertensive heart disease is not usually classified as DCM.

Echo features

The echo assessment of DCM should include a comprehensive assessment of:

- LV dimensions and function (Chapter 11)
- RV dimensions and function (Chapter 15)
- left atrial (LA) dimensions (Chapter 11)
- right atrial dimensions (Chapter 15)
- valvular function (Chapters 13–15).

Examples of DCM are shown in Figures 18.1 and 18.2. The echo study usually cannot identify the aetiology of the DCM.

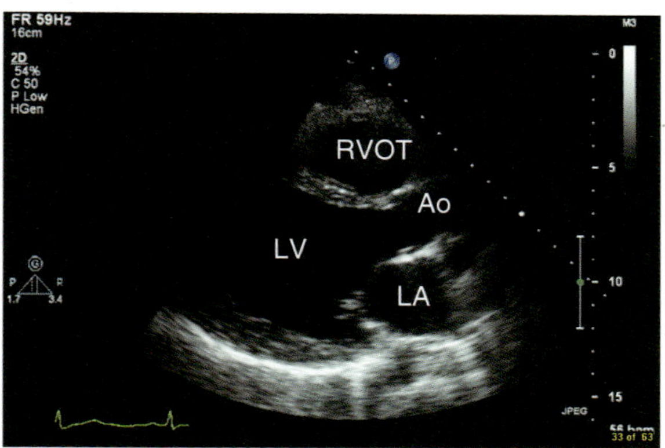

View	Parasternal long axis
Modality	2-D

Fig. 18.1 Dilated cardiomyopathy (Ao = aorta; LA = left atrium; LV = left ventricle; RVOT = right ventricular outflow tract)

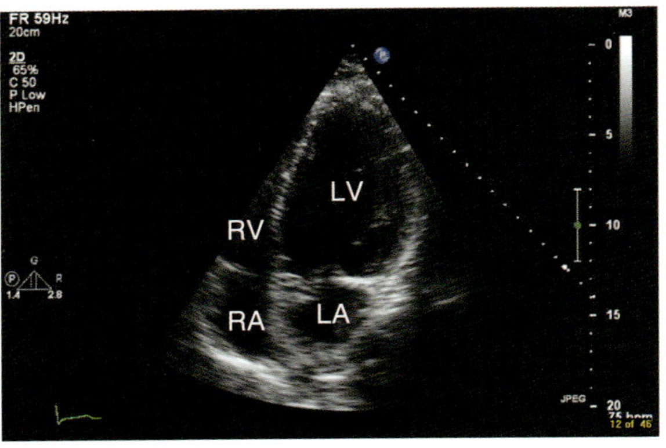

View	Apical 4-chamber
Modality	2-D

Fig. 18.2 Dilated cardiomyopathy (LA = left atrium; LV = left ventricle; RA = right atrium; RV = right ventricle)

APICAL BALLOONING CARDIOMYOPATHY

A rare form of cardiomyopathy, first described in Japan, is apical ballooning or stress cardiomyopathy. It is also known as tako-tsubo ('octopus bottle') cardiomyopathy, named after the characteristic shape of the LV seen in this condition. This cardiomyopathy is most commonly seen in post-menopausal women and is triggered by extreme emotional or clinical stress, which causes a ballooning of the LV apex (Fig. 18.3). Patients present with chest pain and/or heart failure with ECG changes suggestive of an anterior myocardial infarction (but in the absence of coronary disease). In most cases LV function recovers within 2 months of the presenting episode.

Hypertrophic cardiomyopathy

HCM is an autosomal dominant condition affecting 1 in 500 of the population and is a common cause of sudden cardiac death, particularly in the young. The LV hypertrophy in HCM is usually asymmetrical (in contrast to the concentric LV hypertrophy seen in hypertension or aortic stenosis) and systolic function is preserved but diastolic function is impaired.

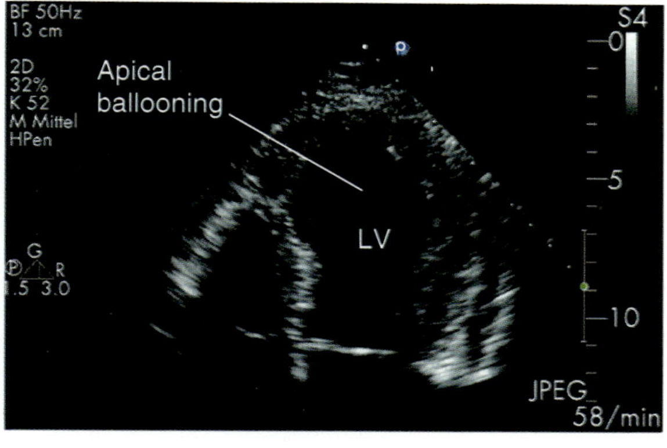

View	Apical 4-chamber
Modality	2-D

Fig. 18.3 Apical ballooning cardiomyopathy (LV = left ventricle) (Reproduced from *Heart*, Nef HM, *et al.* **93**, 1309–15, © 2007, with permission from BMJ Publishing Group Ltd.)

If the hypertrophy is located in the LV outflow tract (LVOT) it may obstruct the flow of blood out of the LV into the aorta – this is hypertrophic *obstructive* cardiomyopathy (HOCM). Another common pattern is apical hypertrophy, which gives the LV cavity a characteristic 'ace of spades' appearance.

Echo features

In HCM, the LV is hypertrophied in the absence of an underlying cause such as hypertension, aortic stenosis or aortic coarctation. In an echo study for HCM look for the following features:

- LV hypertrophy, which is usually asymmetrical (but is sometimes concentric)
- LV systolic and diastolic function (Chapter 11)
- evidence of obstruction (subaortic, midventricular)
- systolic anterior motion of the anterior mitral valve leaflet
- mitral regurgitation.

LV morphology

In HCM, the LV is non-dilated; indeed, the LV cavity is usually small. Assess LV morphology and dimensions looking, in particular, for evidence of asymmetrical hypertrophy (Fig. 18.4). If hypertrophy is present, examine its distribution carefully using multiple views of the LV – short axis views at several levels are particularly useful. Describe the location of the hypertrophy (e.g. apical, LVOT) and its severity (mild/moderate/severe).

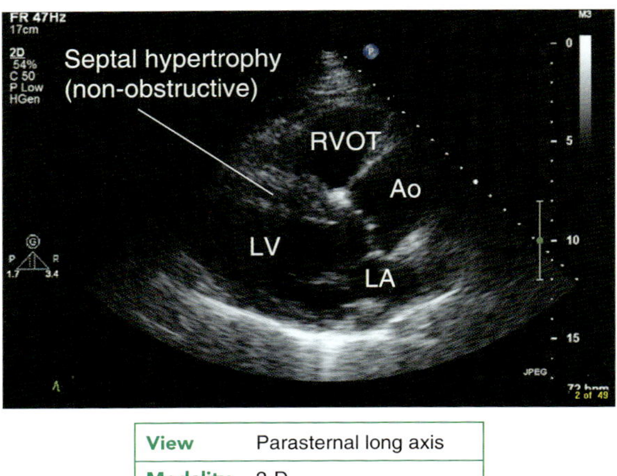

View	Parasternal long axis
Modality	2-D

Fig. 18.4 Asymmetrical septal hypertrophy in hypertrophic cardiomyopathy (Ao = aorta; LA = left atrium; LV = left ventricle; RVOT = right ventricular outflow tract)

Measure LV dimensions, reporting not just the wall thickness in the hypertrophied region but also how it compares to wall thickness in normal regions. For instance, in cases of asymmetrical septal hypertrophy you should quote the ratio between septal and posterior wall thickness as measured on the parasternal long axis view. Assess LV systolic and diastolic function as described in Chapter 11. Assess LA dimensions, which are usually increased.

Historically, an LV wall thickness of ⩾15 mm was thought to indicate HCM. However, more recent genetic studies have shown that HCM can cause milder degrees of hypertrophy. Severe hypertrophy (an LV wall thickness ⩾30 mm) is a risk factor for sudden cardiac death.

Flow obstruction

Assess flow in the LV, looking for any evidence of obstruction (increased flow velocity). Obstruction is most often subaortic, due to systolic anterior motion of the mitral valve leaflets (see below) causing obstruction to flow in

PITFALLS IN THE ECHO ASSESSMENT OF HCM

Difficulties in the echo diagnosis of HCM include:

- Overestimating LV septal thickness by taking a measurement using an oblique cut, or including a moderator band or false tendon in the measurement, leading to a false positive diagnosis of HCM.
- Mistaking the normal variant of sigmoid septum for asymmetrical septal hypertrophy. Sigmoid septum is a prominent bulge or angulation of the septum in the region of the LVOT, commonly seen in older patients. The angulation can make the septum appear hypertrophied, particularly on M-mode, even when the wall thickness is normal.
- Distinguishing between HCM and the normal hypertrophy seen in highly trained athletes. In 'athlete's heart' the LV cavity is dilated (LV end-diastolic diameter (LVEDd) $>$55 mm), in contrast to the small cavity seen in HCM. The LA is not dilated in athlete's heart, unlike in HCM.

the LVOT, but obstruction can sometimes be mid-ventricular. Perform colour Doppler to look for evidence of turbulent LVOT flow, and use continuous wave (CW) Doppler in the apical 5-chamber view to measure any LVOT gradient. You can also use pulsed-wave (PW) Doppler to assess flow in different regions of the LVOT, to distinguish between gradients caused by asymmetrical hypertrophy and any gradient across the aortic valve.

LVOT obstruction is characteristically dynamic, with the rate of increase in flow velocity rising as the velocity increases – this gives the spectral Doppler trace a characteristic 'sabre-shaped' appearance (Fig. 18.5). LVOT obstruction may occur (or increase) with exercise – this is termed latent obstruction and can be assessed by performing an echo Doppler study while the patient undertakes bicycle exercise. HCM can be categorized according to the type of obstruction:

- resting obstruction – gradient $\geqslant$30 mmHg at rest
- latent obstruction – gradient $<$30 mmHg at rest, but $\geqslant$30 mmHg with provocation
- non-obstructive – gradient $<$30 mmHg at rest and with provocation.

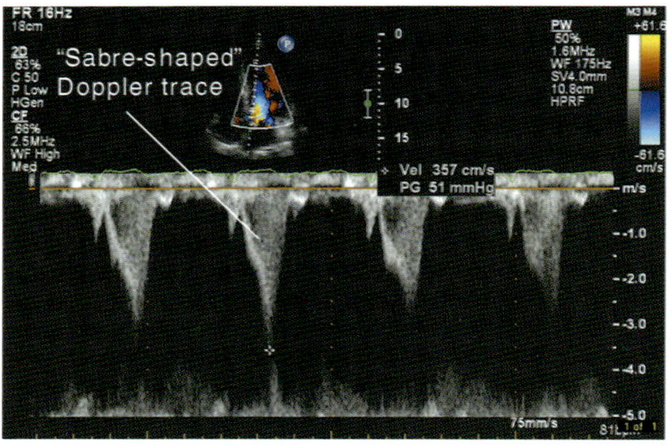

View	Apical 5-chamber
Modality	PW Doppler

Fig. 18.5 Dynamic left ventricular outflow tract obstruction in hypertrophic obstructive cardiomyopathy (PG = pressure gradient; Vel = velocity)

Systolic anterior motion

Inspect the mitral valve for structural abnormalities and look carefully for systolic anterior motion (SAM) of the mitral valve leaflets (Fig. 18.6). SAM is caused by accelerated flow in the LVOT, causing a Venturi effect that

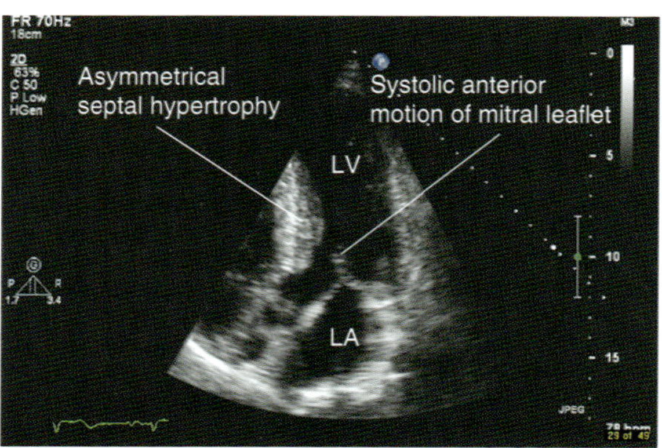

View	Apical 5-chamber
Modality	2-D

Fig. 18.6 Systolic anterior motion in hypertrophic obstructive cardiomyopathy

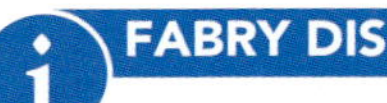

FABRY DISEASE

Fabry disease (also known as Anderson–Fabry disease) is an X-linked lysosomal storage disorder in which glycosphingolipids accumulate in and damage various organs, including the heart. Echo features include:

- LV hypertrophy (usually concentric)
- systolic and/or diastolic dysfunction
- valvular regurgitation (most commonly mitral).

The diagnosis of Fabry disease should be considered in patients with unexplained LV hypertrophy.

'drags' the anterior leaflet towards the septum (causing the leaflet tip to make contact with the septum) during systole. This opens the mitral valve, leading to an eccentric (posteriorly directed) jet of mitral regurgitation into the LA. Assess the degree of mitral regurgitation (Chapter 14).

Isolated ventricular non-compaction cardiomyopathy

Isolated ventricular non-compaction (IVNC), also known as LV non-compaction, is a cardiomyopathy caused by a failure of the normal compaction or 'condensation' process that occurs in the LV myocardium during intrauterine life. The end result is an LV that is heavily trabeculated with deep recesses between the trabeculae. This can cause systolic and/or diastolic dysfunction, and can predispose the patient to thromboembolism and arrhythmias. Some (but not all) cases are familial.

Echo features

Jenni *et al.* (see Further Reading) have described diagnostic criteria for IVNC based upon four echo features:

1. The LV myocardium is two-layered, with a thin (compacted) epicardial layer and a much thicker (non-compacted) endocardial layer that is trabecular with deep endocardial spaces. The ratio between the thickness of the non-compacted (N) and compacted (C) layers should be measured at end-systole, and is characteristically >2 (Fig. 18.7).

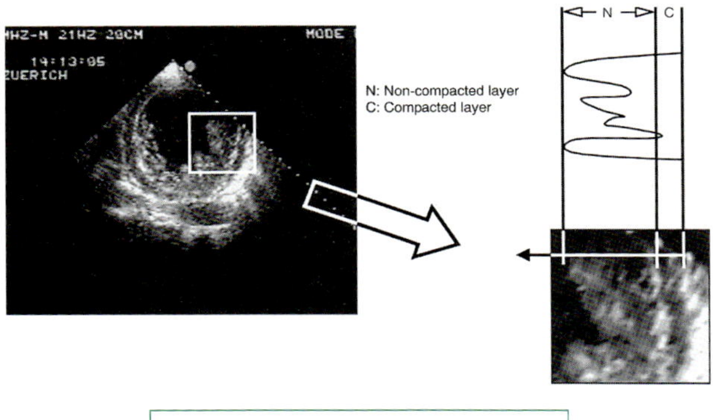

View	Parasternal short axis
Modality	2-D

Fig. 18.7 Isolated ventricular non-compaction cardiomyopathy, showing how to measure the ratio between compacted (C) and non-compacted (N) thickness at end-systole (Reproduced from *Heart*, Jenni R, *et al.* **86**, 666–71, © 2001, with permission from BMJ Publishing Group Ltd.)

2. The non-compacted myocardium is predominantly seen at the apical level and at the mid-ventricular level in the inferior and lateral walls. For the purposes of describing IVNC, a 9-segment LV model is used (rather than the usual 16- or 17-segment model) with a single apical segment and four mid and basal segments (anterior, septal, lateral and inferior).
3. Colour Doppler shows deep perfusion of the inter-trabecular recesses.
4. Other than the abnormalities already described, there should (by definition) be no other cardiac abnormalities.

Restrictive cardiomyopathy

In restrictive cardiomyopathy, the LV is not dilated and its systolic function is normal. However, the LV may be hypertrophied and its diastolic function is impaired, causing myocardial 'stiffness'. Restrictive cardiomyopathy most commonly results from:

- myocardial infiltration, as seen in amyloidosis, haemochromatosis or glycogen storage disease
- endomyocardial fibrosis
- sarcoidosis.

Echo features

A full evaluation of the LV is required, looking in particular at:

- LV dimensions and wall thickness
- LV systolic function (usually normal)
- LV diastolic function (impaired).

The LV myocardium usually appears echo-reflective and 'speckled' in amyloid infiltration, and the endocardium is echo-reflective in endomyocardial fibrosis. Restrictive cardiomyopathy may also involve the RV and both atria are usually significantly dilated as a consequence of elevated ventricular filling pressures.

The distinction between restrictive cardiomyopathy and constrictive pericarditis can be challenging. The distinguishing features of the two conditions are listed in Table 19.5 (p. 268).

Arrhythmogenic right ventricular cardiomyopathy

Arrhythmogenic RV cardiomyopathy or dysplasia (ARVC or ARVD) is a rare hereditary cardiomyopathy, primarily affecting the RV, in which there is loss of myocytes and replacement with fatty/fibrous tissue. Patients may present with ventricular arrhythmias; sudden cardiac death may occur.

Echo features

Inspect the RV carefully, looking for one or more of the following (Fig. 18.8):

- dilatation of the RV (diastolic RVOT dimension >30 mm in parasternal long axis view)
- RV dysfunction (RV wall motion abnormalities, or fractional area change <32 per cent in apical 4-chamber view)
- localised aneurysms of the RV free wall
- thickened, echo-reflective moderator band
- echo-reflective RV myocardium (due to fatty/fibrous tissue).

For more detailed information on echo assessment of the RV, see Chapter 15. The RV is always involved in ARVC but there may be LV abnormalities as well. The echo findings can sometimes be subtle, making the diagnosis of ARVC challenging. Several tests, including cardiac magnetic resonance imaging and endomyocardial biopsy, may be needed to establish the diagnosis.

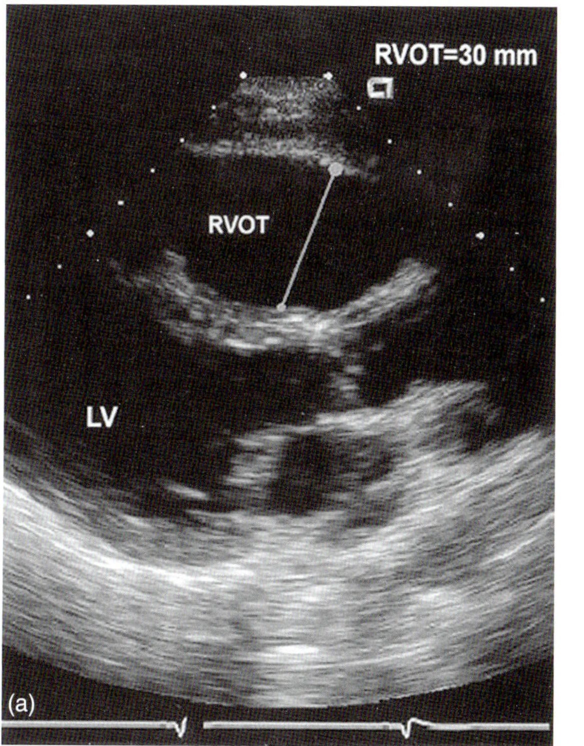

Fig. 18.8 Echo findings in arrhythmogenic right ventricular (RV) cardiomyopathy: (a,b) right ventricular outflow tract (RVOT) enlargement, (c) focal RV apical aneurysm (arrows), (d) excessive trabeculations (arrows), and (e) hyper-reflective moderator band (arrow). AoV = aortic valve; LA = left atrium; LV = left ventricle; RA = right atrium). (Reprinted from *Journal of the American College of Cardiology*, **45**, Yoerger DM, *et al*. Echocardiographic findings in patients meeting task force criteria for arrhythmogenic right ventricular dysplasia, 860–5, © 2005, with permission from Elsevier)

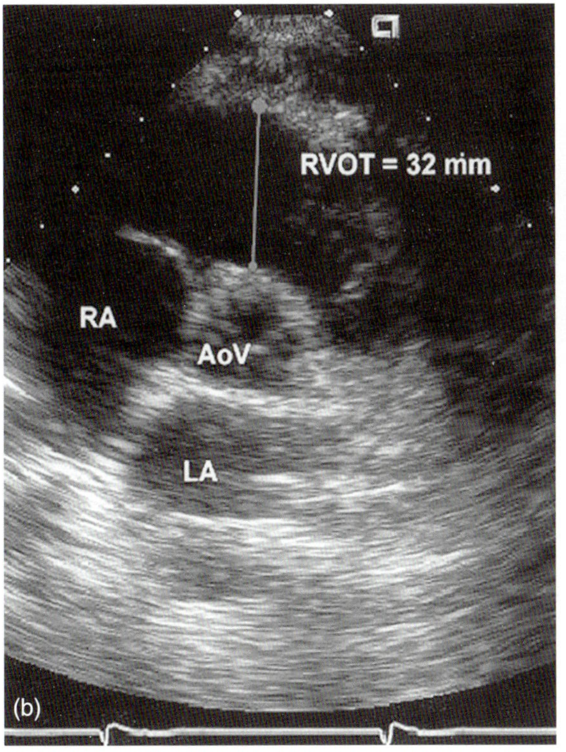

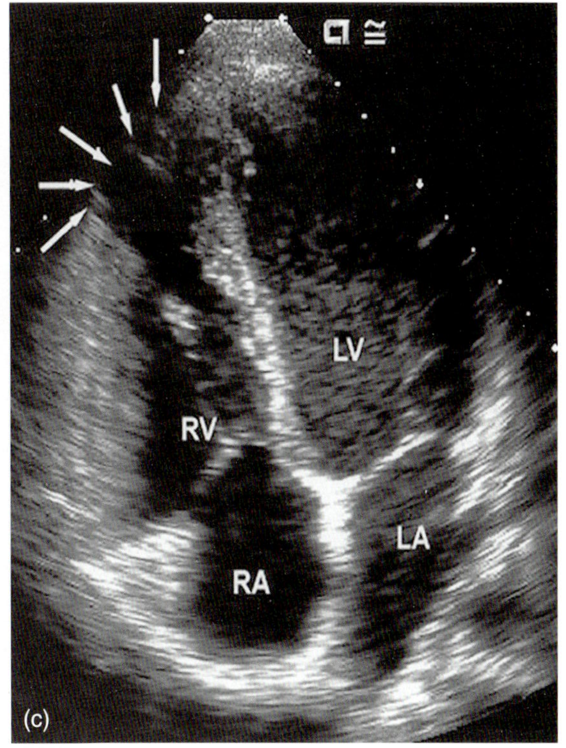

Fig. 18.8 (Continued)

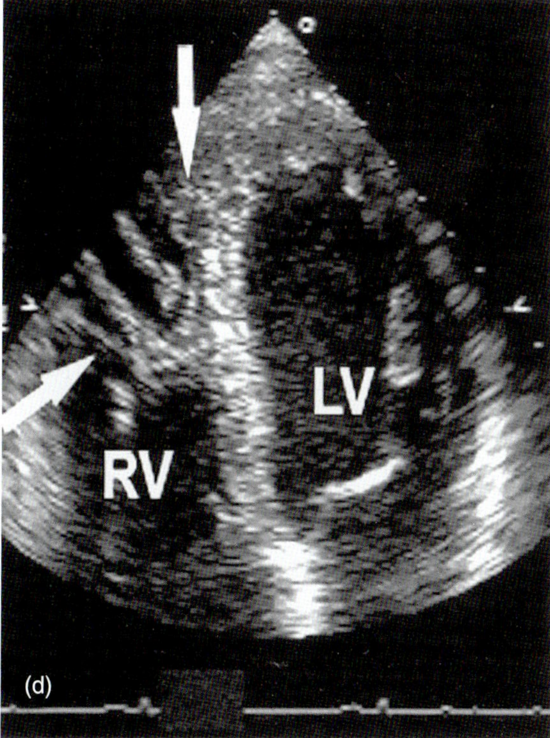

Fig. 18.8 (Continued)

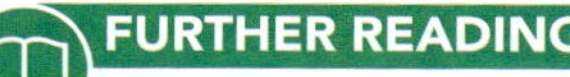

FURTHER READING

Elliott P. Diagnosis and management of dilated cardiomyopathy. *Heart* 2000; **84**: 106–12.

Jenni R, Oechslin E, Schneider J, *et al.* Echocardiographic and pathoanatomical characteristics of isolated left ventricular non-compaction: a step towards classification as a distinct cardiomyopathy. *Heart* 2001; **86**: 666–71.

Jenni R, Oechslin EN, van der Loo B. Isolated ventricular non-compaction of the myocardium in adults. *Heart* 2007; **93**: 11–15.

Maron BJ, McKenna WJ, Danielson GK, *et al.* American College of Cardiology/European Society of Cardiology clinical expert consensus document on hypertrophic cardiomyopathy. *Eur Heart J* 2003; **24**: 1965–91.

Maron BJ, Towbin JA, Thiene G, *et al.* Contemporary definitions and classification of the cardiomyopathies *Circulation* 2006; **113**: 1807–16.

Nef HM, Möllmann H, Elsässer A. Tako-tsubo cardiomyopathy (apical ballooning). *Heart* 2007; **93**: 1309–15.

Nihoyannopoulos P. *British Society of Echocardiography Distance Learning Module 12: Cardiomyopathies.* Accessible from the BSE website (www.bsecho.org).

Richardson P, McKenna W, Bristow M, *et al.* Reports of the 1995 World Health Organization/International Society and Federation of Cardiology task force on the definition and classification of cardiomyopathies. *Circulation* 1996; **93**: 841–2.

Wood MJ, Picard MH. Utility of echocardiography in the evaluation of individuals with cardiomyopathy. *Heart* 2004; **90**: 707–12.

Yoerger DM, Marcus F, Sherrill D. Echocardiographic findings in patients meeting task force criteria for arrhythmogenic right ventricular dysplasia. *J Am Coll Cardiol* 2005; **45**: 860–5.

19 The pericardium

Echo appearances of the normal pericardium

The pericardium is visible in each of the standard imaging planes of the heart and should therefore be examined in each view. As the normal pericardium is thin (1–2 mm) it is not prominent on echo, but may appear as a thin bright line around the heart. The trace of pericardial fluid that is normally present may be visible as a thin black line separating the two layers of the serous pericardium (Fig. 19.1).

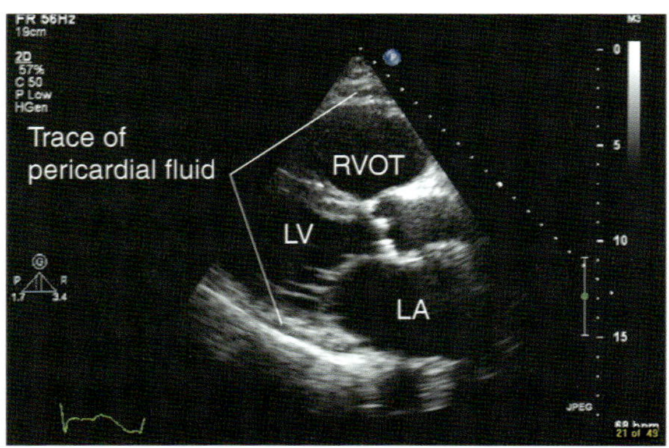

View	Parasternal long axis
Modality	2-D

Fig. 19.1 Trace of pericardial fluid (normal) (LA = left atrium; LV = left ventricle; RVOT = right ventricular outflow tract)

Use 2-D echo to inspect the pericardium in as many views as possible and describe its appearance:

- Does the pericardium appear normal or abnormal?
- Is there thickening of the pericardium?
- Is there pericardial calcification?
- Is there a pericardial effusion? Describe its appearance. How big is it, where is it located and what are its haemodynamic effects?
- Is there evidence of pericardial constriction? What are the haemodynamic effects?
- Are there any pericardial masses?

Pericardial effusion

Any process that causes inflammation or injury to the pericardium can result in a pericardial effusion (Table 19.1).

Table 19.1 Causes of pericardial effusion

Infection	Viral Bacterial (particularly tuberculosis)
Malignant	Primary spread from a local tumour (e.g. lung, breast) Distant metastasis (e.g. melanoma)
Inflammatory	Dressler's syndrome (after myocardial infarction) Uraemia (renal failure) Collagen vascular diseases (e.g. rheumatoid arthritis, systemic lupus erythematosus) Post cardiac surgery Post radiotherapy
Injury/trauma	Post cardiac surgery Aortic dissection Blunt or direct chest trauma
Idiopathic	

Echo assessment of pericardial effusion

Pericardial or pleural?

First of all, be sure what you are assessing. At first glance, pericardial and pleural effusions can appear similar on echo, but there are important distinguishing features. Use 2-D echo in the parasternal long axis view to assess where the effusion lies in relation to the descending aorta. A pericardial effusion will extend just up to the gap in between the left atrium (LA) and the *front* of the descending aorta (Fig. 19.2). In contrast, a pleural effusion extends *behind* the aorta and around the LA (Fig. 19.3). However, bear in mind that some patients will have coexistent pericardial *and* pleural effusions.

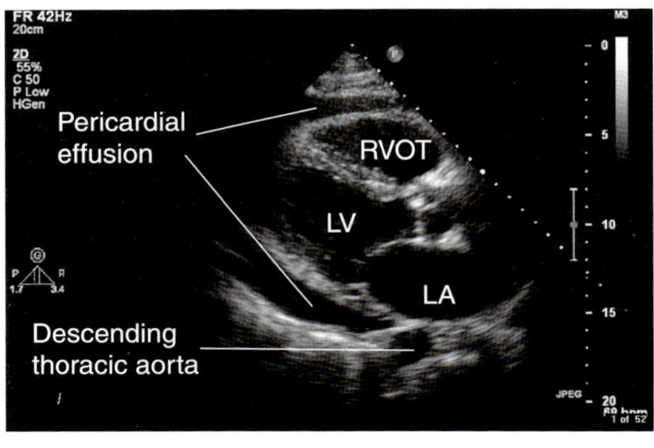

View	Parasternal long axis
Modality	2-D

Fig. 19.2 Pericardial effusion (anterior to descending thoracic aorta) (LA = left atrium; LV = left ventricle; RVOT = right ventricular outflow tract)

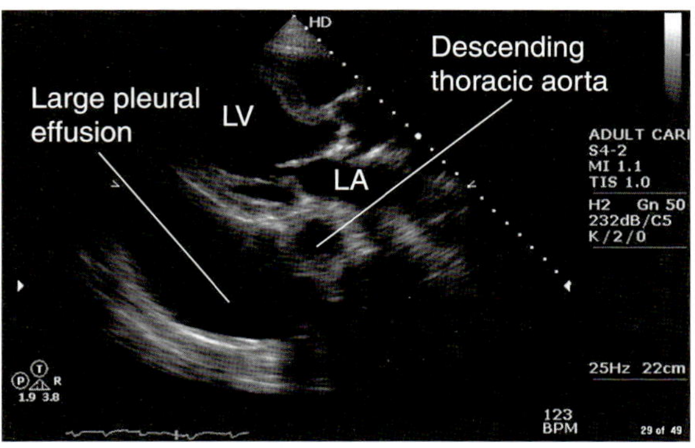

View	Parasternal long axis
Modality	2-D

Fig. 19.3 Pleural effusion (posterior to descending thoracic aorta) (LA = left atrium; LV = left ventricle)

2-D and M-mode

Use 2-D echo to assess the extent of the effusion – is it circumferential, filling the entire pericardium, or localized? If localized, record where the effusion lies in relation to the atria and/or ventricles. Very localized effusions can sometimes be difficult to spot – for instance, if they lie within the oblique sinus – and may only be evident through the compression of adjacent structures (e.g. atria or pulmonary veins). Bear in mind that the patient's position may affect the distribution of the pericardial effusion – for instance, the effusion may localize posteriorly in a supine patient.

Assess the size of the effusion from several different views using 2-D and/or M-mode echo. Record both the depth of the effusion (in cm) and the location where each measurement was taken. The size of an effusion can be gauged by its depth (Table 19.2). It is important to note that effusion size is not the same as clinical severity – small effusions that accumulate quickly can have a greater haemodynamic effect than large effusions that accumulate slowly.

Table 19.2 Pericardial effusion size

	Trace	Small	Moderate	Large
Depth (cm)	<0.5	0.5–1.0	1.0–2.0	>2.0
Volume (mL)	<100	100–250	250–500	>500

It is also possible to estimate the volume of an effusion. In the apical 4-chamber view, you can trace the outline of the pericardium and use the echo machine software to calculate the volume of the entire heart and pericardial effusion. Next, trace the outline of the heart itself and calculate the heart's volume. By subtracting the latter measurement from the former, you are left with the approximate volume of the pericardial effusion.

Pericardial effusions can contain a fluid transudate or exudate, blood or pus. It can be difficult to distinguish between these on echo, and the pericardial fluid will usually look echolucent regardless of its nature. However, there may be strands of fibrin visible within the fluid and these commonly adhere to the outside of the heart. Sometimes masses may be visible within the pericardium (Fig. 19.4). Describe the appearance of any strands or masses, including their size and location.

Once you have assessed the appearances of the pericardial effusion, you should go on to assess its haemodynamic effects to look for evidence that would support a clinical diagnosis of cardiac tamponade (see below).

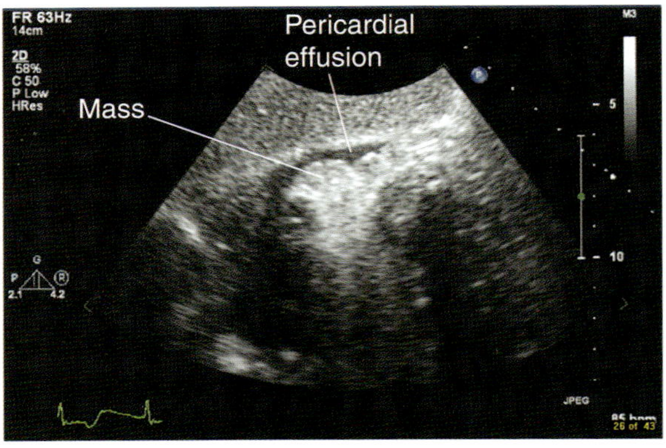

View	Subcostal
Modality	2-D

Fig. 19.4 Mass within a pericardial effusion

Management of pericardial effusion

Patients with pericardial effusion should be investigated as appropriate to determine the underlying cause. Pericardiocentesis is indicated for:

- cardiac tamponade (see below)
- suspected purulent or tuberculous effusions
- effusions measuring >2.0 cm (in diastole).

Pericardiocentesis can be performed for diagnostic purposes for effusions <2.0 cm, but this should only be done by skilled hands in an experienced centre.

Cardiac tamponade

Cardiac tamponade refers to the haemodynamic decompensation that occurs when the pressure within a pericardial effusion compresses the heart. It is a clinical diagnosis indicated by the presence of:

- breathlessness (with clear lungs)
- tachycardia (>100 beats/min)
- hypotension (systolic blood pressure <100 mmHg)
- pulsus paradoxus (>10 mmHg fall in systolic blood pressure during inspiration)

- elevated jugular venous pressure
- quiet heart sounds.

Echo assessment of cardiac tamponade

2-D and M-mode

Use 2-D and M-mode echo to confirm the presence of a pericardial effusion and to assess its extent as described above. Look carefully for signs of chamber collapse during diastole. As pressure within the pericardium rises, the right-sided chambers collapse (at least in part) during diastole (Fig. 19.5). The first chamber to be affected is the right atrium (RA), which is seen to collapse during atrial systole, followed by the right ventricle (beginning with the right ventricular outflow tract, RVOT). Rarely, LA or even left ventricular (LV) collapse may be seen in severe cases.

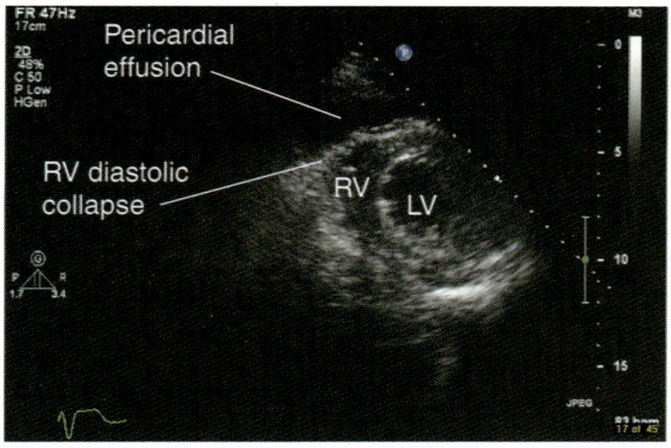

View	Parasternal short axis
Modality	2-D

Fig. 19.5 Cardiac tamponade (right ventricular (RV) diastolic collapse) (LV = left ventricle)

Measure the inferior vena cava (IVC) in the subcostal view, and assess by how much its diameter reduces (if at all) during inspiration. The IVC is normally 1.5–2.5 cm in diameter and this falls by >50 per cent on inspiration. In the presence of tamponade, the IVC dilates and the inspiratory fall in diameter is reduced or absent.

PW Doppler

Use pulsed-wave (PW) Doppler to assess right and left ventricular inflow and look for the exaggerated respiratory variation seen in tamponade. In a normal individual, inspiration increases the flow of blood returning to the right heart and decreases the flow of blood into the left heart; the opposite occurs on expiration. Cardiac tamponade exaggerates this respiratory variation.

To look for this phenomenon, use PW Doppler in the apical 4-chamber view to interrogate tricuspid and mitral inflow. For both valves, measure the maximum and minimum E wave velocities seen during the cardiac cycle (for the tricuspid valve, the maximum will occur during inspiration and the minimum during expiration; vice versa for the mitral valve). The normal respiratory variation in E wave size is <25 per cent for the tricuspid valve and <15 per cent for the mitral valve. In the presence of cardiac tamponade, the same variation occurs but is exaggerated in extent (Fig. 19.6). This is summarized in Table 19.3.

Table 19.3 Respiratory variation in cardiac tamponade

	Normal		Cardiac tamponade	
Tricuspid E wave size				
Inspiration	Maximum	Variation <25%	Maximum	Variation >25%
Expiration	Minimum		Minimum	
Mitral E wave size				
Inspiration	Minimum	Variation <15%	Minimum	Variation >15%
Expiration	Maximum		Maximum	
RVOT V_{max} and VTI				
Inspiration	Maximum	Variation <10%	Maximum	Variation >10%
Expiration	Minimum		Minimum	
LVOT V_{max} and VTI				
Inspiration	Minimum	Variation <10%	Minimum	Variation >10%
Expiration	Maximum		Maximum	

LVOT = left ventricular outflow tract; RVOT = right ventricular outflow tract; V_{max} = peak velocity; VTI = velocity time integral.

Similarly, respiratory variation in ventricular outflow can also be assessed. Use PW Doppler in the parasternal short axis view to interrogate RVOT flow and record both the velocity time integral (VTI) and peak velocity (V_{max}); as with RV inflow, outflow is at its maximum in inspiration and minimum in expiration. In the apical 5-chamber view make the same measurements for the LVOT; as with LV inflow, outflow is at its minimum in inspiration and maximum in expiration. The normal respiratory variability in both parameters is <10 per cent, but is greater in the presence of tamponade.

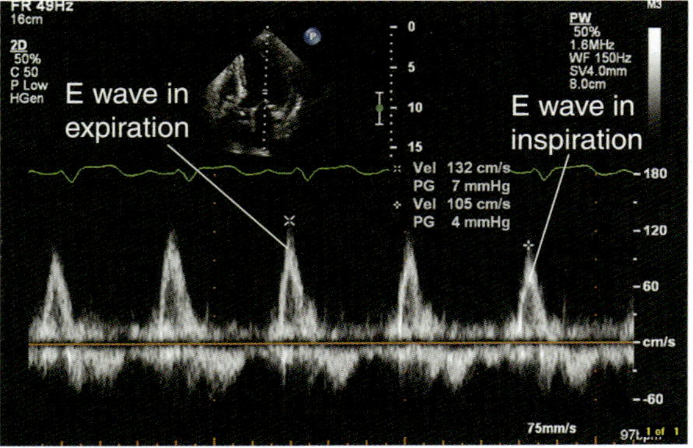

View	Apical 5-chamber
Modality	PW Doppler

Fig. 19.6 Cardiac tamponade (exaggerated respiratory variation in mitral inflow E wave size) (PG = pressure gradient; Vel = velocity)

SAMPLE REPORT

There is a large circumferential pericardial effusion, measuring 3.4 cm adjacent to the right ventricle and 3.2 cm adjacent to the LV. Small fibrin strands are visible adherent to the free wall of the RV. There is diastolic collapse of the right atrium and ventricle. There is exaggerated respiratory variation on Doppler assessment of mitral/tricuspid inflow and pulmonary/aortic outflow. The IVC is dilated with absent inspiratory collapse. The echo findings support the clinical diagnosis of cardiac tamponade.

Management of cardiac tamponade

Cardiac tamponade requires urgent drainage (pericardiocentesis). This is commonly performed via the subxiphisternal approach, and echo is very useful in planning the optimal route to minimize the distance from chest wall to effusion and to avoid intervening structures.

Echo guidance can help determine when the pericardiocentesis needle is correctly located within the pericardium. The needle itself is often difficult to see, and if there is doubt about the needle's position it is possible to instil a small amount of agitated saline (9.5 mL of sterile saline agitated with 0.5 mL of air in a 10 mL syringe, to create a suspension of small air bubbles) through the needle that can be detected by echo screening as bubble contrast within the effusion. If the pericardiocentesis needle has inadvertently punctured the heart, the bubbles will be seen within one of the cardiac chambers instead.

Pericardial constriction

Thickening and fibrosis of the serous pericardium can constrict the heart, like a rigid envelope, impairing filling of the ventricles in diastole. Filling of the heart in early diastole is rapid but then abruptly stops as the diastolic pressure plateaus. The diastolic pressures in the right and left ventricles become equal.

Pericardial constriction can result from pericardial inflammation, often after a long delay, and is most common after tuberculous pericarditis, radiotherapy and cardiac surgery.

Clinical features of pericardial constriction

The clinical features of pericardial constriction (Table 19.4) tend to be vague and the diagnosis is often delayed or missed altogether.

Table 19.4 Clinical features of pericardial constriction

Symptoms	Signs
Fatigue Breathlessness Abdominal swelling and discomfort	Elevated jugular venous pressure Hypotension with low pulse pressure Quiet heart sounds Pleural effusions Hepatomegaly Ascites Peripheral oedema Muscle wasting

Echo assessment of pericardial constriction

2-D and M-mode

Use 2-D and M-mode echo to assess the structure of the pericardium in several different views:

- Is the pericardium thickened? This can be difficult to assess on echo and is more accurately assessed with cardiac computed tomography (CT) or magnetic resonance imaging (MRI).

- Is there any calcification of the pericardium? Is this localized or generalized?

LV dimensions and function will usually be normal. M-mode assessment of the ventricular septum in the parasternal long axis view may show:

- abrupt posterior motion early in diastole, caused by rapid right ventricular diastolic filling, followed by
- little motion in mid-diastole, caused by equalization of right and left ventricular pressures, followed by
- abrupt anterior motion at the end of diastole (after atrial contraction) as there is further RV filling.

There may also be a ventricular septal 'bounce' during inspiration. Increased filling of the RV during inspiration causes the septum to shift over to the left, as the constraints imposed by the pericardium lead to ventricular interdependence. This can be seen as a shift in the ventricular septum towards the LV with inspiration and towards the RV with expiration.

Measure the LA in the parasternal long axis view – it enlarges as a result of the chronically elevated LV diastolic pressure. The RA also enlarges.

Measure the IVC in the subcostal view, and assess how much it collapses during inspiration. The IVC is normally 1.5–2.5 cm in diameter and collapses by >50 per cent on inspiration. In the presence of pericardial constriction, the IVC dilates and inspiratory collapse is reduced or absent.

PW Doppler

Use PW Doppler to assess right and left ventricular inflow and look for exaggerated respiratory variation, as seen in cardiac tamponade (see above).

Look particularly carefully at mitral valve inflow, as recorded by PW Doppler in the apical 4-chamber view. Pericardial constriction causes:

- an exaggeration of the normal E/A ratio (the E wave is larger than normal *and* the A wave is smaller)
- a rapid E-wave deceleration time (normally >160 ms).

Pericardial constriction versus restrictive cardiomyopathy

The differentiation between pericardial constriction and restrictive cardiomyopathy can be challenging and makes a popular topic for echo accreditation examinations! Restrictive cardiomyopathy is discussed in Chapter 18. It shares many of the clinical features of pericardial constriction, so using investigations appropriately to distinguish between the two is important. Table 19.5 lists some of the echo features that can help to distinguish constriction from restriction.

Table 19.5 Pericardial constriction versus restrictive cardiomyopathy

	Pericardial constriction	Restrictive cardiomyopathy
Pericardium	Usually thickened	Normal
Atrial enlargement	Mild-moderate	Moderate-severe
Mitral inflow	E wave respiratory variation >25%	E wave respiratory variation <15 per cent
Tricuspid inflow	E wave respiratory variation >25%	E wave respiratory variation <15 per cent
Ventricular septal motion	Abrupt early diastolic motion	Normal

SAMPLE REPORT

The pericardium appears thickened and calcification is present. Both atria are mildly enlarged. The mitral and tricuspid inflows (E wave) show a variation of >25 per cent between inspiration and expiration. Mitral inflow also shows an exaggerated E/A ratio and a rapid E-wave deceleration time. There is abrupt early diastolic motion of the ventricular septum. The IVC is dilated with reduced inspiratory variation in diameter. There is no pericardial effusion. The echo findings support the clinical diagnosis of pericardial constriction.

Management of pericardial constriction

Surgical intervention (pericardiectomy) is the definitive treatment for permanent pericardial constriction, with a mortality of 6–12 per cent and normalization of haemodynamic parameters in around 60 per cent.

Other pericardial abnormalities

Congenital absence of the pericardium

Congenital absence is a rare abnormality (around 1:10 000) that can affect part (left more commonly than the right) or all of the pericardium. Patients are usually asymptomatic, but it is possible for parts of the heart to become herniated or even strangulated through gaps in the pericardium. With partial absence of the pericardium, herniation of part of the heart may be apparent on 2-D echo. With complete absence of the pericardium, the position of the heart as a whole may be abnormal (usually rotated posteriorly).

Pericardial cysts

Pericardial cysts are discussed on page 291. Small loculated pericardial effusions can be mistaken for congenital cysts.

Pericardial tumours

Pericardial tumours are rare. They can be primary or secondary and include such tumours as lipoma, liposarcoma, mesothelioma and lymphoma. The presence of any pericardial masses should be noted and their appearance described as fully as possible.

FURTHER READING

Hancock EW. Differential diagnosis of restrictive cardiomyopathy and constrictive pericarditis. *Heart* 2001; **86**: 343–9.

Malik I. *British Society of Echocardiography Distance Learning Module 2: The Echo Differentiation of Restriction and Constriction*. Accessible from the BSE website (www.bsecho.org).

Oakley CM. Myocarditis, pericarditis and other pericardial diseases. *Heart* 2000; **84**: 449–54.

Soler-Soler J, Sagristà-Sauleda J, Permanyer-Miralda G. Management of pericardial effusion. *Heart* 2001; **86**: 235–40.

The Task Force on the Diagnosis and Management of Pericardial Diseases of the European Society of Cardiology. Guidelines on the diagnosis and management of pericardial diseases: executive summary. *Eur Heart J* 2004; **25**: 587–610.

20 The aorta

Echo appearances of the normal aorta

The aorta extends all the way from the aortic valve to the point where it bifurcates into the left and right common iliac arteries. Different parts of the aorta are visible in many of the standard transthoracic echo (TTE) views (see Chapter 6):

- left parasternal window
  - parasternal long axis view
  - parasternal short axis view
- right parasternal window
- apical window
  - apical 5-chamber view
  - apical 3-chamber (long axis) view
- subcostal window
- suprasternal window
  - aorta view.

The dimensions of the proximal aorta are measured at four different levels in the parasternal long axis view (Fig. 20.1):

- aortic annulus
- sinuses of Valsalva
- sinotubular junction
- ascending aorta.

The normal ranges for aortic diameter at the level of the sinuses of Valsalva, corrected for body surface area, are shown in the nomograms in Fig. 20.2.

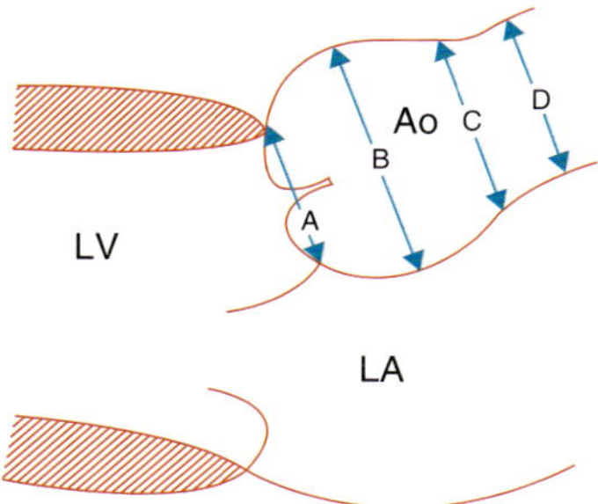

Fig. 20.1 Where to measure the dimensions of the proximal aorta (A = aortic annulus; Ao = aorta; B = sinuses of Valsalva; C = sinotubular junction; D = ascending aorta; LA = left atrium; LV = left ventricle)

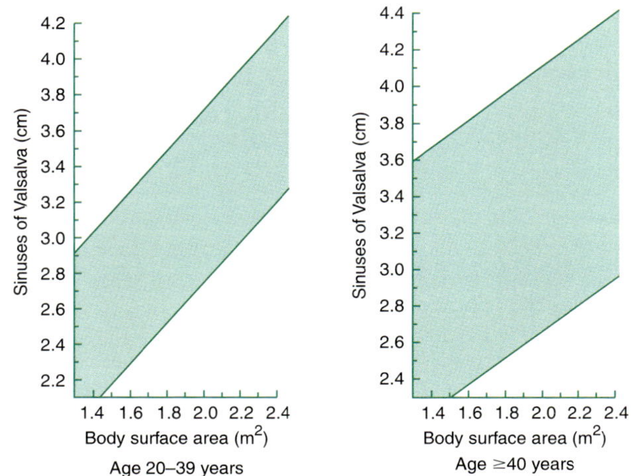

Fig. 20.2 Normal ranges for aortic diameter at the sinuses of Valsalva (Reprinted from Roman MJ, *et al.* Two-dimensional echocardiographic aortic root dimensions in normal adults. *American Journal of Cardiology* **64**, 507–12, © 1989, with permission from Elsevier)

In addition, you can assess the:

- aortic arch in the suprasternal window
- descending thoracic aorta (located behind the left atrium) in the parasternal long axis view
- proximal abdominal aorta in the subcostal view.

For a full echo assessment of the aorta, inspect each part of the aorta and:

- describe its appearance (normal or abnormal)
- comment on any dilatation (stating location and dimensions)
- identify any atheroma or thrombus (stating location, appearance, severity and if it is mobile)
- identify any dissection (stating the entry and exit point and whether there is any thrombus in the false lumen)
- identify any intramural haematoma (stating the location)
- identify any transection (stating the location)
- identify and characterize any aortic coarctation (see p. 305).

Aortic dilatation

Dilatation of the aortic can result from:

- atherosclerosis
- hypertension
- trauma
- post-stenotic (dilatation of the ascending aorta above a stenotic aortic valve).

Aortic dilatation (and dissection) is also more likely in patients with bicuspid aortic valve (p. 303) and correlates with the degree of aortic regurgitation that may be present. Patients with bicuspid aortic valve are 10 times more likely to experience an aortic dissection than those with a normal valve.

A number of connective tissue and inflammatory diseases can cause aortic dilatation:

- Marfan syndrome
- systemic lupus erythematosus
- rheumatoid arthritis
- Reiter syndrome
- syphilitic aortitis.

In aortic dilatation due to Marfan syndrome, the relative proportions of the aortic root (broader at the sinuses of Valsalva, becoming narrower again at the sinotubular junction) are lost and the boundary between the sinuses of Valsalva and the ascending aorta becomes less clear – this is referred to as effacement of the sinotubular junction. Marfan syndrome is discussed on page 316. Localized dilatation of one or more sinuses of Valsalva is called sinus of Valsalva aneurysm (p. 278).

Echo assessment of aortic dilatation

Aortic dilatation can occur in more than one site, so for an aortic assessment it is important to use 2-D (and/or M-mode) echo to measure the aortic dimensions in as many sites as possible (Fig. 20.3):

- aortic annulus
- sinuses of Valsalva
- sinotubular junction
- ascending aorta
- aortic arch
- descending thoracic aorta
- proximal abdominal aorta.

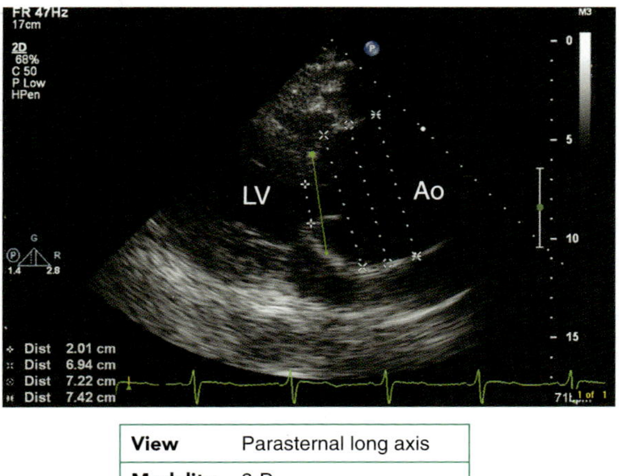

View	Parasternal long axis
Modality	2-D

Fig. 20.3 Severe aortic root dilatation (Ao = aorta; LV = left ventricle)

Look for, and describe, any associated aortic abnormalities:

- atheroma
- thrombus
- dissection
- coarctation.

In cases that involve the aortic root look carefully for the effects on aortic valve structure and function. Dilatation of the aortic root can lead to reduced coaptation between the aortic valve cusps, so look for any distortion of the valve and use Doppler interrogation to assess aortic regurgitation. Remember too that an abnormal aortic valve can sometimes be the *cause* of aortic dilatation (e.g. bicuspid aortic valve, post-stenotic dilatation in aortic stenosis), and a full aortic valve assessment should be performed with this in mind.

Management of aortic dilatation

As the aorta dilates, a potentially catastrophic event such as dissection or rupture becomes increasingly likely. Careful monitoring with surgical intervention at an appropriate time is the key to successful management.

Patients with mild-moderate aortic root dilatation should, where possible, receive treatment with a beta-blocker and undergo echo follow-up every 6–12 months (bearing in mind that the larger an aneurysm, the more quickly it dilates). Elective surgery is usually undertaken if the aortic diameter measures ⩾5.5 cm (some authorities advise a lower threshold of ⩾5.0 cm for patients with Marfan syndrome or bicuspid aortic valve). Rapid dilatation of an aneurysm (⩾1.0 cm/year) is also considered an indication for surgery.

Aortic dissection

If a tear occurs in the intimal layer of the aorta, blood flowing in the aortic lumen can penetrate through to the medial layer to create an extra channel or 'false lumen'. The blood entering the medial layer can propagate proximally or distally within the wall of the aorta. The initial tear ('entry point') can occur anywhere in the aorta, although the vast majority of aortic dissections originate either in the first few centimetres of the ascending aorta or just distal to the origin of the left subclavian artery. Blood flowing in the false lumen can re-enter the 'true' lumen of the aorta through a further intimal tear elsewhere ('exit point'). Aortic dissections are classified according to the region of aorta involved (Table 20.1).

Table 20.1 Classification of aortic dissection

Stanford classification	DeBakey classification
Type A dissections involve the ascending aorta	Type I dissections involve the ascending aorta, arch and descending aorta
Type B dissections do not involve the ascending aorta	Type II dissections are confined to the ascending aorta
	Type III dissections originate distal to the left subclavian artery and are confined to the descending aorta

Aortic dissection can occur in patients with pre-existing aortic dilatation, or conditions that place the aorta under strain or affect the strength of the wall (e.g. hypertension, pregnancy, Marfan syndrome, Ehlers–Danlos syndrome, bicuspid aortic valve, aortic coarctation).

Aortic dissection is a medical emergency, 50 per cent of patients dying within the first 48 h if left untreated. The classical presenting symptom is a sudden-onset 'tearing' interscapular pain. Patients may exhibit a difference in blood pressure (>20 mmHg) between right and left arms. A variety of other clinical features may be seen, depending on the extent of the dissection and whether it impairs the blood supply to other organs.

Echo assessment of aortic dissection

The limited views of TTE mean that a negative study cannot exclude the diagnosis. Additional imaging with transoesophageal echo (TOE) or computed tomography (CT)/magnetic resonance imaging (MRI) may be necessary.

2-D and M-mode

Inspect the aorta from as many views as possible. Remember that the majority of dissections arise in the initial segment of the ascending aorta or just after the left subclavian artery. Look carefully for:

- evidence of aortic dilatation
- evidence of a 'dissection flap'.

A dissection flap is a linear structure within the aorta which is mobile, but its pattern of movement is more erratic than that of the aortic wall (Fig. 20.4). Identify the location of the dissection and try to identify the entry and exit points where possible.

Colour Doppler

Use colour Doppler to assess flow within the true and false lumens – their flow patterns are usually different. Colour Doppler can help to identify the entry and exit points of the false lumen, although it should be noted that there may be multiple entry/exit sites where flow between the true and false lumens can occur.

It can sometimes be difficult to decide which is the true and which is the false lumen, particularly in the descending aorta. The shape of the true

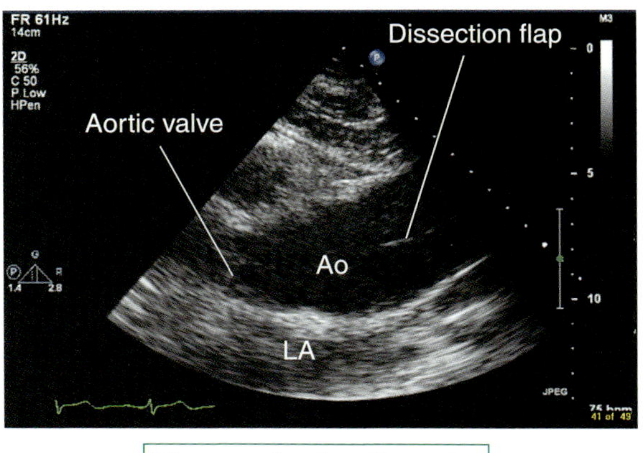

View	Parasternal long axis
Modality	2-D

Fig. 20.4 Aortic dissection in ascending aorta (Ao = aorta; LA = left atrium)

lumen is usually more regular than the false lumen, and the true lumen is more likely to exhibit expansile pulsation during systole.

Blood within the false lumen may start to thrombose, in which case the false lumen may show spontaneous echo contrast or absent flow. The presence of thrombus in the false lumen should be noted in your report.

Associated features

TTE is useful in identifying complications of aortic dissection:

- **Aortic regurgitation** – if the dissection involves the aortic root, the normal structure of the aortic valve can be distorted causing regurgitation.
- **Myocardial ischaemia/infarction** – involvement of the coronary arteries (most commonly the right coronary artery) can lead to ischaemia/infarction, evidenced by left ventricular regional wall motion abnormalities.
- **Pericardial effusion/cardiac tamponade** – rupture of the dissection into the pericardial space causes a haemorrhagic pericardial effusion and/or tamponade.

PITFALLS IN THE ECHO ASSESSMENT OF AORTIC DISSECTION

- False negative diagnosis – a normal TTE study does not exclude an aortic dissection.
- False positive diagnosis – echo artefact within the aortic lumen can be mistaken for dissection. Typical causes of artefact include reverberation or beam-width artefact (p. 28). Artefacts usually lack the chaotic motion seen with a dissection flap.
- In a patient with acute chest pain and left ventricular wall motion abnormality, always check for aortic dissection as a potential cause of the myocardial ischaemia/infarction.

SAMPLE REPORT

The aortic root is dilated (diameter 5.8 cm at the level of the sinuses of Valsalva). There is a linear echogenic structure with erratic movement arising in the aortic root and extending to the descending aorta, just distal to the origin of the left subclavian artery, indicative of an aortic dissection flap. A false lumen is noted containing blood flow on colour Doppler, with an entry point at the sinotubular junction. There is poor apposition of the aortic valve cusps and moderate aortic regurgitation. There is no pericardial effusion. Left ventricular function is normal. The appearances indicate an aortic dissection (Stanford Type A) with a dilated aortic root and moderate aortic regurgitation.

Management of aortic dissection

Patients with aortic dissection may be critically ill and haemodynamically compromised, requiring urgent stabilization. Dissections involving the ascending aorta are managed with urgent surgical intervention. Dissections confined to the descending aorta are usually managed pharmacologically (e.g. assiduous control of hypertension), with surgery being reserved for any complications (e.g. rupture) that may occur.

INTRAMURAL HAEMATOMA

Intramural haematoma can present with similar symptoms to aortic dissection and is managed similarly. However, in intramural haematoma there is bleeding into the aortic medial layer not from the aortic lumen but from vessels that supply the aorta itself – there is therefore no communication between the blood in the aorta and in the haematoma. Intramural haematoma can nevertheless lead to aortic dissection or rupture. On echo, an intramural haematoma appears as an echogenic 'mass' within the wall of the aorta, between the intimal and adventitial layers.

Sinus of Valsalva aneurysm

Just above the level of the aortic valve lie the three sinuses of Valsalva, each one corresponding to one of the aortic valve cusps (right coronary, left coronary and non-coronary). Although any of the sinuses of Valsalva can develop aneurysmal dilatation, the right sinus is affected most commonly (around two-thirds of cases) and the non-coronary sinus in around a quarter of cases; the left sinus is seldom affected.

Sinus of Valsalva aneurysm can be congenital, occurring as a result of an abnormality of the aortic media and elastic tissue, leading to dilatation of a single sinus. Congenital aneurysms can become elongated and are classically described as having a 'windsock' appearance on echo. Acquired causes include atherosclerosis, endocarditis, cystic medial necrosis, chest trauma and syphilis. Acquired cases often affect all three sinuses. Sinus of Valsalva aneurysm is seen in around 10 per cent of patients with Marfan syndrome.

Sinus of Valsalva aneurysm can lead to:

- aortic regurgitation
- compression or distortion of local structures (e.g. coronary arteries, right ventricular outflow tract, conduction system)
- rupture of the aneurysm into an adjacent structure (most commonly the right ventricle or right atrium, or more rarely into the left heart chambers, pulmonary artery or pericardium).

Echo assessment of sinus of Valsalva aneurysm includes:

- measurement of aortic root dimensions
- description of the sinus(es) involved

- assessment of aortic valve structure and function, looking in particular for aortic regurgitation
- looking for evidence of compression or distortion of any neighbouring structures by the aneurysm
- assessment of whether rupture is present, which chamber is involved, and what the haemodynamic effects are
- looking for associated abnormalities (ventricular septal defect, bicuspid aortic valve).

Repair of a ruptured sinus of Valsalva aneurysm can be performed surgically or percutaneously, using an occluder device. Unruptured aneurysms can be repaired surgically, although the optimal timing of such surgery is controversial.

Aortic atheroma

Atherosclerotic plaques can form in the aorta, particularly in patients with vascular disease elsewhere (e.g. coronary artery disease, cerebrovascular disease, peripheral vascular disease). Aortic atheroma is seen in the descending aorta more frequently than in the ascending aorta, and is best studied with TOE (but it may be seen during TTE studies too).

Clinical features of aortic atheroma

Aortic atheroma is commonly an incidental finding and in itself is therefore often asymptomatic. However, it can be a source for arterial emboli downstream of the plaque, causing stroke and/or peripheral emboli. Atheromatous disease of the aorta can also be a precursor to dilatation of the aorta and/or to aortic dissection (see above).

Patients with aortic atheroma may have atheromatous disease elsewhere in the arterial system, and this can cause symptoms, e.g.:

- coronary artery disease – causing angina and/or acute coronary syndromes
- cerebrovascular disease – causing transient ischaemic attacks and/or stroke
- peripheral vascular disease – causing intermittent claudication.

Review patients with aortic atheroma for symptoms and signs of vascular disease, and also for major treatable risk factors for vascular disease:

- hyperlipidaemia
- tobacco consumption

- diabetes mellitus
- hypertension.

Echo assessment of aortic atheroma

Use 2-D echo to examine the aorta for the presence of atheroma. If atheroma is present, describe its location:

- aortic root
- ascending aorta
- aortic arch
- descending thoracic aorta
- abdominal aorta.

Describe the appearance of the atheroma:

- Is there any calcification of the atheroma?
- Is there protrusion of the atheroma into the lumen of the vessel? How thick is any protruding plaque?
- Is the atheroma mobile?
- Is the atheromatous plaque ulcerated?

Finally, you should grade the extent of any aortic atheroma as mild, moderate or severe. Although these gradings are not clearly defined, it is reasonable to regard plaque disease that is mobile, ulcerated and/or protruding with a thickness of 5 mm or more as 'severe'.

SAMPLE REPORT

There is mild calcified atheromatous plaque visible in the ascending aorta, and moderate calcified plaque in the aortic arch, protruding into the aortic lumen with a thickness up to 3 mm. The atheromatous plaque is not mobile.

Management of aortic atheroma

Counsel patients with aortic atheroma about risk factor management (e.g. quitting smoking, dietary modification). Drug treatment with an antiplatelet drug (e.g. aspirin) and a statin is often appropriate. Atheroma associated with aortic dilatation or dissection may require surgical intervention.

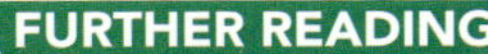

FURTHER READING

Anderson RH. Clinical anatomy of the aortic root. *Heart* 2000; **84**: 670–3.

Erbel R, Eggebrecht H. Aortic dimensions and the risk of dissection. *Heart* 2006; **92**: 137–42.

Nataf P, Lansac E. Dilation of the thoracic aorta: medical and surgical management. *Heart* 2006; **92**: 1345–52.

The Task Force on Aortic Dissection, European Society of Cardiology. Diagnosis and management of aortic dissection. *Eur Heart J* 2001; **22**: 1642–81.

Von Kodolitsch Y, Robinson PN. Marfan syndrome: an update of genetics, medical and surgical management. *Heart* 2007; **93**: 755–60.

21 Cardiac masses

The finding of a cardiac mass often has significant clinical implications and therefore apparent masses need careful echo evaluation to determine, as far as possible, their likely nature. Some harmless structures, such as the right ventricular (RV) moderator band, can give the appearance of a mass, and so it is particularly important to try to distinguish a mass that it pathological from one that is a normal variant. Cardiac masses on echo can result from:

- tumours
  - primary cardiac tumours
    - benign
    - malignant
  - secondary cardiac tumours
- thrombus
- vegetations
- normal variants and other conditions
  - moderator band
  - Lambl's excrescences
  - Eustachian valve
  - Chiari network
  - lipomatous hypertrophy of the interatrial septum
  - dilated vessels
  - cysts
  - implanted devices.

Tumours

The echo assessment of a cardiac tumour should include a description of its:

- Size (measure its dimensions)
- Location
- Shape (e.g. spherical, pedunculated, papillary, flat)

- Surface appearance (e.g. regular, irregular, multilobular)
- Texture (e.g. solid, layered, cystic, calcified, heterogeneous)
- Mobility (mobile or fixed)
- Associated features (local invasion, pericardial effusion).

Because echo does not allow for a *precise* diagnosis, it is generally more appropriate to report a cardiac mass as being, for example, 'suggestive of a myxoma' than as a 'definite' myxoma.

The characteristics of the commonest tumours, and the features that distinguish them from other cardiac masses, are described below.

Primary cardiac tumours

Primary cardiac tumours are those that arise from the heart itself. They are rare (1 in 2000 autopsies) and 75 per cent are benign (Table 21.1).

Table 21.1 Primary cardiac tumours

Benign (75 per cent)	Malignant (25 per cent)
Myxoma	Angiosarcoma
Papillary fibroelastoma	Rhabdomyosarcoma
Lipoma	
Haemangioma	
Teratoma	
Rhabdomyoma	
Fibroma	

Primary cardiac tumours can present with systemic features such as fever and weight loss, or more specifically with:

- Embolism – either of part the tumour itself or adherent thrombus
- Obstruction – usually of a valve orifice or outflow tract
- Arrhythmias – either tachyarrhythmias, such as ventricular tachycardia, or atrioventricular block.

Cardiac tumours can also be found incidentally during echo studies for other indications.

Myxoma

Myxoma is the commonest primary cardiac tumour, accounting for 50 per cent of cases, and is commoner in women. It is typically diagnosed between the ages of 50 and 70 years. Myxomas are usually (but not always) solitary: 75–80 per cent are found in the left atrium (LA), 15–20 per cent in the right atrium (RA), and rarely in the ventricles.

Around 10 per cent of myxomas are familial (autosomal dominant), and these are more commonly multiple and found in the ventricles. Familial myxomas tend to present at a younger age. There can be associated abnormalities such as facial freckling and endocrine tumours, and such syndromes are grouped together as a 'Carney complex'. Other myxoma syndromes include NAME syndrome and LAMB syndrome. Screening of first-degree relatives is appropriate in suspected familial cases.

Myxomas are attached to the heart by a pedunculated stalk – in the case of atrial myxomas, they attach to the interatrial septum at the fossa ovalis (Fig. 21.1). The echo appearances of a myxoma are of a well-defined mass, which is often mobile, and the pedicle may be visible. The tumour itself appears heterogeneous and may contain small areas of lucency and occasionally speckles of calcium. Transthoracic echo (TTE) is usually adequate for making the diagnosis, but transoesophageal echo (TOE) has a greater sensitivity and specificity and provides a more detailed assessment of the myxoma.

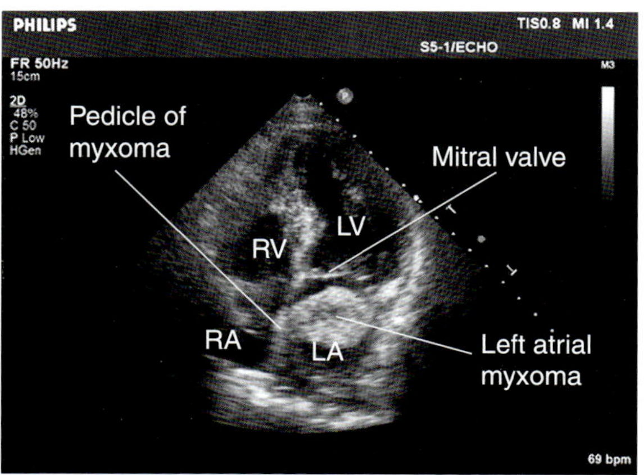

View	Apical 4-chamber
Modality	2-D

Fig. 21.1 Left atrial myxoma (LA = left atrium; LV = left ventricle; RA = right atrium; RV = right ventricle) (Figure reproduced with permission of Philips)

The echo assessment of a myxoma should include all the standard parameters discussed above, together with a Doppler assessment of the myxoma's haemodynamic effects (e.g. obstruction of the mitral valve orifice, causing functional mitral stenosis).

SAMPLE REPORT

The LA contains a mass attached to the interatrial atrial septum via a pedicle. The mass is approximately spherical, measuring 1.6 cm by 1.4 cm, and has an irregular surface and a heterogeneous texture with areas of lucency and of calcification. The mass is mobile but is not causing any obstruction to mitral valve flow. No other intracardiac masses are seen. The appearances are suggestive of a left atrial myxoma.

Surgical resection of the myxoma is the treatment of choice. Following resection, longer-term follow-up is appropriate to monitor for tumour recurrence (particularly in familial cases, where the recurrence rate is 20 per cent).

Other benign cardiac tumours

Papillary fibroelastoma is a small (<1.5 cm) benign valvular tumour, attached to the downstream side of the aortic or mitral valve. They account for 10 per cent of primary cardiac tumours. They are usually found incidentally during echo, cardiac surgery or post mortem, and their similarity to vegetations can lead to a mistaken diagnosis of infective endocarditis. The tumours can embolize and surgical resection should therefore be considered.

Lipomas are usually seen beneath the epicardium. Cardiac magnetic resonance imaging (MRI) is a useful technique to confirm the diagnosis. Lipomas are distinct from lipomatous hypertrophy of the interatrial septum (see below).

Haemangioma is a rare benign vascular tumour which can occur in any chamber.

Rhabdomyoma is the commonest cardiac tumour seen in infants and children. It is usually multiple and found in the ventricles. It is commonly associated with tuberous sclerosis.

Fibromas are also commonest in infants and children, and mainly affect the interventricular septum. Fibromas are up to 10 cm in diameter and appear heterogeneous with multifocal calcification on echo. They often cause obstruction and arrhythmias.

Teratomas are germ cell tumours found in infants and children that usually affect the pericardium and are associated with a pericardial effusion. Echo shows a complex cystic mass within the pericardium and usually on the right side of the heart.

Malignant primary cardiac tumours

Malignant tumours make up 25 per cent of primary cardiac tumours and the vast majority are sarcomas. There are various types of cardiac sarcoma, including angiosarcoma (the commonest), rhabdomyosarcoma, malignant fibrous histiocytoma and osteosarcoma.

Angiosarcomas almost always affect the RA (in contrast to the other sarcomas) and they occur more commonly in men, usually in the age range 30–50 years. Patients often present with symptoms of right heart obstruction and, because pericardial involvement is common, cardiac tamponade. On echo the mass is broad based, often arises near the junction of the inferior cava with the RA, and may be invasive.

Primary cardiac lymphomas are usually non-Hodgkin lymphomas. Although it is not unusual for the heart to be affected as a consequence of lymphoma elsewhere, primary cardiac lymphoma (i.e. confined to the heart and pericardium alone) is very rare, although it is more frequent in acquired immunodeficiency syndrome and in immunosuppressed transplant recipients. Echo reveals masses, most commonly affecting the right heart, often with a pericardial effusion.

Secondary cardiac tumours

Secondary cardiac tumours are those that have arisen elsewhere in the body and have metastasized to the heart (Fig. 21.2). They are much commoner than primary cardiac tumours (1 in 100 autopsies) but only 10 per cent cause symptoms or signs during life. The tumours that metastasize to the heart most frequently include melanoma, lymphoma and leukaemia, bronchial carcinoma and breast carcinoma. Symptomatic patients usually present with arrhythmias or heart failure, and may have pericardial effusion.

Echo most commonly shows epicardial thickening, although the myocardium and endocardium can also be involved, often with pericardial effusion. Tumours can also spread to the heart directly along vessels – renal cell carcinoma can invade the heart via the inferior vena cava, and bronchial carcinoma via the pulmonary veins.

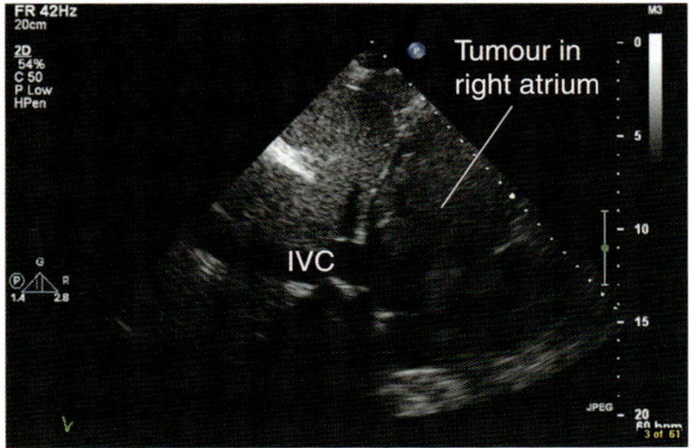

View	Subcostal
Modality	2-D

Fig. 21.2 Large secondary tumour within right atrium (IVC = inferior vena cava)

Thrombus

Cardiac thrombus is more likely to form when:

1. there is stasis (or slow flow) of blood
2. there is abnormal endocardium (allowing thrombus to attach)
3. the blood is hypercoagulable (making it more likely to clot).

Thrombus formation is therefore more likely in the LA in atrial fibrillation (AF), when there is a loss of normal atrial contraction, and in the left ventricle (LV) following myocardial infarction, when reduced contractility predisposes to thrombus formation (particularly if there is aneurysm formation). The presence of an intracardiac device, such as a prosthetic valve or a pacing wire, can also act as a focus for thrombosis. Where there is a high risk of thrombosis (or where a thrombus has already formed) anticoagulation with a drug such as warfarin is used.

When you suspect you have found a cardiac thrombus, it is important to ask yourself, 'What is the substrate?'. In other words, what is the underlying abnormality that has allowed the thrombus to form? If you cannot find a substrate, you should reassess whether are you observing a thrombus or a different type of cardiac mass. For instance, LV thrombus formation would be very unusual in the presence of a structurally normal LV with good function.

Echo assessment of thrombus

The echo assessment of a cardiac thrombus should include a description of its:

- size (measure its dimensions)
- location
- shape (e.g. flat, protruding, spherical)
- surface appearance (e.g. regular, irregular)
- texture (e.g. solid, layered, calcified)
- mobility (mobile or fixed)
- associated features (e.g. dilated LA, LV aneurysm).

Compared with a myxoma, a thrombus usually has a more irregular shape. Thrombus usually attaches to the endocardium via a broad base rather than a pedicle, and is consequently less mobile. A large proportion of LA thrombi are within the LA appendage, which can be difficult to inspect fully on TTE. The appendage is, however, clearly seen on TOE. It is important to try to distinguish between thrombus and the pectinate muscles, the normal muscle ridges found on the walls of both atria and the appendage. Pectinate muscles are immobile and run in bands; thrombus is usually more rounded and mobile.

Stasis of blood within the heart (and sometimes even the aorta) can be evident as 'spontaneous echo contrast'. This has the appearance of a swirling 'cloud' of tiny particles, hence it is sometimes referred to as 'smoke'. Although it is most often (and mostly clearly) seen during TOE studies, it can also be observed during TTE. Spontaneous contrast is caused by echo reflections from aggregations of red blood cells moving at low velocity, and it is most often observed in the LA in patients in AF, particularly if they also have mitral stenosis. It indicates an increased risk of thrombus formation.

Thrombus in the LV normally occurs in association with an area of wall motion abnormality and/or aneurysm formation, commonly the apex (Fig. 21.3). The echo texture of the thrombus is usually distinct from the adjacent myocardium. With the passage of time, the thrombus may become organized and layered, and there may be associated calcification. TTE is better than TOE for the detection of ventricular thrombus, as the ventricle is closer to the probe on TTE imaging.

Thrombus in the right heart is less commonly found, and may represent a thromboembolism that has arisen in the peripheral veins and is 'in transit' to becoming a pulmonary embolism. Another cause of right heart thrombi is the presence of devices such as pacing/defibrillator leads or intravascular catheters, which can act as a focus for thrombus formation.

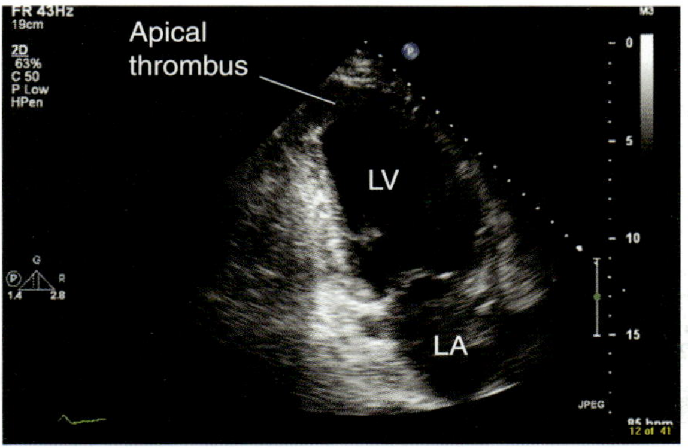

View	Apical 2-chamber
Modality	2-D

Fig. 21.3 Left ventricular apical thrombus (LA = left atrium; LV = left ventricle)

SAMPLE REPORT

The LV contains an immobile mass at its apex. The mass is 1.8 cm across and 0.8 cm deep, and has a regular surface and a layered texture. There is no calcification. The underlying apical segments of the LV are akinetic. The appearances are suggestive of a mural thrombus at the LV apex, secondary to an apical infarct.

Vegetations

Vegetations are discussed more fully in Chapter 17. Vegetations are usually irregular in shape, mobile and attached to valve leaflets on the upstream side (in contrast with papillary fibroelastoma, which attaches downstream). Infective endocarditis can also cause abscesses, which also have the appearance of cardiac masses. As well as the echo features, the clinical context is important in distinguishing between vegetations and other causes of cardiac masses.

Normal variants and other conditions

Moderator band

The moderator band is a prominent muscular ridge of tissue that runs across the RV and is particularly well seen from the apical window. It can be mistaken for a cardiac mass. Similarly, 'false chords' in the LV (and even the papillary muscles) can inadvertently be mistaken for abnormal masses.

Lambl's excrescences

Lambl's excrescences are small filamentous strands on the ventricular side of the aortic valve. They are a normal finding in the elderly and are thought to arise from 'wear and tear' at the edges of the cusps. On echo they can be mistaken for papillary fibroelastomas, but are usually smaller.

Eustachian valve

The Eustachian valve is a membranous embryological remnant – its role in fetal life is to direct oxygenated blood towards the foramen ovale and away from the tricuspid valve. In adult life it is usually seen as a thin flap at the junction of the inferior vena cava with the RA. The size and mobility of the Eustachian valve is very variable between individuals, but this represents normal variation.

Chiari network

A Chiari network is an embryological remnant of the sinus venosus and forms a net-like web across the RA in around in 2 per cent of the population. It has no clinical significance, although it can make passage of right heart catheters more difficult.

Lipomatous hypertrophy of the interatrial septum

Lipomatous hypertrophy of the interatrial septum is characterized by an accumulation of non-encapsulated fatty tissue within the interatrial septum. It has an incidence of between 1 per cent and 8 per cent and is commoner with increasing age. Although usually asymptomatic, associations with arrhythmias have been reported. The characteristic echo appearances are:

- marked thickening of the interatrial septum (⩾15 mm)
- echogenic appearance of the lipomatous tissue
- sparing of the fossa ovalis (giving a dumbbell appearance).

Dilated vessels

A **dilated coronary sinus** can give the appearance of a cystic mass behind the heart (Fig. 21.4). Enlargement of the coronary sinus usually occurs as a result of anomalous drainage of a *left-sided* superior vena cava. This can be confirmed by an injection of agitated saline into a left arm vein – the bubbles will be seen to fill the coronary sinus, followed by the RA.

An **aneurysmal coronary artery** can also give the appearance of a cardiac cystic mass along the route of the coronary arteries. The right coronary

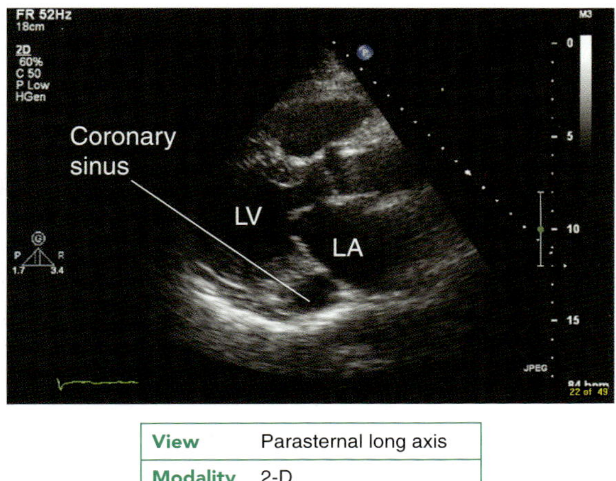

View	Parasternal long axis
Modality	2-D

Fig. 21.4 Dilated coronary sinus (LA = left atrium; LV = left ventricle)

artery is more commonly affected than the left. The diagnosis can be confirmed by coronary angiography or cardiac computed tomography (CT)/magnetic resonance imaging (MRI).

Cysts

Pericardial cysts are a benign abnormality that are usually congenital but have also been reported following cardiac surgery. They are most commonly located at the right cardiophrenic angle. Most are asymptomatic and discovered incidentally, but some can present with compressive symptoms. On echo they have the appearance of an oval cavity, rather like a loculated pericardial effusion, and are commonly 1–5 cm in size. Management options include observation, percutaneous drainage and surgical resection.

Implanted devices

At first sight, implanted devices can sometimes have the appearance of a cardiac mass. The diagnosis is usually clarified simply by asking the patient about any past cardiac procedures. Devices than can cause confusion include:

- pacemaker and defibrillator leads (in RV and RA)
- intravascular catheters
- prosthetic valves
- atrial septal occluder devices
- LV assist device.

FURTHER READING

Grebenc ML, de Christenson MLR, Burke AP, *et al.* Primary cardiac and pericardial neoplasms: radiologic-pathologic correlation. *Radiographics* 2000; **20**: 1073–103.

Joshi J. *British Society of Echocardiography Distance Learning Module 5: Tumours and Infiltrative Processes.* Accessible from the BSE website (www.bsecho.org).

Nadra I, Dawson D, Schmitz SA, *et al.* Lipomatous hypertrophy of the interatrial septum: a commonly misdiagnosed mass often leading to unnecessary cardiac surgery. *Heart* 2004; **90**: e66.

Patel J, Park C, Michaels J, *et al.* Pericardial cyst: case reports and a literature review. *Echocardiography* 2004; **21**: 269–72.

Shapiro LM. Cardiac tumours: diagnosis and management. *Heart* 2001; **85**: 218–22.

22 Congenital heart disease

This book is concerned with *adult* echocardiography, and so the congenital abnormalities described in this chapter are primarily those that may be encountered in adult patients, often following surgical or percutaneous correction. A detailed discussion of congenital heart disease is beyond the scope of this book but a number of excellent reference works are available for further reading.

Atrial septal defect

Atrial septal defect (ASD) is the commonest form of congenital heart disease seen in adults. The commonest form of defect is the **secundum ASD**, accounting for two-thirds of cases, in which the fossa ovalis is absent, leaving a defect in the centre of the interatrial septum. **Primum ASD** is rarer and causes a defect in the inferior interatrial septum, often associated with a cleft anterior mitral valve leaflet. **Sinus venosus ASD** is also rare and is found near to where the superior or inferior vena cava joins the right atrium (RA). It is associated with partial anomalous pulmonary venous drainage, in which one or more pulmonary veins drain directly into the RA (or one of the vena cavae) instead of the left atrium (LA).

An ASD can also be acquired as a result of deliberate puncture of the interatrial septum during balloon mitral valvuloplasty or left-sided electrophysiological procedures, or accidental puncture during right heart catheterization or pacing.

Clinical features of atrial septal defect

ASD can remain asymptomatic for many years and may present late in adult life. It can also be an incidental finding. The clinical features are summarized in Table 22.1. In advanced cases, the increased pulmonary blood flow with an ASD eventually leads to pulmonary hypertension and right heart failure.

Table 22.1 Clinical features of atrial septal defect

Symptoms	Signs
May be asymptomatic Breathlessness Recurrent respiratory infections Palpitations (atrial fibrillation) Paradoxical embolism	Atrial fibrillation can occur Wide fixed splitting of the second heart sound Systolic (flow) murmur in pulmonary area Right heart failure (advanced cases)

Echo assessment of atrial septal defect

The best transthoracic view of the interatrial septum is obtained from the **subcostal window**, although the septum can also be seen from the apical window (4-chamber view) and the parasternal window (short axis view, aortic valve level). In each view, use 2-D echo to assess the structure of the interatrial septum:

- Does the interatrial septum appear normal or is there any aneurysm formation (see box)?
- Is there any echo dropout in the septum to indicate a defect? In the apical view, it is not unusual to see areas of 'apparent' dropout in the interatrial septum, which is quite a long way from the probe, so be careful not to report dropout as an ASD unless you can also see it in other views and/or you also have further supporting evidence.
- Assess right atrial and ventricular size/function – are they dilated as a consequence of a left-to-right shunt? Is there evidence of right heart volume overload (paradoxical motion of the interventricular septum)?

Use colour Doppler to check for the presence of flow across the defect. Flow across an ASD is normally from left to right, mainly during diastole, and also in systole (Fig. 22.1).

In the subcostal view, use pulsed-wave (PW) Doppler to assess flow across the defect.

If you identify an ASD, comment on its size and location (secundum, primum or sinus venosus), and be sure to check for any associated abnormalities (e.g. cleft anterior mitral valve leaflet). Check also for the presence of tricuspid and/or pulmonary regurgitation and, where possible,

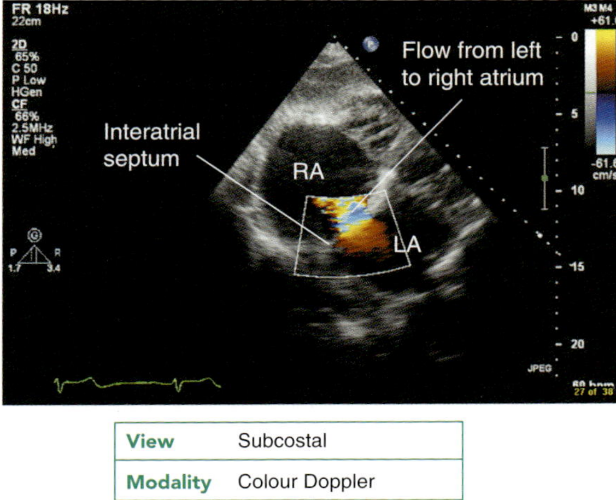

View	Subcostal
Modality	Colour Doppler

Fig. 22.1 Secundum atrial septal defect (LA = left atrium; RA = right atrium)

assess pulmonary artery pressure in case pulmonary hypertension has developed. Perform a shunt calculation to estimate the shunt ratio (see box).

SHUNT CALCULATIONS

Normally the stroke volume of the right heart equals that of the left. However, the presence of a left-to-right shunt such as an ASD means that a portion of the blood that would normally leave the left heart with each heartbeat instead enters the right heart, and is pumped through the lungs before returning to the left heart again. Thus in the presence of a left-to-right shunt the stroke volume of the right heart is greater than that of the left, and the ratio between the two is a measure of the severity of shunting. The ratio is often referred to as Qp/Qs, where Qp is pulmonary blood flow and Qs is systemic blood flow. To calculate the shunt ratio:

- In the parasternal short axis view (aortic valve level), measure the diameter of the right ventricular outflow tract (RVOT) in cm, then use this to calculate the cross-sectional area (CSA) of the RVOT in cm^2:

$$CSA_{RVOT} = 0.785 \times (\text{RVOT diameter})^2$$

- In the same view, measure the velocity time integral (VTI) of flow in the RVOT (using PW Doppler) to give VTI_{RVOT}, in cm.
- The stroke volume in the RVOT (SV_{RVOT}), in mL/beat, can then be calculated from:

$$SV_{RVOT} = CSA_{RVOT} \times VTI_{RVOT}$$

- In the parasternal long axis view, measure the diameter of the LVOT in cm, then use this to calculate the CSA of the LVOT in cm^2:

$$CSA_{LVOT} = 0.785 \times (\text{LVOT diameter})^2$$

- In the apical 5-chamber view, measure the VTI of flow in the LVOT (using PW Doppler) to give VTI_{LVOT}, in cm.
- The stroke volume in the LVOT (SV_{LVOT}), in mL/beat, can then be calculated from:

$$SV_{LVOT} = CSA_{LVOT} \times VTI_{LVOT}$$

The shunt ratio is the ratio of SV_{RVOT} to SV_{LVOT} which, in the presence of a left-to-right shunt, will be greater than 1. A significant limitation to shunt calculations is that they are heavily dependent on an accurate measurement of RVOT and LVOT diameter – as the calculation involves squaring these measurements, even a small inaccuracy in measurement can lead to a large error in the final result.

If there is doubt about the presence of an ASD, it may be necessary to perform an 'agitated' saline contrast study as for patent foramen ovale (PFO) (see box). Although transthoracic echo (TTE) can often detect evidence of an ASD, transoesophageal echo (TOE) will usually be required to assess an ASD in detail (or to rule out an ASD if clinical suspicion remains after a normal TTE). Sinus venosus defects can be very difficult to visualize on TTE.

ATRIAL SEPTAL ANEURYSM

Atrial septal aneurysms are thought to have a prevalence of around 1 per cent. They are defined as a bulge or deformation of the interatrial septum protruding at least 10 mm into the right or left atrium (or, if mobile, swinging by at least 10 mm from side to side) and with a diameter across their base of at least 15 mm. They have been reported to be associated with ASD and PFO (and also with mitral valve prolapse) and are also thought to be a potential cardiac source of emboli.

Management of atrial septal defect

An ASD can be closed percutaneously or surgically. Percutaneous closure is performed for secundum ASDs if there is an adequate rim of tissue around the defect to allow deployment of a septal occluder device without impinging on nearby structures. Surgical closure requires a thoracotomy to open one of the atria and suture a patch (made from Dacron or from the patient's own pericardium) over the defect.

Echo assessment following repair

Using the same views as for unrepaired ASD:

- comment on the presence of a septal occluder device or patch
- check for any residual shunt
- assess right heart size and function
- assess pulmonary artery pressure.

ASD AND 3-D ECHO

3-D echo can be helpful in the assessment of congenital heart disease and has been of particular value in assessing ASDs, providing information on the morphology of the interatrial septum and the surrounding structures. It has also been used to guide device closure.

Patent foramen ovale

In utero, the foramen ovale is a flap-like structure that permits shunting of blood directly from the RA to the LA. The flap normally closes after birth, when LA pressure rises, and becomes sealed within 12 months. However, in around

25 per cent of the general population the foramen does not close completely and the resulting PFO is a potential conduit between right and left atria.

Clinical features of patent foramen ovale

In the majority of people PFO causes no problems and no direct clinical findings, but in a small number it can be a cause of stroke (allowing a clot to pass from the venous to the arterial side of the circulation: 'paradoxical embolism') and is also associated with decompression illness in scuba divers (paradoxical gas embolism). There is also a higher incidence of PFO among patients with migraines.

Echo assessment of patent foramen ovale

With the echo probe in the **apical window**, obtain a 4-chamber view and visualize the interatrial septum.

Use colour Doppler to check for the presence of any flow across the interatrial septum. Asking the patient to perform and then release a Valsalva manoeuvre (deep breath in and 'bear down') can momentarily open up a PFO and reveal a brief jet of right-to-left flow.

Next, move the probe to the subcostal window (which usually allows a better view of the interatrial septum, as it is seen face on) and inspect the interatrial septum again using colour Doppler, repeating the Valsalva manoeuvre as necessary.

It may be necessary to go on to perform an 'agitated' saline bubble contrast study (see p. 93). Although TTE can sometimes detect a PFO, TOE is regarded as the investigation of choice.

Management of patent foramen ovale

PFO is common and requires no treatment if it is an incidental finding. For patients who have had a stroke as a result of paradoxical embolism, treatment with aspirin or warfarin is usually considered. Some patients may also be candidates for PFO repair, which can be undertaken either percutaneously (using a PFO occluder device) or surgically. The role of PFO closure in the treatment of migraine remains controversial.

Echo assessment following repair

Using the same views as for unrepaired PFO:

- comment on the presence of a septal occluder device or patch
- check for any residual shunt.

Ventricular septal defect

The interventricular septum has two parts: the muscular septum and the thinner, fibrous membranous septum (which lies just below the aortic valve). A ventricular septal defect (VSD) permits flow directly between left and right ventricles, and can be a congenital abnormality (indeed, VSD is the commonest congenital heart defect) or can be acquired as a complication of myocardial infarction (p. 147).

VSDs can be categorized according to their location as:

- **(Peri-)membranous VSD** – the commonest type, located in the membranous part of the septum below the aortic valve. It is well seen in the parasternal long axis view.
- **Muscular VSD** – found in the muscular part of the septum. Muscular VSDs can be multiple ('Swiss cheese septum').
- **Inlet VSD** – also known as canal-type or posterior VSD, this is found posterior to the tricuspid septal leaflet and may be associated with an atrioventricular canal defect. It is well seen in the apical 4-chamber view.
- **Subpulmonary VSD** – also known as supracristal, outlet or doubly committed VSD, this type is uncommon, and lies just below the aortic and pulmonary valves. It is well seen on the parasternal short axis view. This type of VSD is commonly associated with aortic regurgitation due to prolapse of the right coronary cusp of the aortic valve.

A large VSD may present with heart failure in infancy; small VSDs are usually asymptomatic. VSDs cause a pansystolic murmur at the lower left sternal edge, and as a general rule the smaller the defect the louder the murmur. The left-to-right shunting of blood can lead to pulmonary hypertension which can cause reversal of the shunt (Eisenmenger syndrome, see box). Decisions on VSD closure can be complex and should take into account symptoms, the presence of heart failure, the degree of shunting and the presence of pulmonary hypertension.

Echo assessment of ventricular septal defect

The interventricular septum should be inspected in as many views as possible. Use 2-D echo to assess the structure of the interventricular septum:

- Is there any echo dropout in the septum to indicate a defect? Describe the type of VSD according to its location ((peri-)membranous, muscular, inlet or subpulmonary). Assess whether multiple defects are present

- Measure the size of the VSD
- Assess RV size and function – is it dilated as a consequence of a left-to-right shunt?
- Assess LA size – is it dilated as a result of volume overload?
- Assess LV size and function (usually normal).

Use colour Doppler to check for the presence of flow across the interventricular septum into the RV (Fig. 22.2).

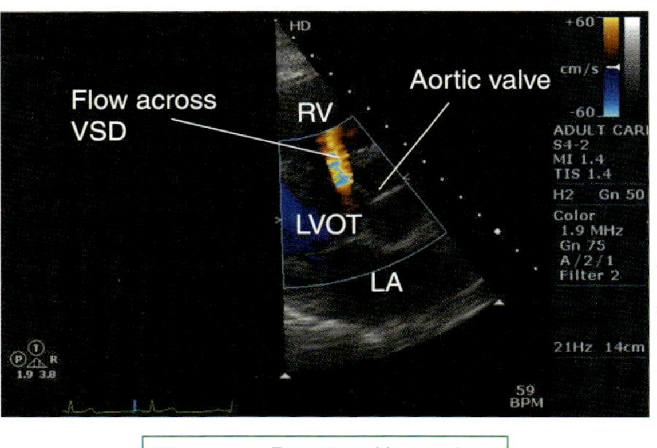

View	Parasternal long axis
Modality	Colour Doppler

Fig. 22.2 Ventricular septal defect (VSD) (LA = left atrium; LVOT = left ventricular outflow tract; RV = right ventricle)

In the subcostal view, use continuous wave (CW) and pulsed-wave (PW) Doppler to assess flow across the defect. There is usually a high-velocity jet from left to right ventricle during systole, with lower velocity flow during diastole.

If you identify a VSD, check for any associated abnormalities (e.g. aortic cusp prolapse, aortic regurgitation). Check also for the presence of tricuspid and/or pulmonary regurgitation and, where possible, assess pulmonary artery pressure in case pulmonary hypertension has developed. Perform a shunt calculation to estimate the shunt ratio.

Echo assessment following repair

Using the same views as for unrepaired VSD:

- comment on the presence of a septal patch
- check for any residual shunt

- check for aortic regurgitation (after closure of outflow tract VSD)
- assess left heart size and function
- assess right heart size and function
- assess pulmonary artery pressure.

Persistent ductus arteriosus

Persistent ductus arteriosus (PDA) is also sometimes referred to as *patent* ductus arteriosus. In the fetus, the ductus arteriosus acts as a shunt connecting the pulmonary artery (at the junction of the main and left pulmonary arteries) to the aortic arch (just after the origin of the left subclavian artery). This allows most (90 per cent) of the blood pumped by the RV to reach the systemic circulation directly, bypassing the lungs. The ductus arteriosus normally starts to close immediately after birth, and is normally fully closed within a few days, leaving behind just a cord-like remnant (the ligamentum arteriosum).

Failure of the ductus arteriosus to close means that a left-to-right shunt persists between the aortic arch and the pulmonary artery, with blood flow from the high-pressure aorta to the lower-pressure pulmonary artery. This leads to excessive blood flow through the pulmonary circulation and, in the longer term, can cause pulmonary hypertension.

Clinical features of persistent ductus arteriosus

Neonates with PDA are usually asymptomatic, but may sometimes have difficulty feeding or failure to thrive. The clinical features of PDA may include tachycardia, a wide pulse pressure and bounding pulse, a continuous systolic–diastolic 'machinery murmur', clubbing, and cyanosis.

Echo assessment of persistent ductus arteriosus

With the echo probe in the **suprasternal window**, obtain an aorta view to visualize the PDA as it arises from the aortic arch.

Use colour Doppler to assess flow in the aorta, looking in particular for evidence of a PDA arising just beyond the origin of the left subclavian artery.

Next, move the probe to the left parasternal window and tilt the probe to obtain a **parasternal RVOT view**, or rotate it to obtain a **parasternal short axis view at the aortic valve level**.

In either of these views, use colour Doppler to assess flow in the pulmonary artery, looking in particular for evidence of blood flow into the pulmonary artery via a PDA (Fig. 22.3).

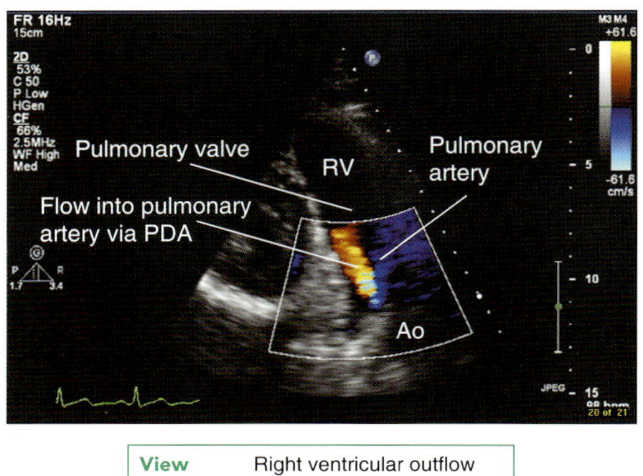

View	Right ventricular outflow
Modality	Colour Doppler

Fig. 22.3 Persistent ductus arteriosus (PDA) (Ao = aorta; RV = right ventricle)

Look carefully for any knock-on effects of the shunt on the rest of the heart, such as the development of pulmonary hypertension and right heart dilatation.

Management of persistent ductus arteriosus

Premature neonates with PDA can be treated with prostaglandin inhibitors (e.g. intravenous indometacin). Invasive techniques to close the PDA include the use of percutaneous closure devices or surgical ligation.

The presence of a PDA can sometimes be advantageous, for example in transposition of the great vessels (when it allows oxygenated blood to reach the systemic circulation) and under these circumstances the PDA can be kept open by giving prostaglandins.

Echo assessment following repair

Using the same views as for unrepaired PDA:

- check for any residual shunt
- assess right heart size and function
- assess pulmonary artery pressure.

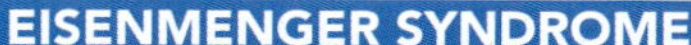

EISENMENGER SYNDROME

The presence of a left-to-right shunt (such as an ASD, VSD or PDA) allows blood to pass directly from the left side of the circulation to the right, increasing the volume of blood flowing through the pulmonary circulation. This leads to an increased pressure within the pulmonary vessels (pulmonary hypertension) and, over time, the vessels develop an increasing resistance to blood flow. This leads to a back pressure on the right heart and, gradually, the right-sided pressures rise and begin to equal and then exceed the pressures found in the left heart. As this occurs, the left-to-right shunt reverses, causing blood to start shunting from right to left instead. At this point, the patient is said to have developed Eisenmenger syndrome (or reaction). This means that a portion of the venous (deoxygenated) blood entering the right heart starts crossing directly into the left heart, bypassing the lungs, and reducing the overall oxygen content in the arterial circulation. Clinically, the patient develops cyanosis, a blue discoloration of the skin and tongue, together with breathlessness and a fall in exercise capacity.

Bicuspid aortic valve

A bicuspid aortic valve has two functioning cusps, usually of unequal size, with just a single line of coaptation. Pseudobicuspid valves have three cusps, but fusion of two of the cusps ('functionally' bicuspid). There is a strong association with aortic coarctation (p. 305), a bicuspid aortic valve being present in at least 50 per cent of cases.

The prevalence of bicuspid aortic valve is 1–2 per cent of the population, and it is thought to be responsible for around half of cases of severe aortic stenosis in adults. The stenotic process is similar to that seen in calcific degeneration, but occurs at a younger age. Fibrosis typically starts in a patient's teens, with gradual calcification from their thirties onwards. Patients who require surgery for stenosis of a bicuspid aortic valve do so on average 5 years earlier than those with calcific degeneration of a tricuspid aortic valve.

Bicuspid aortic valve is often asymptomatic, but with the onset of valve dysfunction patients may develop clinical features of aortic stenosis or regurgitation. Patients are also at risk of aortic root dilatation and infective endocarditis. Clinical examination often reveals a systolic ejection click, and features of aortic stenosis or regurgitation may be present.

Once a bicuspid aortic valve has been diagnosed, serial follow-up echo is required to monitor for the onset of aortic valve dysfunction and/or aortic root dilatation, which should be managed as appropriate.

Echo assessment of bicuspid aortic valve

- In the parasternal long and short axis (aortic valve level) views, use 2-D echo to:
  - assess the appearances and dimensions of the aortic valve (Fig. 22.4). Fibrosis and calcification of a bicuspid aortic valve can distort the valve, making recognition of its bicuspid nature difficult on echocardiography
  - look for evidence of cusp fusion (pseudobicuspid valve) – the line where the cusps are fused is called a raphe. Describe which cusps are fused
  - look at the closure line of the aortic valve in the parasternal long axis view – M-mode imaging is best for this. A bicuspid valve will usually have an eccentric closure line (i.e. no longer in the middle of the aortic annulus)
  - assess aortic root dimensions.
- Use colour Doppler to look for evidence of aortic regurgitation.

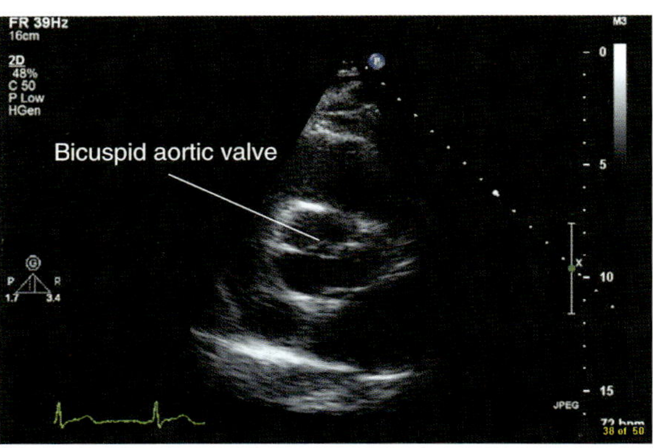

View	Parasternal short axis (aortic valve level)
Modality	2-D

Fig. 22.4 Bicuspid aortic valve

- Use CW and PW Doppler to assess flow through the aortic valve and assess the severity of any aortic stenosis or regurgitation (Chapter 13).

Perform a complete echo study, looking in particular for evidence of associated aortic coarctation.

Subvalvar and supravalvar aortic stenosis

The echo assessment of aortic stenosis is discussed in Chapter 13, p. 151.

Aortic coarctation

Aortic coarctation is a narrowing of the aorta that most commonly occurs just distal to the origin of the left subclavian artery. It accounts for 5–10 per cent of congenital heart disease and occurs more commonly in men.

Clinical features of aortic coarctation

Children with aortic coarctation may present with heart failure or problems resulting from reduced arterial perfusion to the lower half of the body. Adults with aortic coarctation are often asymptomatic and the diagnosis is made during assessment of hypertension or as an incidental finding (Table 22.2). Patients may have the clinical features of an associated condition such as bicuspid aortic valve or Turner syndrome.

Table 22.2 Clinical features of aortic coarctation

Symptoms	Signs
Often asymptomatic	Hypertension Systolic murmur Weak femoral pulse Radio-femoral delay (femoral pulse occurs after radial)

Echo assessment of aortic coarctation

With the echo probe in the **suprasternal window**, obtain an aorta view to visualize the aortic arch.

- Use 2-D echo to assess the appearances and dimensions of the aortic arch. Aortic coarctation is seen most commonly just distal to the origin of the left subclavian artery. There may be dilatation of the aorta on either side of the coarctation.

- Use colour Doppler to assess flow in the aorta, looking in particular for evidence of high-velocity or turbulent flow in the region of a suspected coarctation.
- Use CW and PW Doppler to assess flow in the descending aorta using CW Doppler, looking for evidence of increased flow velocity through the coarctation. The CW Doppler trace in Fig. 22.5 shows a velocity of 3.5 m/s in the descending aorta in a patient with aortic coarctation. Use PW Doppler to measure flow velocity proximal to the coarctation, and use the modified Bernoulli equation to calculate the gradient across the coarctation:

$$\Delta P = 4(V_2^2 - V_1^2)$$

where: ΔP=peak gradient across coarctation, in mmHg; V_2=peak velocity across coarctation, in m/s (CW Doppler); and V_1=peak velocity proximal to coarctation, in m/s (PW Doppler).

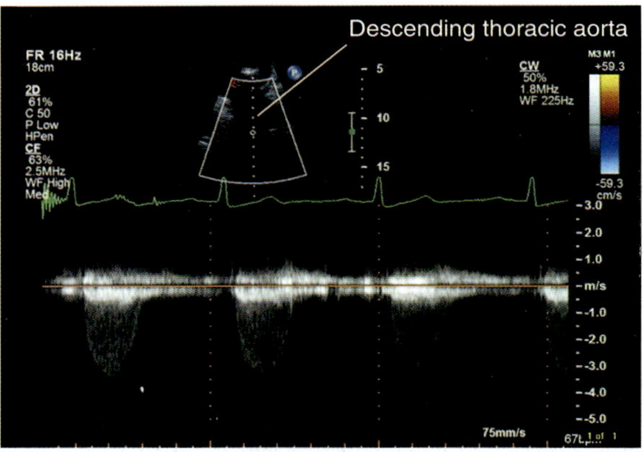

View	Suprasternal
Modality	CW Doppler

Fig. 22.5 Aortic coarctation – continuous wave (CW) Doppler study from suprasternal window

Perform a complete echo study to look carefully for any other abnormalities that can be associated with, or result from, aortic coarctation, including:

- bicuspid aortic valve (present in at least 50 per cent of cases)
- subvalvar aortic stenosis
- VSD

- LV hypertrophy (LVH) or dysfunction (as a consequence of hypertension).

Management of aortic coarctation

Aortic coarctation can be managed by surgical excision of the area of coarctation (followed either by end-to-end anastomosis of the aorta, or with the use of a graft to bridge the resulting gap). It can also be managed percutaneously by angioplasty and/or stenting of the coarctation.

Echo assessment following repair

Following correction, patients with aortic coarctation require lifelong follow-up with annual echo studies. Using the same views as for unrepaired coarctation:

- measure any residual gradient
- check for the development of any dilatation of the aorta.

In addition:

- assess any LVH (patients may remain hypertensive)
- assess any associated abnormalities such as bicuspid aortic valve.

Subvalvar, valvar and supravalvar pulmonary stenosis

The echo assessment of pulmonary stenosis is discussed in Chapter 15, p. 209.

Ebstein's anomaly

In Ebstein's anomaly the tricuspid valve (specifically the septal and posterior leaflets) is displaced towards the RV apex. As a result, part of the RV becomes 'atrialized' – although it becomes part of the RA, it still contracts with the RV, which impairs the haemodynamic function of the right heart and tends to exacerbate the tricuspid regurgitation that is usually present (and ranges in severity from mild to severe). There are several associated conditions:

- ASD and VSD
- pulmonary stenosis
- accessory pathway (Wolff–Parkinson–White syndrome).

When Ebstein's anomaly presents in adult life, it can be with:

- breathlessness and fatigue
- tricuspid regurgitation
- right heart failure

- cyanosis
- palpitations.

Echo assessment of Ebstein's anomaly

The tricuspid valve can be studied in:

- left parasternal window
  - parasternal right ventricular inflow view
  - parasternal short axis view
- apical window
  - apical 4-chamber view
- subcostal window
  - subcostal long axis view.

2-D

Use 2-D echo to assess the structure of the tricuspid valve:

- Is the tricuspid valve position normal or is it displaced apically (in Ebstein's anomaly the tricuspid valve plane is displaced at least 1 cm towards the RV apex, in comparison with the mitral valve plane)?
- Are the tricuspid valve leaflets morphologically normal or abnormal? Do the leaflets coapt normally or eccentrically?
- Is the RA dilated?
- Is the RV dilated? Is RV function impaired?

Colour Doppler

Use colour Doppler to:

- assess the severity of tricuspid regurgitation
- look for shunts (see 'Associated features' below).

CW and PW Doppler

Use CW Doppler to obtain a trace of regurgitant flow through the tricuspid valve. You should obtain traces from the apex and from at least one other position, such as the parasternal short axis or RV inflow views. Assess the severity of tricuspid regurgitation and calculate pulmonary artery systolic pressure.

Associated features

A number of conditions can be associated with Ebstein's anomaly, so perform a complete echo study to look for them:

- ASD
- PFO (as a consequence of RA dilatation)

- VSD
- pulmonary stenosis.

Management of Ebstein's anomaly

The management of Ebstein's anomaly includes the treatment of any RV failure and arrhythmias. Surgical options include tricuspid valve repair (or sometimes replacement), resection of the atrialized portion of the RV, and correction of any shunts.

Tetralogy of Fallot

Tetralogy of Fallot (ToF) accounts for 3.5 per cent of cases of congenital heart disease and, as the word 'tetralogy' suggests, consists of four key abnormalities:

- VSD
- overriding aorta (Fig. 22.6)
- RVOT obstruction
- RV hypertrophy.

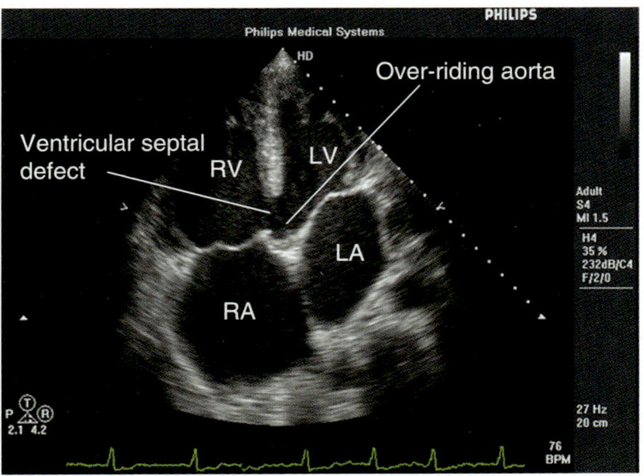

View	Apical 4-chamber
Modality	2-D

Fig. 22.6 Tetralogy of Fallot (LA = left atrium; LV = left ventricle; RA = right atrium; RV = right ventricle) (Figure reproduced with permission of Philips)

The RVOT obstruction can be due to narrowing of the muscular part (infundibulum) of the RVOT that leads into the pulmonary artery, or affecting the pulmonary valve itself (where there can be a degree of cusp tethering). RV hypertrophy develops in response to the pressure overload that results from the RVOT obstruction.

In some cases ToF may be diagnosed *in utero* with fetal ultrasound scanning. After birth, the clinical severity depends primarily upon how severe the RVOT obstruction is. Neonates may present with failure to thrive and/or cyanosis, although cyanotic episodes may not appear until later. The clinical features include a harsh ejection systolic murmur in the pulmonary area, cyanosis and clubbing.

Management and echo follow-up in tetralogy of Fallot

It's very rare to see adults with untreated ToF, as fewer than 10 per cent of patients with untreated ToF survive to the age of 20 years. As a result, almost all the adults seen with a history of ToF will have undergone surgical correction. ToF is usually treated with primary repair (closing the VSD and relieving the RVOT obstruction) before the age of 1 year. However, where necessary it is possible to perform a modified Blalock–Taussig shunt procedure (placing a graft between the subclavian artery and the pulmonary artery) as a palliative measure – this does not fully correct the ToF, but it does increase blood flow to the pulmonary circulation.

Following primary ToF repair in childhood, survival at 30 years is over 90 per cent. As a result, there are now many adults with previous ToF repair who need follow-up. The key problems to assess during echo follow-up include:

- pulmonary regurgitation
- severity of any residual RVOT obstruction
- any shunting across a residual VSD.

Pulmonary regurgitation is common following repair and this can lead to RV dilatation and dysfunction (and a risk of ventricular tachycardia). It is therefore important to assess the degree of any pulmonary regurgitation, in addition to assessing the impact of this on RV dimensions and function (Chapter 15). Any residual RVOT obstruction should be quantified with Doppler studies. Use colour Doppler to detect any shunting across a residual VSD and then go on to assess the degree of shunting.

It should be noted that although echo plays an important role in follow-up after ToF repair, cardiac magnetic resonance imaging can provide more detailed information about residual right heart abnormalities.

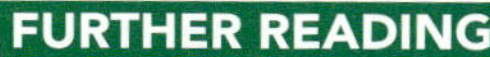

FURTHER READING

Brickner ME, Hillis LD, Lange RA. Congenital heart disease in adults: first of two parts. *N Engl J Med* 2000; **342**: 256–63.

Brickner ME, Hillis LD, Lange RA. Congenital heart disease in adults: second of two parts. *N Engl J Med* 2000; **342**: 334–42.

Li W. *British Society of Echocardiography Distance Learning Module 9: Adult Congenital Heart Disease*. Accessible from the BSE website (www.bsecho.org).

Shinebourne EA, Babu-Narayan SV, Carvalho JS. Tetralogy of Fallot: from fetus to adult. *Heart* 2006; **92**: 1353–9.

The Task Force on the Management of Grown Up Congenital Heart Disease of the European Society of Cardiology. Management of grown up congenital heart disease. *Eur Heart J* 2003; **24**: 1035–84.

23 Common echo requests

A number of echo requests crop up commonly, such as 'Breathlessness ?cause' and 'Stroke ?cardiac source of emboli'. This chapter considers some of the requests you will see most often and discusses the key points that you need to consider in each case.

Breathlessness

Breathlessness is a common symptom that has a multitude of possible causes. In many cases the clinician will want the sonographer to look for evidence of heart failure (systolic or diastolic), but it is important to be alert to a broad range of possible diagnoses as you perform the echo study. Even if you do find evidence of left ventricular (LV) dysfunction, remember that an individual patient can have more than one contributing factor for their symptoms. Common causes of breathlessness are listed below:

- **Heart failure**:
  - Measure left and right ventricular dimensions.
  - Assess left and right ventricular systolic function.
  - Check for LV diastolic dysfunction.
  - Describe any regional wall motion abnormalities.
  - Check for associated valvular disease.
- **Valvular disease**:
  - Assess valvular structure and function.
  - Assess chamber dimensions and function.
  - Assess pulmonary artery pressure (if possible).
- **Ischaemic heart disease**:
  - Are there any regional wall motion abnormalities?
  - Consider stress echo.

- **Lung disease**:
  - Assess right ventricular (RV) dimensions and function.
  - Assess pulmonary artery pressure (if possible).
  - Is there any evidence of pulmonary embolism?

Remain alert to non-cardiac causes of breathlessness that might nonetheless be detected on echo, such as a pleural effusion (Fig. 19.3, p. 260).

Arrhythmias

Echo is frequently requested in patients with arrhythmias to check for associated structural heart disease. Although the heart will often prove to be structurally normal, it is nonetheless important to perform a full echo study as there are several possible abnormalities that may be found. It is helpful to have as much detail as possible about the nature of the arrhythmia to help guide the echo study. An echo should be part of the assessment of patients with sustained (or non-sustained) supraventricular or ventricular tachyarrhythmias. It is not usually helpful in those with isolated supraventricular or ventricular ectopic beats, in the absence of any other features.

Atrial fibrillation

Atrial fibrillation (AF) is the commonest sustained arrhythmia, affecting 0.5 per cent of the adult population (and 10 per cent of those aged over 75 years). Many conditions can cause AF (Table 23.1), and an echo may reveal evidence of these, in particular:

- valvular heart disease
- cardiomyopathy
- LV hypertrophy (LVH) in hypertension
- right heart abnormalities in pulmonary disease or pulmonary embolism
- pericardial disease.

Table 23.1 Causes of atrial fibrillation

Ischaemic heart disease	Pulmonary disease
Valvular heart disease	Pulmonary embolism
Hypertension	Pneumonia
Cardiomyopathy	Pericarditis
Myocarditis	'Lone' atrial fibrillation (no identified cause)
Alcohol	
Thyrotoxicosis	

Longstanding AF leads to dilatation of the left and right atria (Fig. 23.1), but be sure to check for other causes of atrial enlargement such as mitral/tricuspid valve disease or restrictive cardiomyopathy. Atrial enlargement indicates a lower success rate for cardioversion (see below).

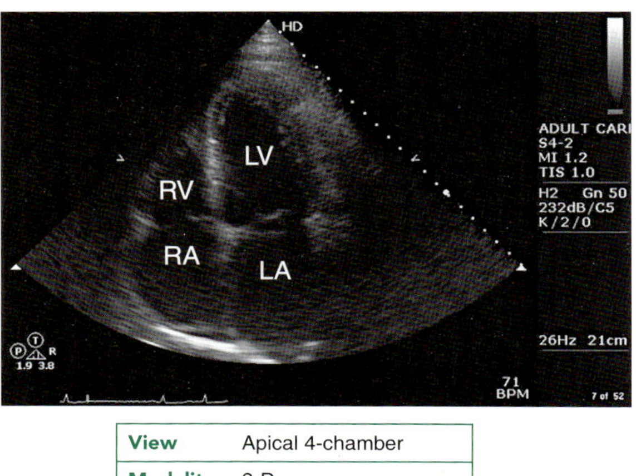

View	Apical 4-chamber
Modality	2-D

Fig. 23.1 Dilated atria in longstanding atrial fibrillation (LA = left atrium; LV = left ventricle; RA = right atrium; RV = right ventricle)

AF is a risk factor for embolic stroke and patients at high risk should be considered for anticoagulation with warfarin. Echo indicators of high stroke risk include the presence of valve disease or impaired LV function (clinical indicators include heart failure, previous stroke/transient ischaemic attack (TIA) or peripheral embolic events, or, in those aged 75 years or over, the presence of hypertension, diabetes or vascular disease).

Cardioversion of persistent AF back to sinus rhythm should be considered in patients where the procedure is likely to succeed (and sinus rhythm maintained in the longer term). The presence of structural heart disease on echo (such as a left atrium (LA) $>$ 5.5 cm or mitral stenosis) suggests a lower likelihood of successful cardioversion.

If cardioversion is going to be undertaken for a patient who has been in AF for longer than 48 h, it is important to minimize the risk of embolism either by arranging therapeutic anticoagulation for at least 3 weeks prior to the cardioversion, or by performing a transoesophageal echo (TOE) to rule out intracardiac thrombus – this is called TOE-guided cardioversion. If there is no thrombus present, the cardioversion is normally carried out with heparin cover, and the patient treated with warfarin for 4 weeks afterwards.

Ventricular arrhythmias

Ventricular tachycardia and/or fibrillation commonly result from underlying structural heart disease. Echo should therefore be part of the assessment of patients who have had, or are regarded as being at high risk of, ventricular arrhythmias, looking in particular for evidence of:

- myocardial infarction/ischaemia
- valvular heart disease (in particular, mitral valve prolapse)
- cardiomyopathy (e.g. hypertrophic cardiomyopathy, dilated cardiomyopathy, arrhythmogenic RV cardiomyopathy).

A full assessment of both LV and RV dimensions, morphology and function is required. If myocardial ischaemia is suspected, a stress echo study may be required (Chapter 8).

One treatment option for patients at risk of ventricular arrhythmias is an implantable cardioverter defibrillator (ICD) device, and the accurate measurement of LV ejection fraction plays a key role in identifying patients most likely to benefit from ICD implantation.

Ejection systolic murmur

An ejection systolic murmur begins after the first heart sound, rises in intensity to reach a peak during systole, and then falls in intensity to end before the second heart sound (Fig. 23.2). The murmur is also described as 'diamond-shaped' or 'crescendo-decrescendo'. Causes of an ejection systolic murmur include:

- aortic stenosis
- bicuspid aortic valve

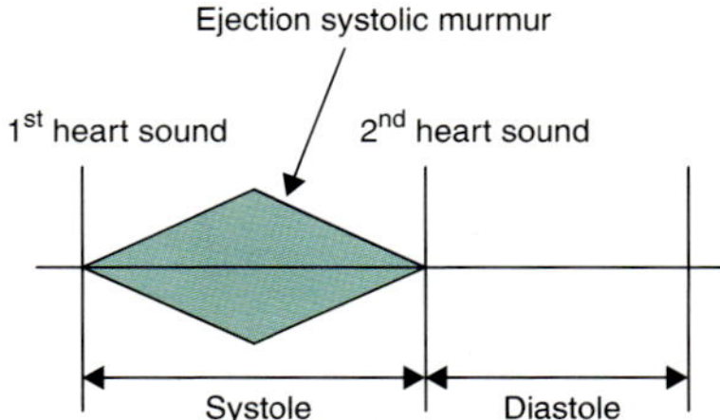

Fig. 23.2 Ejection systolic murmur

- pulmonary stenosis
- hypertrophic obstructive cardiomyopathy.

Remember that aortic and pulmonary stenosis can occur not just at the valve but also with obstruction to outflow at a subvalvular or supravalvular level.

'Ejection systolic murmur cause?' is a common echo request and must include a search for all these structural abnormalities. If no structural heart disease is found, the murmur is likely to be a result of increased flow across a normal aortic or pulmonary valve, as seen in hyperdynamic flow states (e.g. exercise, anaemia, pregnancy, thyrotoxicosis), and is termed an 'innocent' murmur.

Hypertension

Hypertension is arbitrarily defined as a blood pressure >140/90 mmHg and is a major risk factor for cardiovascular disease. In 95 per cent of cases hypertension is idiopathic, but in 5 per cent there is an identifiable underlying cause such as renal disease, metabolic/endocrine abnormalities or coarctation of the aorta.

Echo assessment is appropriate for patients with suspected hypertensive heart disease, but not as a routine screening tool in uncomplicated hypertension. When performing an echo in hypertension, look for aortic coarctation (Chapter 22) and for end-organ damage as a consequence of the hypertension:

- LVH and diastolic dysfunction
- LV dilatation and systolic dysfunction
- Aortic root dilatation and aortic regurgitation.

You should calculate LV mass in patients found to have LVH (p. 118). LVH is a significant independent risk factor for cardiovascular morbidity and mortality.

Collagen abnormalities

Marfan syndrome is a genetic condition with an autosomal dominant pattern of inheritance (although in a quarter of cases there is no family history, i.e. a new mutation) and an incidence of 2–3 per 10 000 population. Patients with Marfan syndrome have an abnormality of fibrillin, a constituent of connective tissue, and this can cause abnormalities affecting the musculoskeletal and cardiovascular systems, and also the skin and eyes.

The diagnosis of Marfan syndrome is based on the Ghent criteria, which require the presence of 'major' criteria in two organ systems and a 'minor' criterion in a third system. Major cardiovascular criteria include:

- aortic root dilatation
- dissection of the ascending aorta.

Minor cardiovascular criteria include:

- mitral valve prolapse
- mitral valve calcification (<40 years)
- pulmonary artery dilatation
- dilatation/dissection of the descending aorta.

Echo therefore plays an important role in the diagnosis of Marfan syndrome. It is also essential in follow-up; patients with Marfan syndrome require regular echo monitoring with particular attention to the aortic root, which should be measured at the level of the aortic annulus, the sinuses of Valsalva (which is where dilatation usually begins), the sinotubular junction and the ascending aorta. Measurements should be compared with normal range nomograms which take into account the patient's age and body surface area. For follow-up studies, it is important to ensure that the measurements are reproducible and therefore can be compared from one study to the next. Echo follow-up should occur at least annually in adults (and every 6–12 months in children).

The risk of aortic dissection is related to the aortic diameter, and the risk of rupture is particularly high if the aortic root diameter exceeds 5.5 cm. Treatment with beta-blockers should be considered if any degree of aortic dilatation is present, and surgical referral should be made if the aortic root diameter exceeds 5.0–5.5 cm in an adult (or 5.0 cm in a child). Decisions on the timing of surgery may also be influenced by the rate of aortic dilatation or a family history of aortic dissection. For details on the risks of pregnancy in Marfan syndrome, see below.

Ehlers–Danlos syndrome is a group of genetic disorders, classified into six subgroups, characterized by collagen abnormalities. Some patients develop mitral valve prolapse and echo assessment is important if this is suspected. Patients with the Ehlers–Danlos vascular subtype (type IV) are prone to develop arterial aneurysms that can include the aorta, and a screening echo to assess the aortic root and arch is appropriate.

Renal failure

The echo assessment of patients with chronic renal failure should include a full assessment of LV dimensions, and systolic and diastolic function. Hypertension is common in chronic renal failure and may be associated with LVH. Both systolic and diastolic dysfunction may be impaired.

Amyloidosis refers to a group of conditions in which amyloid protein builds up in tissues, including the kidney and the heart. Patients with amyloid-related renal failure may therefore show signs of cardiac amyloid on echo (p. 252).

Mitral annular calcification is a frequent finding in chronic renal failure, and its presence is associated with a poor prognosis. It is recognized as a calcified (echodense) area at the junction of the posterior mitral valve leaflet and atrioventricular groove (Fig. 23.3).

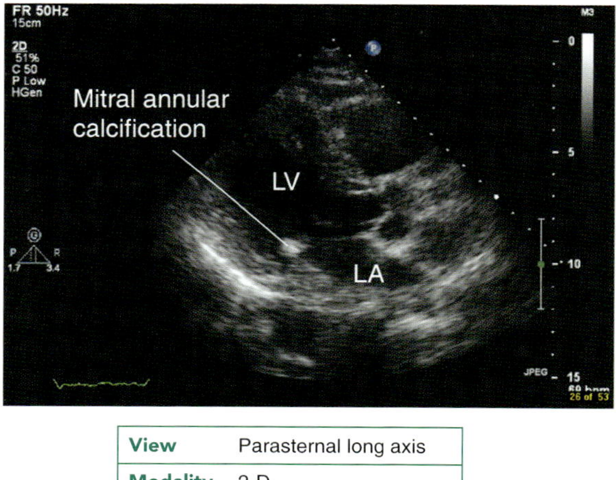

View	Parasternal long axis
Modality	2-D

Fig. 23.3 Mitral annular calcification (LA = left atrium; LV = left ventricle)

Uraemia is a consequence of renal failure and can cause uraemic pericarditis, in which pericardial effusion (and possibly cardiac tamponade) may occur.

Coronary artery disease (CAD) is the commonest cause of death in patients with chronic renal failure, and its detection (and treatment) prior to renal transplantation is important. Dobutamine stress echo (DSE, Chapter 8) has proven a valuable technique for detecting CAD in these patients (and is superior to exercise treadmill testing). It also provides information on prognosis – the greater the extent of myocardial ischaemia (percentage of ischaemic segments) during DSE, the greater the risk of premature death.

Stroke

In patients who have had a TIA or an embolic stroke or a peripheral arterial embolism, an echo is commonly requested to check whether there is a cardiac source of emboli. However, the yield of such studies is low, particularly in the absence of any other features in the history, examination or ECG that point towards a cardiac abnormality. The use of echo to assess for an embolic source varies from centre to centre, but a transthoracic echo (TTE) is often requested in patients who are younger than 50 years of age or if clinical evaluation is suggestive of an underlying cardiac abnormality. The diagnostic yield of transoesophageal echo (TOE) is better than that of TTE, and TOE is often considered in younger patients (<50 years), or if there is ongoing clinical suspicion of a cardiac source of emboli after a normal TTE, or if an abnormality found on TTE requires more detailed evaluation.

Echo may identify a direct source of emboli:

- LV thrombus
- LA thrombus (especially LA appendage)
- left heart tumour (e.g. myxoma)
- infective endocarditis
- aortic atheroma.

Alternatively, echo may find a condition associated with an increased risk of emboli:

- atrial septal aneurysm
- patent foramen ovale/atrial septal defect (paradoxical embolism)
- ventricular septal defect (with pulmonary hypertension)
- acute myocardial infarction
- dilated cardiomyopathy
- mitral stenosis
- prosthetic heart valve.

One of the commonest cardiac causes of emboli is AF. Although this is diagnosed with an ECG rather than an echo, an echo is nonetheless important in the assessment of patients with this condition (see above).

Pregnancy

Echo provides a safe and effective means of assessing the heart during pregnancy. Pregnant patients may require an echo to assess known pre-existing cardiac problems, or as a diagnostic investigation in the case of new symptoms (e.g. breathlessness) or signs (e.g. murmurs). It is important to be aware of the normal cardiovascular changes in pregnancy and the effect that these changes can have on those with prior cardiac conditions.

During a normal pregnancy, cardiac output increases by around 40 per cent, because of a rise in both heart rate and stroke volume, reaching a peak towards the end of the second trimester. Cardiac output then remains on a plateau until the time of delivery, at which point there is a further increase (due to an increase in venous return to the heart, relief of pressure on the inferior vena cava, and the return of blood from the contracted uterus to the circulation) before gradually returning to normal over the next 2 weeks.

The 'volume overload' of pregnancy leads to an increase in LV end-systolic and end-diastolic diameters, and also an increase in LV mass. There is also an increase in valve orifice area of all four valves, increasing the likelihood of valvular regurgitation.

Pre-existing dilated cardiomyopathy is poorly tolerated during pregnancy, with a high maternal mortality rate, particularly if the patient has moderate/severe symptoms or an ejection fraction $<$20 per cent. A cardiomyopathy can also develop as a consequence of pregnancy (**peripartum cardiomyopathy**, defined as an ejection fraction $<$45 per cent occurring in the last months of pregnancy or within 5 months of delivery). Although fetal outcome is generally good, maternal mortality can be high. It is particularly important to assess the risk of recurrence in future pregnancies – persistently abnormal LV function 1 year after pregnancy predicts a high (20 per cent) risk of mortality in a subsequent pregnancy.

'Innocent' flow-related heart murmurs are common in pregnancy, and are a frequent reason for echo referrals. However, not all murmurs in pregnancy are benign, and structural valvular disease must be identified and assessed carefully. Obstructive cardiac lesions such as mitral stenosis and aortic stenosis (and also hypertrophic obstructive cardiomyopathy) can be very poorly tolerated and require careful clinical and echo assessment.

Patients with Marfan syndrome (see above) have a 1 per cent risk of aortic dissection during pregnancy, even if the aortic dimensions are initially normal. This risk is much higher is the aortic root is dilated $>$4 cm (or is rapidly dilating), or if there is cardiac involvement or a poor family history. Monthly clinical assessment and echo are appropriate, with the full involvement of a multidisciplinary specialist team (particularly at the time of delivery). Beta-blockers should be continued throughout pregnancy.

Patients with pre-existing congenital heart disease should receive appropriate assessment and counselling before planning a pregnancy. Some conditions are very high risk – patients with Eisenmenger syndrome, for example, have a maternal mortality of around 40 per cent and are advised to avoid pregnancy (and indeed pulmonary hypertension, whatever the cause, generally presents a high risk in pregnancy). A detailed discussion of the risks of pregnancy in different congenital heart problems is beyond the scope of this book, but helpful guidance is available (see Further Reading).

FURTHER READING

Chambers JB, de Belder MA, Moore D. Echocardiography in stroke and transient ischaemic attack. *Heart* 1997; **78** (suppl 1): 2–6.

Dean JCS. Management of Marfan syndrome. *Heart* 2002; **88**: 97–103.

Douglas PS, Khandheria B, Stainback RF, *et al.* ACCF/ASE/ACEP/ASNC/SCAI/SCCT/SCMR 2007 Appropriateness criteria for transthoracic and transesophageal echocardiography. *J Am Coll Cardiol* 2007; **50**: 187–204.

Feringa HHH, Bax JJ, Schouten O. Ischemic heart disease in renal transplant candidates: towards non-invasive approaches for preoperative risk stratification. *Eur J Echocardiogr* 2005; **6**: 313–16.

Thorne SA. Pregnancy in heart disease. *Heart* 2005; **90**: 450–6.

Appendix 1 Echo resources

TEXTBOOKS

Introductory handbooks

Kaddoura S. *Echo Made Easy*, 2nd edn. Edinburgh: Churchill Livingstone, 2009. ISBN-13: 978-0443103636.

Leeson P, Mitchell AR, Becher H. *Echocardiography*. Oxford: Oxford University Press, 2007. ISBN-13: 978-0199215751.

Rimington H, Chambers J. *Echocardiography: A Practical Guide for Reporting*, 2nd edn. Oxford: Informa Healthcare, 2007. ISBN-13: 978-1841846347.

Comprehensive reference books

Feigenbaum H, Armstrong WF, Ryan T. *Feigenbaum's Echocardiography*, 6th edn. Philadelphia: Lippincott Williams & Wilkins, 2004. ISBN-13: 978-0781731980.

Jae KO, Seward JB, Tajik AJ. *The Echo Manual*, 3rd edn. Philadelphia: Lippincott Williams & Wilkins, 2006. ISBN-13: 978-0781748537.

Otto CM. *Textbook of Clinical Echocardiography*, 3rd edn. Edinburgh: Elsevier Saunders, 2004. ISBN-13: 978-0721607894.

JOURNALS

Cardiovascular Ultrasound (online journal): www.cardiovascularultrasound.com

Echo: The Journal of the British Society of Echocardiography: www.bsecho.org

Echocardiography: A Journal of Cardiovascular Ultrasound and Allied Techniques: www.blackwell-synergy.com/loi/echo

European Journal of Echocardiography: http://ejechocard.oxfordjournals.org

Journal of the American Society of Echocardiography: http://journals.elsevierhealth.com/periodicals/ymje

KEY GUIDELINES

Key guidance published by the British Society of Echocardiography (BSE) and available from its website (www.bsecho.org):

- *Clinical Indications for Echocardiography*
- *A Minimum Dataset for a Standard Adult Transthoracic Echocardiogram*
- *Recommendations for Standard Adult Transthoracic Echocardiography*
- *Recommended Views for a Standard Adult Transthoracic Echo.*

Posters published by the BSE and British Heart Foundation (details can be obtained from the BSE):

- Echocardiography: guidelines for chamber quantification
- Echocardiography: guidelines for valve quantification.

Cerqueira MD, Weissman NJ, Dilsizian V, *et al.* Standardized myocardial segmentation and nomenclature for tomographic imaging of the heart. *Circulation* 2002; **105**: 539–42.

Douglas PS, Khandheria B, Stainback RF, *et al.* ACCF/ASE/ACEP/ASNC/SCAI/SCCT/SCMR 2007 Appropriateness criteria for transthoracic and transesophageal echocardiography. *J Am Coll Cardiol* 2007; **50**: 187–204.

Douglas PS, Khandheria B, Stainback RF, *et al.* ACCF/ASE/ACEP/AHA/ASNC/SCAI/SCCT/SCMR 2008 Appropriateness criteria for stress echocardiography. *J Am Coll Cardiol* 2006; **51**: 1127–47.

Lang RM, Bierig M, Devereux RB, *et al.* Recommendations for Chamber Quantification: A Report from the American Society of Echocardiography's Guidelines and Standards Committee and the Chamber Quantification Writing Group, Developed in Conjunction with the European Association of Echocardiography, a Branch of the European Society of Cardiology. *J Am Soc Echocardiogr* 2005; **18**: 1440–63.

The Task Force on the Management of Valvular Heart Disease of the European Society of Cardiology. Guidelines on the management of valvular heart disease. *Eur Heart J* 2007; **28**: 230–68.

Zoghbi WA, Enriquez-Sarano M, Foster E, *et al.* American Society of Echocardiography: Recommendations for evaluation of the severity of native valvular regurgitation with two-dimensional and Doppler echocardiography. *J Am Soc Echocardiogr* 2003; **16**: 777–802.

SOCIETIES

American Society of Echocardiography
2100, Gateway Centre Boulevard
Suite 310
Morrisville NC 27560
United States of America

Tel: +919 861 5574
Fax: +919 882 9900
Website: www.asecho.org

British Society of Echocardiography
10-16, Tiller Road
Docklands Business Centre
London E14 8PX
United Kingdom

Tel: 020 7345 5185
Fax: 020 7345 5186
Website: www.bsecho.org

European Association of Echocardiography
European Society of Cardiology
The European Heart House
2035, Route des Colles
BP 179 – Les Templiers
F-06903 Sophia Antipolis
France

Tel: +33.4.92.94.76.00
Fax: +33.4.92.94.76.01
Website: www.escardio.org/bodies/associations/EAE

WEBSITES

In addition to the websites already listed above, the following sites contain material of interest to anyone learning or practising echocardiography:

E-chocardiography Journal: www2.umdnj.edu/~shindler

Echocardiology.org: www.echocardiology.org

Wikiecho: www.wikiecho.com

Yahoo! Discussion Group – Cardiovascular Ultrasound:
http://health.groups.yahoo.com/group/echocardiography

Yale Atlas of Echocardiography:
http://info.med.yale.edu/intmed/cardio/echo_atlas/contents.

Appendix 2 Help with the next edition

We would like to know what should be included (or omitted!) in the next edition of *Making Sense of Echocardiography*. Please write with your comments or suggestions to:

Dr Andrew R. Houghton
Making Sense of Echocardiography
c/o Hodder Arnold (Publishers)
338 Euston Road
London NW1 3BH

We will acknowledge all suggestions that are used.

Index